OBSTETRICS
and
GYNECOLOGY
the clinical core

RALPH M. WYNN, M.D.

PROFESSOR OF OBSTETRICS AND GYNECOLOGY
STATE UNIVERSITY OF NEW YORK
HEALTH SCIENCES CENTER AT BROOKLYN
Formerly Professor of Obstetrics and Gynecology
University of New Mexico School of Medicine

OBSTETRICS
and
GYNECOLOGY
the clinical core

FIFTH EDITION

With the assistance of:
Francis W. Byrn, M.D.
David K. Guardia, M.D.
Luis A. Izquierdo, M.D.
Thomas V. Sedlacek, M.D.

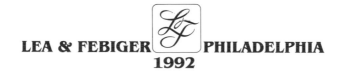

LEA & FEBIGER PHILADELPHIA
1992

LEA & FEBIGER
Box 3024
200 Chester Field Parkway
Malvern, PA 19355 U.S.A.
(215) 251-2230

Executive Editor: Darlene Barela Cooke
Project Editor: Jessica Howie Martin
Production Manager: Thomas J. Colaiezzi

First Edition 1974
Reprinted 1975
Second Edition 1979
Reprinted 1980, 1981,1982
Third Edition 1983
Reprinted 1983, 1985
Fourth Edition 1988
Fifth Edition, 1992

Library of Congress Cataloging-in-Publication Data

Wynn, Ralph M.
  Obstetrics and gynecology: the clinical core / Ralph M. Wynn,
5th ed.
    p.   cm.
  Includes index.
  ISBN 0-8121-1565-1
  1. Gynecology. 2. Obstetrics. II. Title
  [DNLM: 1. Curriculum. 2. Genital Diseases, Female.
3. Obstetrics.   WQ 100 W988o]
RG101.W96 1992
618—dc20
DNLM/DLC
for Library of Congress   92-13526
                                                       CIP

> Reprints of chapters may be purchased from Lea & Febiger in quantities of 100 or more.
> Contact Sally Grande in the Sales Department

PRINTED IN THE UNITED STATES OF AMERICA

Print number : 4 3 2 1

TO
THE MEDICAL STUDENTS AND RESIDENTS
WHOM I HAVE HAD THE PRIVILEGE TO TEACH
DURING THE PAST THIRD OF A CENTURY

PREFACE

Education may be defined as planned change in behavior of the student over a period of time. Medical educators, in common with their colleagues in other fields, must therefore select experiences and teach them as rapidly and efficiently as possible to the level of performance described as acceptable behavior. The planning of medical curricula, including the process of selection, design, and sequential arrangement of instructional units, requires a rationale and thus cannot be left to chance.

A curriculum should be based on four educational principles: development of objectives, preparation of an entry test, construction of a set of learning activities, and formulation of procedures for evaluation of the results. A core curriculum defines the criteria for minimal competence required of all medical students. It provides at least three major advantages in the educational process. First, it reduces the amount of purely factual material to be learned. Second, it identifies the requisite knowledge and skill for all medical students. Third, it increases the time available for elective studies in the basic or clinical sciences.

The availability of a core curriculum that details the data base frees the teacher from the task of mere dissemination of information and allows him time for influencing attitudes and demonstrating skills. In a modern curriculum the student may proceed at his or her own rate to accomplish the educational objectives of the core and may devote more time to mastering areas of difficulty. The faster learner may pursue areas in depth or proceed to other areas. The construction of a core curriculum in obstetrics and gynecology is thus a step toward increased flexibility in the undergraduate medical curriculum. It spells out the minimal needs of every physician for knowledge and skills in obstetrics and gynecology and allows time for additional electives or special tracks for students who choose a career in this field.

A good textbook is probably the fastest means of transmitting a large body of knowledge. The skilled reader can control his or her rate of learning and can read the printed page more rapidly than any lecturer can deliver the same material intelligibly. As self-instructional media and synopses increase in quality and as retrieval of information from handbooks and other reference sources improves, the classic textbook, which struggles in vain to be both instructionally sound and encyclopedic, will gradually disappear. Quite different is the student text based on educational principles. It seldom presents new knowledge. Instead, it offers the available knowledge to the student in a selective, sequential, simplified presentation.

Although I have enlisted the aid of several colleagues in the preparation of this edition, the final writing of the entire text is mine and I therefore accept full responsibility for the selection and arrangement in sequence of the material. I have attempted to make the definitions of terms in this text consistent with the recommendations of the Committee on Terminology of the American College of Obstetricians and Gynecologists wherever possible.

The fifth edition of this textbook is the most extensive revision since the volume first appeared in 1974. The text has always conformed to the Instructional Objectives for a Clinical Curriculum in Obstetrics and Gynecology, prepared under the auspices of the Association of Professors of Gynecology and Obstetrics. The fifth and most recent edition of those objectives expanded the scope of the subject matter, which was divided into 6 instructional units and 56 objectives. The fifth edition of this textbook follows the format of 6 units and only a slightly larger number of chapters (60). The textbook thus can be used to supplement the objectives with maximal ease.

For the fifth edition, I have had the assistance of fourteen colleagues, four of whom made major contributions to the text. In alphabetical order, Dr. Francis Byrn critically reviewed the material on gynecologic endocrinology and infertility, Dr. David Guardia on general gynecology, Dr. Luis Izquierdo on obstetrics and perinatal medicine, and Dr. Thomas Sedlacek on gynecologic oncology. To these four academic obstetrician-gynecologists I express my deep appreciation.

I am happy to acknowledge the following additional contributors, who are members of the faculty of the University of New Mexico School of Medicine. In alphabetic order, they are: Dr. Frederick Clevenger for contributing material on shock; Dr. Luis Curet for reviewing the material on diabetes, the initiation of labor, maternal physiology, and preeclampsia; Dr. William Dail for reviewing the section on gross anatomy; Dr. Raymond Doberneck for revising the material dealing with the breast; Dr. Maxine Dorin for expanding the sections on urogynecology and human sexuality; Dr. Robert Kelley for reviewing the material on embryology; Dr. Karen Knieriem for revising and expanding the section on obstetric anesthesia; Dr. J. Robert Willson for adding a section on the aging woman; and Dr. Gordon Wolf for contributing new material on gonadotropins and neuroendocrinology.

As he has done in all prior editions of this textbook, Dr. Leon Chesley has made numerous scholarly suggestions, all of which were incorporated into the relevant sections of the text, particularly those dealing with maternal physiology and hypertensive disorders in pregnancy. The timely appearance of this edition is due again in large measure to the cooperation and efficiency of Mr. Thomas J. Colaiezzi, Darlene Barela Cooke, Jessica Howie Martin, and their colleagues at Lea & Febiger.

RALPH M. WYNN, M.D.
BROOKLYN, NEW YORK

CONTRIBUTORS

Francis W. Byrn, M.D.

Assistant Professor of Obstetrics and Gynecology, University of New Mexico

Leon C. Chesley, Ph.D.

Professor Emeritus of Obstetrics and Gynecology, State University of New York Health Sciences Center at Brooklyn

Frederick W. Clevenger, M.D.

Assistant Professor of Surgery, University of New Mexico

Luis B. Curet, M.D.

Professor of Obstetrics and Gynecology, University of New Mexico

William G. Dail, Ph.D.

Professor of Anatomy, University of New Mexico

Raymond C. Doberneck, M.D.

Professor of Surgery, University of New Mexico

Maxine H. Dorin, M.D.

Assistant Professor of Obstetrics and Gynecology, University of New Mexico

David K. Guardia, M.D.

Assistant Professor of Obstetrics and Gynecology, University of New Mexico

Luis A. Izquierdo, M.D.

Assistant Professor of Obstetrics and Gynecology, University of New Mexico

Robert O. Kelley, Ph.D

Professor and Chairman of Anatomy, University of New Mexico

Karen Knieriem, M.D., Ph.D.

Associate Professor of Anesthesiology, University of New Mexico

Thomas V. Sedlacek, M.D.

Chairman, Department of Gynecology, The Graduate Hospital, Philadelphia, Pennsylvania

J. Robert Willson, M.D.

Adjunct Professor of Obstetrics and Gynecology, University of New Mexico

Gordon C. Wolf, Ph.D., M.D.

Assistant Professor of Obstetrics and Gynecology, University of New Mexico.

CONTENTS

U N I T   III

UNIT IV

UNIT V

UNIT VI

HUMAN SEXUALITY 349

NOTES ON THE USE OF THIS TEXT AND SUGGESTIONS FOR FURTHER READING

This core text defines only the data base required for minimal competence in the cognitive domain of obstetrics and gynecology. Detailed information, illustrative material, and references must be sought in standard textbooks, specialized treatises, and periodicals. Audiovisual aids, lectures, conferences, rounds, and clinical experiences with patients are required to achieve educational objectives in the affective and psychomotor (skills) domains. The basic reproductive biology included in this volume should provide the student with essential information for successful completion of an entry test for a clerkship in obstetrics and gynecology.

A list of standard reference texts follows. These books are to be supplemented, as necessary, with articles from the current literature.

General Obstetrics and Fetal-Maternal Medicine

Creasy, R, and Resnik, R.: Maternal-Fetal Medicine: Principles and Practice, 2nd ed. Philadelphia, W.B. Saunders, 1989.

Cunningham, F.G., et al.: Williams Obstetrics, 18th ed. Norwalk, CT, Appleton & Lange, 1989.

Evans, M., et al.: Fetal Diagnosis & Therapy: Science, Ethics, and the Law. Philadelphia, J.B. Lippincott Co. 1988.

Scott, J.R., et al. (eds.): Danforth's Obstetrics and Gynecology. Philadelphia, J.B. Lippincott Co., 1990.

Zuspan, F.P., and Quilligan, E.J.: Douglas-Stromme's Operative obstetrics, 5th ed. Norwalk, CT, Appleton & Lange, 1988.

General Gynecology

Droegemueller, W., et al. Comprehensive Gynecology, 2nd ed. St. Louis, Mosby/Yearbook Inc., 1991.

Jones, H.W. et al.: Novak's Texbook of Gynecology, 11th ed. Baltimore, The Williams and Wilkins Co., 1988.

Scott, J.R., et al. (eds.): Danforth's Obstetrics and Gynecology. Philadelphia, J.B. Lippincott Co., 1990.

Gynecologic Endocrinology and Infertility

Speroff, L., et al.: Clinical Gynecologic Endocrinology and Infertility, 4th ed. Baltimore, The Williams and Wilkins Co., 1989.

Yen, S.S.C., and Jaffe , R.B.: Reproductive Endocrinology, 3rd ed. Philadelphia, W.B. Saunders Co., 1991.

Gynecologic Oncology

Di Saia, P., and Creasman, W.: Clinical Gynecologic Oncology, 4th ed. St. Louis, Mosby/Yearbook Inc., 1992.

Basic Reproductive Sciences and Gynecologic Pathology

Clemente, C.D. (ed.): Gray's Anatomy of the Human Body, 30th ed. Philadelphia, Lea & Febiger, 1985.

Kurman, R.J. ed.: Blaustein's Pathology of the Female Genital Tract, 3rd. ed., New York, Springer-Verlag New York, Inc., 1987.

Moore, K.L.: The Developing Human: Clinically Oriented Embryology, 4th ed. Philadelphia, W.B. Saunders Co., 1988.

O'Rahilly, R. and Mueller, F.: Human Embryology & Teratology, Baltimore, Urban & Schwarzenberg, 1991.

Woodburne, R.T. & Burkel, W.E. Essentials of Human Anatomy, 8th ed. New York, Oxford University Press, 1988.

Wynn, R.M. and Jollie, W.P. (eds.): Biology of the Uterus, 2nd ed., New York, Plenum Pub., 1989.

I

HISTORY, ANATOMY, AND PHYSICAL EXAMINATION

1
CHAPTER

THE GYNECOLOGIC AND OBSTETRIC HISTORY

AGE OF PATIENT

The patient's age is a most important factor in the evaluation of gynecologic signs and symptoms. For example, in the childbearing age the most important causes of uterine bleeding are associated with disorders of reproduction. In postmenopausal women, carcinomas of the genital tract figure prominently in differential diagnosis, whereas in adolescent girls the cause of abnormal uterine bleeding is much more likely to be endocrine.

OBSTETRIC HISTORY

Gravidity is synonymous with pregnancy and a gravida is a pregnant woman. A primigravida, or gravida 1, is a woman who is pregnant for the first time. A secundigravida is a woman in her second pregnancy. A multigravida is a pregnant woman who has been pregnant several times. The numeric designation of gravidity is not altered by plural gestation. For example, a patient who is pregnant for the first time with twins is gravida 1, and she becomes gravida 2 during her second pregnancy.

Parity is the state of having given birth to an infant weighing 500 g or more, alive or dead. When the weight of the infant is not known, an estimated gestational length of 20 weeks or more, calculated from the first day of the last menstrual period, may be used to establish parity. For purposes of defining parity, plural gestations are counted the same as singleton pregnancies.

A primipara is a woman who has given birth for the first time to an infant or infants, alive or dead, weighing 500 g or more. A primigravida is often incorrectly designated a primipara. A multipara is a woman who has given birth two or more times to an infant or infants weighing 500 g or more, alive or dead. The designation "grand" multipara is often applied to a woman who has given birth seven or more times to an infant or infants weighing 500 g or more.

There are two common methods of summarizing the obstetric history. The first identifies only gravidity, parity, and the number of abortions. For example, a woman who has had two term pregnancies, one of which was a twin pregnancy, and one abortion, and is now pregnant would be gravida 4, para 2, ab 1. Abortions should be recorded as spontaneous or induced (medically indicated or elective). The second method uses four digits to indicate, respectively, the number of term pregnancies, premature deliveries, abortions, and living children. The history of the gravida 4, para 2, ab 1 just described would be abbreviated in the four-digit system as 2-0-1-3. A woman whose only pregnancy terminated in premature quintuplets, all of whom survived, would be designated gravida 1, para 1, ab 0 according to the first system, and 0-1-0-5 according to the second.

A parturient is a woman in the process of giving birth. A puerpera is a woman who has given birth during the preceding 42 days.

GYNECOLOGIC HISTORY

CHIEF COMPLAINT AND PRESENT ILLNESS

The chief complaint is the basic reason why the patient is seeking medical attention. In arriving at a diagnosis, it is often profitable to use the patient's own words in describing her chief complaint. Clinical acumen and experience often are required to discern the real reason behind the alleged chief complaint. For example, lack of sexual satisfaction often may present as vulvar pruritus, or a fear of cancer may be expressed as concern over a trivial vaginal discharge.

The present illness should be described in detail. Listening to the patient carefully without undue direction of the questioning usually provides most of the pertinent diagnostic information. In obtaining a gynecologic history, the physician should elicit details of the following signs and symptoms: changes or abnormalities in uterine bleeding; pain in the lower abdomen, flank, vagina, or external genitalia; a lesion on the external genitalia or a palpable mass in the pelvis; a change in the quality or quantity of vaginal discharge; changes in gastrointestinal or urinary habits; protrusion of the vaginal wall; and infertility.

MENSTRUAL HISTORY

When the major complaint involves a change or abnormality in uterine bleeding, a detailed menstrual history should be obtained. When the chief complaint and present illness are not related primarily to vaginal bleeding, an abbreviated menstrual history should be recorded after the present illness.

The menstrual history should include the age of onset of menstrual periods (menarche), the interval between the periods, the duration of flow, the amount of flow as measured by the number of pads or tampons used, the date of onset of the last normal menstrual period (LNMP), and the date of onset of the preceding menstrual period (PMP). A formula for recording menarche, interval between periods in days, and duration of flow in days is exemplified by $14 \times 28 \times 4$, which indicates that menarche occurred at age 14, the first day of the period follows the first day of the preceding period by 28 days, and the duration of flow is 4 days. Dysmenorrhea (painful periods) and signs and symptoms of premenstrual tension should be recorded as part of the menstrual history.

Primary dysmenorrhea (essential, or functional, dysmenorrhea) is menstrual pain in the absence of a recognized pelvic lesion (p. 340). Secondary dysmenorrhea is menstrual pain caused by demonstrable pelvic disease.

Premenstrual syndrome is a condition characterized by increased nervousness, irritability, emotional instability, depression, frequent headaches, and edema. The syndrome may include painful swelling of the breasts, abdominal bloating, nausea, vomiting, fatigue, and a variety of other complaints. Premenstrual syndrome occurs during the 7 to 10 days preceding menstruation and usually disappears a few hours after the onset of menstrual flow (p. 347).

In older women, the date of the last menstrual period (menopause) and a history of associated symptoms such as hot flashes and sweating should be elicited. The menopause refers strictly to the cessation of menstrual function, whereas the climacteric is the period of a woman's life characterized by cessation of menses as well as vasomotor changes and a variety of endocrine, somatic, and psychic readjustments (p. 341 and 342).

In an adult woman, the relation of changes in uterine bleeding to use of exogenous hormones including oral contraceptives and postmenopausal replacement should be clarified. Changes in menstrual patterns should be distinguished from uterine bleeding unrelated to the menses.

Menorrhagia is excessive (hypermenorrhea) or prolonged menstrual bleeding, whereas metrorrhagia is irregular acyclic uterine bleeding. Menometrorrhagia is irregular or excessive uterine bleeding during menstruation as well as between menstrual periods. Menometrorrhagia may be a sign of a variety of diseases and is not a diagnostic entity.

Hypomenorrhea is a diminution in the amount of flow or a shortening of the duration of menstruation. Oligomenorrhea is a reduction of the frequency of menstruation, in which the interval between the cycles is longer than 38 days but less than three months. The opposite of oligomenorrhea is polymenorrhea, which is abnormally frequent menstruation.

Abnormalities of bleeding confined to the menses are often of endocrine origin, whereas intermenstrual bleeding suggests other lesions, including benign and malignant neoplasms. Bleeding after contact (intercourse or douching) should always suggest a malignant lesion, most often cervical cancer.

PAIN

Pain should be described in terms of location, onset, and character. The history should note whether the pain is diffuse or localized, sharp or dull, constant or intermittent, mild or severe; whether it is abdominal, pelvic, vaginal, or lumbar; and whether it radiates to the thighs or is referred to the shoulder. Pain referred to the low back or buttocks is often associated with diseases of the cervix, urethra, or lower portions of the bladder and rectum. Pain localized to the lower abdomen may arise from the uterus or vagina. Adnexal pain is usually referred to the lower abdominal quadrants and often radiates down the medial aspect of the thigh. Dysmenorrhea and dyspareunia should be recorded at this point. The pain should be described as acute or chronic, and its onset as sudden or gradual. If a precipitating event is ascertained, it should be recorded along with associated signs and symptoms of urinary tract or gastrointestinal disease, such as nausea, vomiting, dysuria, chills, and fever. The sequence of events preceding and following the onset of pain should be described meticulously and recorded chronologically. Any factors that ameliorate or aggravate the discomfort should be noted.

OTHER COMPLAINTS

In the description of vaginal discharge, its relation to menses and coitus and the response to therapy should be noted. It must be recognized that vaginal discharge may stem from a primary lesion of the vulva, cervix, or corpus.

In obtaining a history of urinary incontinence it is necessary to differentiate stress incontinence (loss of urine upon increase in intraabdominal pressure, as in straining and coughing) from frequency and urgency with dribbling unrelated to stress and from total incontinence, which is a more or less constant loss of urine. In eliciting a history of fecal incontinence, the physician should document obstetric injuries and gynecologic procedures of possible etiologic importance.

Various complaints referable to pelvic relaxation are common in parous women. The history is of paramount importance in these patients because treatment is based more on symptoms than on purely anatomic defects.

RECORDING THE HISTORY

Table 1–1 and 3–1 and 3–2 in Chapter 3 are useful guides to recording the obstetric and gynecologic history and physical examination in institutions that employ this conventional method of obtaining these data. In institutions that use the problem-oriented record, the same information must be elicited but is generally recorded in the following four categories: objective data, subjective data, assessment, and plan.

THE MEDICAL RECORD

Excellent medical records are invaluable in medicolegal defense. According to the Department of Professional Liability of the American College of Obstetricians and Gynecologists, good medical records must be accurate, objective, timely, comprehensive,

TABLE 1–1. GYNECOLOGIC AND OBSTETRIC HISTORY

I. Age, Parity, and Day of Onset of Last Normal Menstrual Period

II. Chief Complaint

III. Present Illness

   A. Bleeding

      1. Change in interval, duration, and amount of menstrual bleeding

      2. Intermenstrual bleeding

      3. Contact bleeding

      4. Postmenopausal bleeding

      5. Relation to exogenous steroids

   B. Pain

      1. Location

      2. Relation to menses

      3. Radiation

      4. Character

   C. Mass

      1. Location

      2. Time when first identified

      3. Rate of growth

      4. Pain, discomfort, pruritus, discharge, or bleeding

      5. Relation to menses

   D. Vaginal discharge

      1. Color, odor, and consistency

      2. Onset, duration, and quantity

      3. Pain or pruritus

   E. Urinary and gastrointestinal symptoms

      1. Frequency, urgency, dysuria, urinary incontinence, and hematuria

      2. Diarrhea, constipation, tenesmus, fecal incontinence, and rectal bleeding

   F. Protrusion through the vagina

      1. Sensation of mass falling out

      2. Difficulty in emptying bowel

      3. Stress incontinence of urine

      4. Relaxed vaginal outlet

   G. Infertility

      1. Female factors (endometrial biopsy, hysterosalpingography, laparoscopy)

      2. Male factors (semen analysis)

      3. Factors shared by both partners

IV. Menstrual History

   A. Age of menarche

   B. Character of early cycles

   C. Interval between normal periods

   D. Amount and duration of normal periods

   E. Associated signs and symptoms

   F. Days of onset of last normal menstrual period and prior normal menstrual period

   G. Premenstrual signs and symptoms

   H. Abnormalities of uterine bleeding

   I. Hypomenorrhea or amenorrhea

   J. Relation to oral contraceptives

   K. Menopause

      1. Date of last menses

      2. Climacteric signs and symptoms

V. Obstetric History

   A. Dates of deliveries

   B. Lengths of gestations

   C. Complications during pregnancy (bleeding, headache, edema)

   D. Durations of labors

   E. Methods of deliveries (spontaneous, forceps, cesarean section) and complications

   F. Weight, sex, and condition of infants at delivery

   G. Number and health of children now alive

   H. Postpartum complications

   I. Abortions

      1. Spontaneous

      2. Medically indicated

      3. Elective

VI. Contraceptive History

   A. Types of contraceptives used

   B. Duration of use

   C. Reason for choice

   D. Satisfaction with method

   E. Effectiveness of method

   F. Undesirable side effects

VII. Sexual History

   A. Age at first coitus and number of sexual partners

   B. Regularity and type of sexual activity

   C. Libido, satisfaction, and orgasm

   D. Dyspareunia, frigidity, and other sexual problems such as premature ejaculation

   E. Sexual preference (homosexual, heterosexual, bisexual)

   F. Sexually transmitted diseases.

VIII. Medical History

   A. Diabetes

   B. Hypertension

   C. Cardiac disease

   D. Renal disease

   E. Syphilis

   F. Tuberculosis

   G. Epilepsy

   H. Exposure to rubella

   I. Allergies

   J. Present medications

IX. Surgical History

   A. Dates of operations and transfusions

   B. Surgeons and hospitals where performed

   C. Diagnoses

   D. Results

X. Family History

   A. Twinning

   B. Hereditary diseases

XI. Social History

   A. Tobacco

   B. Alcohol

   C. Drugs

   D. Occupation

   E. Hobbies and recreational activities

legible, and unaltered. In addition, effective communication with the patient serves to decrease the likelihood of legal action in the event of an unsuccessful outcome of treatment. Such communication involves: establishment of a healthy rapport with the patient and family; display of respect for the patient as a person; projection of the image of an ally; accurate reporting of the symptoms and history; disclosure of all relevant facts; explanation of any alternatives and reservations; assurance that the patient and family comprehend; answers to all questions; acquisition of valid consent; and provision of adequate follow-up.

2
CHAPTER

ANATOMY OF THE FEMALE PELVIS AND PERINEUM

The abdominopelvic cavity is a space enclosed by the bones, muscles, and fasciae of the abdominal and pelvic walls, from the diaphragm superiorly to the pelvic diaphragm inferiorly. The perineum is the outlet of the pelvis, specifically those structures inferior to the pelvic diaphragm. Knowledge of the bones, ligaments, and muscles that provide the boundaries and landmarks for this region is prerequisite to understanding the structures located in these areas.

THE PELVIS

The bony pelvis is composed of the right and left hip bones, sacrum, and coccyx (Fig. 2–1). Each hip bone (os coxae) is composed of a pubis, ischium, and ilium. The two pubic bones are joined anteroinferiorly at the symphysis pubis. The two ischiopubic rami extend posterolaterally from the symphysis to the ischial tuberosities. The ischial spine is located superior to the ischial tuberosity; the concavity between these two structures is the lesser sciatic notch (Fig. 2–2). The greater sciatic notch is directly superior to the ischial spine and is formed principally by the ilium. The greater and lesser sciatic notches are converted to foramina by the sacrospinous and sacrotuberous ligaments. Each ilium has an auricular

facet for its articulation with the sacrum, and anterosuperior to the pelvic brim the bone forms a fan-shaped concavity called the iliac fossa. The obturator foramen is formed by the ischium and pubis. Except for a small opening anteriorly and superiorly called the obturator canal, the foramen is closed by the tough obturator membrane.

The sacrum, composed of five fused vertebrae, has a concave pelvic, or anterior, surface. It is roughly triangular in shape. The base, formed by the body of the first sacral vertebra, has right and left alae that extend laterally to articulate with the ilia at the sacroiliac joints. The anterior border of the base is the promontory of the sacrum. There are four pairs of sacral foramina (anterior and posterior) for the passage of ventral and dorsal rami of spinal nerves from the vertebral canal.

The coccyx also is triangular in shape and is composed of 3 to 5 pieces. The first piece has prominent transverse processes that are joined to the sacrum by ligaments.

The pelvic brim is the boundary between the major and minor pelvis. From anteroinferior to posterosuperior, the brim is composed of the symphysis pubis, the pubic crest, the iliopectineal line (the arcuate is the ilial part of this line), the anterior border of the ala, and the promontory. The major pelvis is superior to the pelvic brim and is formed by the iliac fossae and alae of the

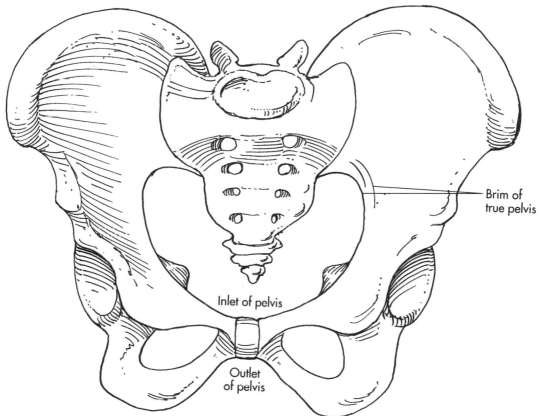

Brim of true pelvis

Inlet of pelvis

Outlet of pelvis

FIG. 2—1. Female pelvis. Anterior aspect.

sacrum. The minor pelvis is inferior to the pelvic brim and is bound by the inner surfaces of the sacrum, coccyx, ischium, pubis, and part of the ilium. In the minor pelvis are found the greater and lesser sciatic foramina, the obturator foramen with its obturator membrane, and the anterior sacral foramina.

In a living subject who is standing, the anterior superior iliac spines and the antero-superior part of the symphysis pubis are in a vertical plane. The anterosuperior part of the symphysis pubis and the tip of the coccyx are in a horizontal plane.

There are four important articulations: the lumbosacral and sacrococcygeal, the sacroiliac joints, and the symphysis pubis. The lumbosacral joint has a thick interver-tebral disc and a strong iliolumbar ligament extending from the transverse processes of L-5 to the iliac crest. The ligaments prevent axial rotation and keep L-5 from sliding anteriorly on the sacrum. The sacrococ-

cygeal joint allows the coccyx to move posteriorly during defecation and parturi-tion. The sacroiliac joints are large and involve the medial surface of the ilium posterior to the iliac fossa and the auricular facet of the sacrum. The joint is strength-ened by the interosseous sacroiliac, dorsal sacral, and iliolumbar ligaments, which, along with the sacrotuberous and sacro-spinous ligaments, resist anterior rotation of the sacrum when the weight of the body is imposed on the lumbosacral joint. The two hip bones are united anteriorly by fibrocar-tilage at the symphysis pubis (Fig. 2—3).

In the female pelvis, as compared with that of the male, the bones are lighter, the joints smaller, the sacrum wider and shorter, the ischial tuberosities everted rather than inverted, the angle of the greater sciatic notch larger, the coccyx more posteriorly directed, the angle of the pubic arch greater (90° or more rather than about 60° for the male), and the pelvic diameters greater. The

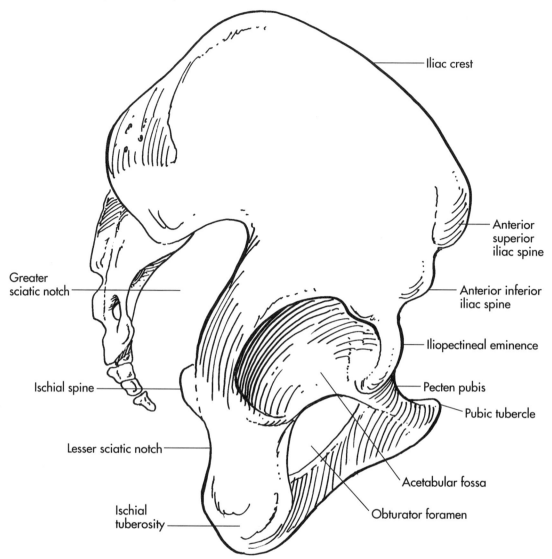

Iliac crest

Anterior superior iliac spine

Anterior inferior iliac spine

Iliopectineal eminence

Pecten pubis

Pubic tubercle

Greater sciatic notch

Ischial spine

Lesser sciatic notch

Ischial tuberosity

Acetabular fossa

Obturator foramen

FIG. 2−2. Right hip bone with sacrum and coccyx. External or lateral surface. (From Benninghoff and Goerttler. 1975.)

principal diameters of the inlet (pelvic brim) are the anteroposterior or conjugate between the superior end of the symphysis pubis and the promontory of the sacrum (10.5 to 11 cm) and the transverse, which is the greatest width across the inlet (13.5 cm). These diameters are about 0.5 cm greater in the female than in the male. The principal diameters of the outlet are the anteroposterior, from the inferior edge of the symphysis pubis to the tip of the coccyx (9 to 11 cm), and the transverse, between the two ischial tuberosities (11 cm). The diameters of the outlet are about 2.5 cm greater in the female than the male. There is an angle of about 60° between the conjugate line of the inlet and the horizontal plane, and one of about 15° between the anteroposterior line of the outlet and the horizontal plane in the female (Figs. 2−4 and 2−5).

The abdominopelvic cavity is separated from the perineum by the pelvic diaphragm, which stretches across the pelvis like a hammock. The pelvic diaphragm is formed by the levator ani and coccygeus from each half of the pelvis, which join in a continuous

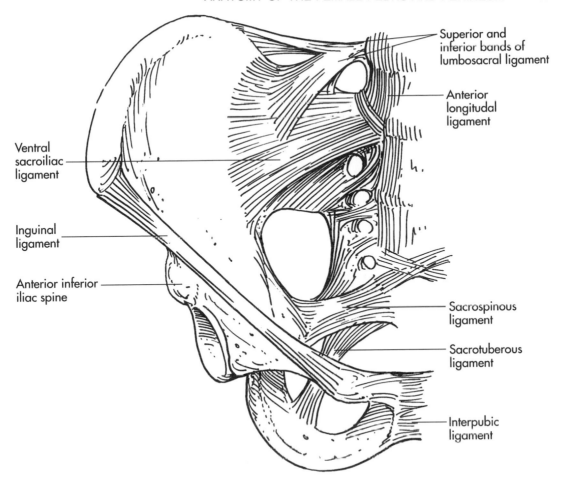

FIG. 2–3. The joints and ligaments of the right half of the pelvis. Anterior superior aspect.

line posteriorly from the junction of the rectum and anal canal to the coccyx. Anteriorly the two sheets of muscle are separated by a space sometimes called the genital hiatus. The human coccygeus is unimportant, comprising merely a few strands of muscle coating the internal surface of the sacrospinous ligament. The levator ani, however, is very important and essential for the functional integrity of both the pelvis and perineum (Fig. 2–6).

The anterolateral walls of the minor pelvis are covered almost entirely by the obturator internus muscles, which originate from the obturator membrane and the pelvic surfaces of the pubis, ischium, and even part of the ilium (Fig. 2–7). Its fibers converge on the lesser sciatic notch before making a right-angle turn to pass out of the pelvis into the

gluteal region. The internal surface of this muscle is coated with the thick obturator fascia.

Each levator ani comprises a pubococcygeus and an iliococcygeus. The pubococcygeus originates from the posterior surface of the pubis along an oblique line extending from the lower border of the symphysis pubis to the obturator canal. Functionally, it is two muscles, a medial part called the puborectalis and a lateral part called the pubococcygeus proper. The fibers of the puborectalis extend posteriorly; some insert into the side of the vagina (pubovaginalis), and others into the perineal body and the external anal sphincter; the remainder meet with their fellows from the opposite side posterior to the junction of the rectum and anal canal to form a rectal sling. This sling is

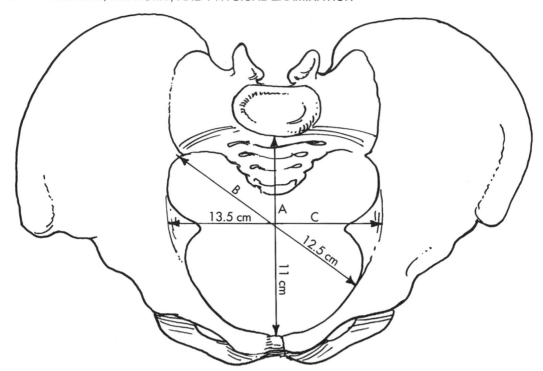

FIG. 2–4. Diameters of superior aperture of lesser pelvis (female). *A*, Anteroposterior or conjugate diameter. *B*, Oblique diameter. *C*, Transverse diameter.

responsible for the 90° angle between the ampulla of the rectum and the anal canal. Its integrity is important for both voluntary and involuntary control of the bowel. Fibers of the pubococcygeus interdigitate with those from the opposite side in a raphe extending from the junction of the rectum and anal canal to the coccyx.

The iliococcygeus is the second major component of the levator ani. It originates from a thickening of the obturator fascia that extends between the ischial spine posteriorly and the pubis, just anterior to the obturator canal. This thickened line is called the arcus tendineus, or tendinous arch of the levator ani. Fibers originating from the arch sweep posteriorly and medially to insert with those of the pubococcygeus in the anococcygeal raphe and coccyx. Some of the fibers of the iliococcygeus join the longitudinal coat of muscle around the anal canal. Although the pelvic diaphragm usually functions without conscious control, it is composed of striated muscle and is a voluntary muscle innervated by the anterior branches of the ventral rami of S-3 and S-4. Its principal function is to support the pelvic viscera and maintain the 90° angle at the junction between the rectum and anal canal.

THE PERINEUM

The perineum is the outlet of the pelvis; it includes all structures inferior to the pelvic diaphragm. On the surface, it is the floor of the groove between the thighs and buttocks and therefore includes the external genitalia and anus. When the thighs are spread and the skin removed, this surface becomes a diamond-shaped area bounded anteriorly by the symphysis pubis and arcuate pubic ligament, anterolaterally by the ischiopubic rami, laterally by the ischial tuberosities, posterolaterally by the sacrotuberous ligaments, and posteriorly by the tip of the coccyx. The perineum is a three-dimensional space bounded superomedially by the pelvic diaphragm, laterally by the obturator fascia, and inferiorly by the skin covering the diamond-shaped area previously described.

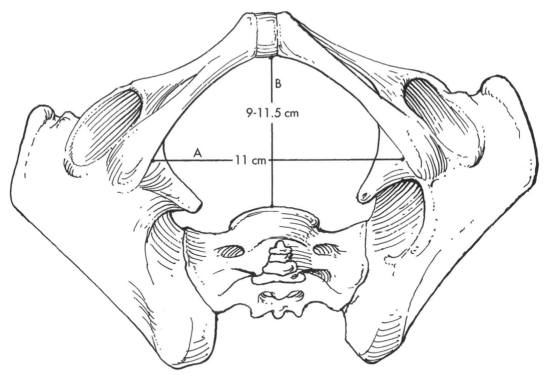

FIG. 2−5. Diameters of inferior aperture of lesser pelvis (female). *A,* Transverse diameter. *B,* Anteroposterior diameter.

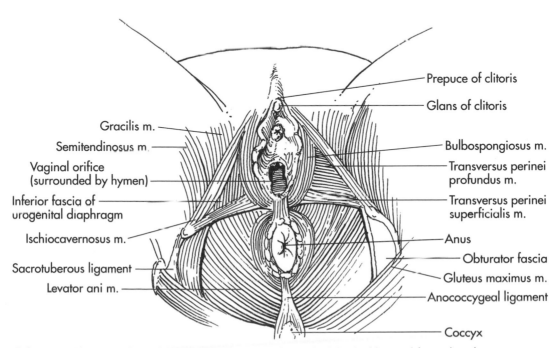

Gracilis m.

Semitendinosus m.

Vaginal orifice (surrounded by hymen)

Inferior fascia of urogenital diaphragm

Ischiocavernosus m.

Sacrotuberous ligament

Levator ani m.

Prepuce of clitoris

Glans of clitoris

Bulbospongiosus m.

Transversus perinei profundus m.

Transversus perinei superficialis m.

Anus

Obturator fascia

Gluteus maximus m.

Anococcygeal ligament

Coccyx

FIG. 2−6. Muscles of the female perineum. The fat pad of the ischiorectal fossa has been removed to reveal the levator ani muscle.

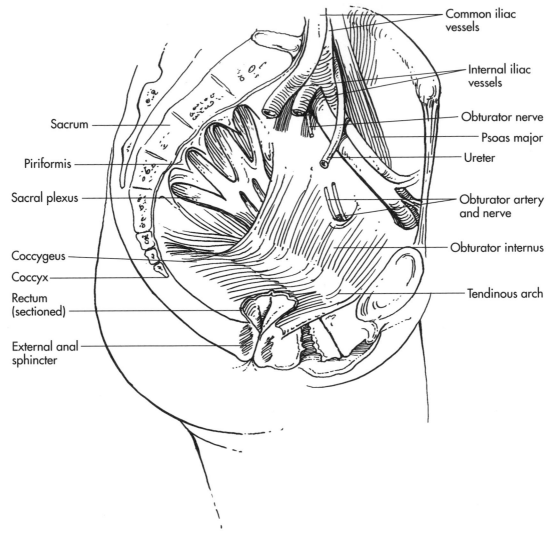

FIG. 2–7. Interior of the female pelvis in a sagittal section, showing the muscles of the left lateral wall, the obturator fascia, and the tendinous arch of the levator ani muscle.

The diamond-shaped perineum is divided into an anterior urogenital triangle and a posterior anal triangle by an arbitrary line drawn between the ischial tuberosities. The urogenital diaphragm is a thin sheet of muscle stretching between the two ischiopubic rami, covered on its superior and inferior surfaces with fascia. By definition, it is in the perineum, because it is just inferior to the pelvic diaphragm; it also is in the urogenital triangle, that is, anterior to the line between the ischial tuberosities. The anal triangle comprises the anus, external anal sphincter, ischiorectal fossae, and the vessels and nerves supplying them. These structures also are in the perineum, because

they are inferior to the pelvic diaphragm.

There are three parts to the external anal sphincter: subcutaneous, superficial, and deep. The subcutaneous part, formed by a few circular fibers, causes the wrinkled appearance of the anal verge. The superficial part is fusiform, extending from the tip of the coccyx and anococcygeal raphe to the perineal body, which is a large mass of connective tissue interposed between the anus and anal canal posteriorly and the urogenital diaphragm and inferior part of the vagina anteriorly. The superficial part of the external anal sphincter is infiltrated by longitudinal fibers of the anal canal. The deep part of the sphincter comprises a thick, circular mass of fibers that mingle superiorly with the puborectalis portion of the levator ani. Anteriorly, some of these fibers interdigitate with the superficial transverse perineus muscle. As does the pelvic diaphragm, the anal sphincter consists of voluntary muscle but functions without conscious control. The rectum and anal canal are coated by two layers of smooth muscle, an inner circular and an outer longitudinal. The circular layer is particularly thick at the end of the anal canal, where it forms the internal anal sphincter.

The ischiorectal fossae are fat-filled, wedge-shaped spaces located on either side of the anal canal and sphincter. The boundaries of the fossae are: anteriorly, the base of the urogenital diaphragm; laterally, the fascia covering the obturator internus muscle; mediosuperiorly, the levator ani of the pelvic diaphragm; inferiorly, the skin; and posteriorly, the sacrotuberous ligament.

Inferior rectal nerves and vessels course medially across each ischiorectal fossa from the pudendal canal in the lateral wall to the anal sphincter. They are branches of the pudendal nerve and internal pudendal vessels, which originate in the pelvis. To gain access to the perineum, they pass out of the pelvis into the gluteal area via the greater sciatic foramen, course around the ischial spine and sacrospinous ligament, and enter the perineum through the lesser sciatic foramen. From the lesser sciatic foramen posteriorly to the posterolateral corners of the urogenital diaphragm, the pudendal vessels and nerves lie in a canal formed by a split in the obturator fascia. The inferior rectal nerves and vessels are branches that pass through the wall of the pudendal canal to supply the fat of the ischiorectal fossa as well as the terminal part of the digestive tube with its sphincter. Because the pudendal canal follows a precise course, it is fairly easy to effect a perineal block by injecting an anesthetic agent into the area.

THE EXTERNAL GENITALIA

The external genital organs of the female (pudendum, or vulva) are located principally in the urogenital triangle but extend on to the lower abdominal wall (Fig. 2–8). The mons pubis is a fatty fibrous pad of connective tissue anterior to the pubis; its skin is covered with hair after puberty. The labia majora begin at the mons, where their medial margins are united by a low ridge of skin, the anterior commissure. They diminish in size posteriorly and are joined again by a low ridge of skin anterior to the anus, the posterior commissure. The labia majora are sparsely covered with hair laterally, but their medial surfaces are smooth and moist. The pudendal cleft is the space separating the labia majora. The clitoris is the homologue of the penis; much of it is hidden behind the posteroinferior part of the mons in the anterior part of the pudendal cleft. The labia minora are a pair of thin folds of skin devoid of fat. In the nullipara they usually are hidden by the labia majora. Anteriorly, each labium minus divides into a medial and lateral fold. The medial folds from the two sides join to form the frenulum, which connects to the glans of the clitoris. The lateral folds join to cover the surface of the clitoris and its glans as the prepuce. Posteriorly, the labia minora pass on either side of the orifice of the vagina, diminish in size, and end by joining about 1 cm posterior to the vaginal orifice in a transverse ridge called the frenulum labiorum. The vestibule is the space between the labia minora; into it open the vagina, urethra, and ducts of the greater vestibular glands. The vaginal orifice opens in the middle of the vestibule, and the urethra terminates just anterior to it, about 2.5 cm posterior to the clitoris. The ducts of the greater vestibular glands empty into the vaginal orifice posterolaterally, just distal to the hymen. The vestibular fossa is the area between the vaginal orifice and the frenulum labiorum.

The superficial fascia of the urogenital triangle, with its superficial and deep perineal pouches, is continuous with Scarpa's fascia of the abdomen. The integument over the abdominal wall may be divided into skin and tela subcutanea. The skin is composed of the epidermis and dermis; the tela comprises the panniculus adiposus and a deeper membranous layer, the stratum fibrosum. In the lower, anterior abdominal wall, the panniculus adiposus is called Camper's fascia; the particularly well developed stratum fibrosum is called Scarpa's fascia. Inferiorly Scarpa's fascia attaches to the fascia lata of

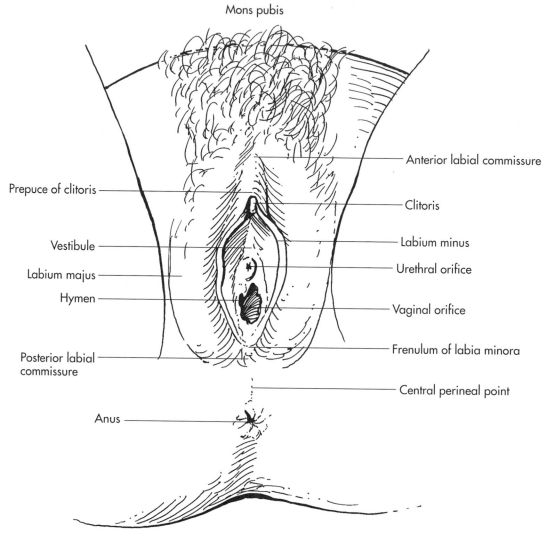

FIG. 2–8. The female external genitalia. The labia majora and labia minora have been drawn apart.

the thigh in a curved line from the two anterior superior iliac spines to the pubic tubercles. From the pubic tubercles, the lines of attachment follow the ischiopubic rami posterolaterally to the posterior border of the urogenital diaphragm, from which it doubles back anteriorly over its inferior surface as the perineal membrane. Scarpa's fascia of the abdominal wall changes its name to Colles' fascia of the perineum as it passes from the pubic tubercle to the ischiopubic ramus. Scarpa's fascia condenses in the midline over the anterior surface of the rectus sheath to form the fundiform ligament, which extends inferiorly to join the

suspensory ligament of the clitoris, which arises directly from the symphysis pubis.

The perineal membrane is the superior boundary of the superficial perineal pouch. Colles' fascia limits this space inferiorly. The other boundaries are formed by the attachments of Colles' fascia laterally to the ischiopubic rami and posteriorly to the posterior border of the urogenital diaphragm. Medially the pouch is interrupted by the opening for the vagina; thus, Colles' fascia is continuous with the connective tissue that forms the core of the labia minora. Anteriorly, the superficial perineal pouch (of the perineum) is continuous with the space just deep to

Scarpa's fascia (of the abdominal wall). Openings between the two spaces occur on either side of the fundiform ligament through the so-called abdominolabial meatuses. These openings are bounded medially by the fundiform ligament, posteriorly by the pubic bones, laterally by the pubic tubercles, and anteriorly by the bridge of Scarpa's fascia between the pubic tubercles and fundiform ligament. The abdominolabial meatuses are filled by the digital processes of fat that extend from the superficial inguinal rings into the labia majora. Each process of fat is accompanied by minute blood vessels and the structures emerging from the inguinal canal, namely, the ilioinguinal nerve, which supplies the anterior part of the labium, and the round ligament of the uterus, which attaches to its skin.

The superficial perineal pouch is a potential space between the perineal membrane and the superficial perineal fascia (Colles'). It is filled with the crura of the clitoris, the bulbs of the vestibule, the greater vestibular glands, three pairs of superficial perineal muscles, and the superficial perineal vessels and nerves. The crura are elongated, tapered columns of erectile tissue attached to the ischium and perineal membrane and are continuous anteriorly at the inferior part of the symphysis pubis with the corpora cavernosa of the clitoris. The bulbs of the vestibule are elongated, pyriform masses of erectile tissue attached to the perineal membrane on either side of the vaginal orifice. Anteriorly each bulb tapers and joins its fellow from the opposite side to form the slender anterior commissure of the bulbs. The greater vestibular glands are located posteriorly under the vestibular bulbs next to the perineal membrane. Their small ducts lead to the groove between the hymen and the labium minus. There are three pairs of superficial perineal muscles: the bulbospongiosus, the ischiocavernosus, and the superficial transverse perinei. Each bulbospongiosus attaches to the perineal body posteriorly and the perineal membrane anteriorly. Each ischiocavernosus muscle attaches to both the perineal membrane and the ischiopubic ramus. Its fibers cover the crus of the clitoris. The superficial transverse perinei muscles are very small and occasionally even absent. They originate from the ischial tuberosities and extend medially as narrow bands to insert in the anterior part of the perineal body and to interdigitate with the fibers of the bulbospongiosus muscle. The area is supplied by perineal branches of the internal pudendal vessels, which emerge from the anterior ends of the pudendal canals and divide into medial and lateral labial branches. Small transverse perineal arteries arise from the medial labial arteries and course toward the perineal body and posterior parts of the bulbs of the vestibule. Branches of the perineal nerves with the same names follow similar courses. The area is supplied in addition by the perineal branches of the two posterior femoral cutaneous nerves.

The deep perineal pouch is essentially the urogenital diaphragm with its fascias and the structures that pass through it. It is bounded inferiorly by the perineal membrane, which forms the superior boundary of the superficial perineal pouch, and superiorly by the fascia on the pelvic surface of the urogenital diaphragm. The contents of the deep perineal pouch include a segment of the vagina with the urethra partially embedded in its anterior wall, the sphincter urethrae and deep transverse perinei muscles, the dorsal nerves of the clitoris, the internal pudendal vessels, and the arteries to the bulb of the vagina. The sphincter urethrae is a thin layer of muscle fibers that encircle the urethra and extend between the two ischiopubic rami. The deep transverse perinei are thin bands of muscle stretching between the two ischial tuberosities; they parallel the superficial transverse perinei lying in the superficial perineal pouch. The dorsal nerves of the clitoris and the internal pudendal vessels enter the deep perineal pouch from the pudendal canals on each side. The dorsal nerves course along the sides of the ischiopubic rami, pierce the perineal membrane, and then lie on the dorsal surface of the crura and body of the clitoris all the way to its glans. The internal pudendal arteries also enter the deep perineal pouch from the pudendal canals and follow a course similar to that of the dorsal nerves of the clitoris. Each artery sends a branch, the artery to the bulb, medially to pierce the perineal membrane and enter the bulbs of the vagina on their deep surfaces. The internal pudendal arteries next send deep (profunda) branches through the perineal membrane to supply their respective crura. Finally the internal pudendal arteries themselves pierce the perineal membrane and parallel the dorsal nerves of the clitoris on the crura and body of the clitoris. These are the dorsal arteries of the clitoris.

Superior to the pelvic diaphragm are located the urinary bladder, the female internal genitalia, the rectum, and the nerves and vessels supplying both the pelvis and perineum. The urinary bladder (vesica urinaria) has four surfaces: one superior, two inferolateral, and one inferoposterior. The superior surface is roughly triangular and is located between the two ureters, which enter it posterolaterally, and the urachus, which is anterior in the midline. The sigmoid colon or ileum lies on the peritoneum covering the superior surface. The inferolateral surfaces of the bladder lie against the pubic bones, the obturator internus muscles, and the levator ani. The inferoposterior surface of the bladder (base) lies against the anterior wall of the vagina. The bladder is surrounded by vesical fascia, which is continuous with the extraperitoneal connective tissue. A well developed vesical plexus of veins lies in the fascia and separates the urinary bladder from the retropubic space.

Each ureter is about 25 cm long; half of it is in the abdomen and half in the pelvis. The ureter enters the pelvis at the bifurcation of the common iliac artery, descends anterior to the internal iliac artery, and crosses inferior to the uterine artery before entering the wall of the bladder. As the ureter passes inferior to the uterine artery, it frequently lies next to the lateral fornix of the vagina, but this anatomic relation may be only unilateral because the superior part of the vagina is often displaced considerably from the midline of the body.

The ureters do not go directly through the wall of the bladder; instead they angle from the point where they enter inferiorly and medially in an oblique fashion. Each ureter enters the lumen of the bladder about 2 cm posterolateral to the opening of the urethra and about 2 cm from the orifice of the other ureter. Thus a small triangle called the trigone of the bladder is formed by the openings of the three ducts. The surface of the mucosa over the trigone is relatively smooth, whereas it is wrinkled elsewhere when the bladder is empty. The interureteric fold is a prominent ridge between the openings of the two ureters.

The female urethra is about 4 cm long. It passes from the neck of the bladder through the urogenital diaphragm to open in the vestibule just anterior to the vagina about 2.5 cm posterior to the glans of the clitoris. The distal end of the urethra is embedded in the anterior wall of the vagina. This relatively fixed relation is the reason it is occasionally injured during parturition or irritated by coitus.

The rectum is the part of the digestive tract between the sigmoid, or pelvic, colon and the anal canal. It begins where the sigmoid colon loses its mesentery, just anterior to the body of the third sacral vertebra. Although the word "rectum" means "straight," its 12-cm length follows the curvature of the sacrum and coccyx. The entire rectum may be considered a retroperitoneal structure, but peritoneum covers its proximal third on the anterior and lateral surfaces, and its middle third on the anterior surface. The distal third, where it dilates to form the ampulla, is inferior to the peritoneum. Where the peritoneum covers the anterior and lateral surfaces of the proximal part of the rectum, pararectal fossae are formed on both sides. In addition to the curvature caused by the concavity of the sacrum, the rectum has three lateral curvatures. A prominent indentation of its right wall occurs at the bottom of the rectouterine pouch, and two smaller indentations of its left wall occur about 2 cm proximal and 2 cm distal to this point. These indentations produce the transverse folds (plicae transversales) or shelves that project into the lumen of the bowel. The large right plica may form a partial obstruction to the insertion of a proctoscope.

The rectum ends at its junction with the anal canal, about 4 cm anterior to the tip of the coccyx. There the digestive tube makes a 90° turn as a result of the pull of the puborectal portion of the levator ani. The anal canal is only about 2.5 to 3.5 cm long. Its superior part has 5 to 10 permanent longitudinal ridges called anal columns, which unite at their distal ends by semilunar folds, the anal valves. Together the ends of the anal columns and the anal valves form the circular, serrated pectinate line around the lumen. The pectinate line is an important landmark. Superior to it the epithelium is composed of columnar cells; its arterial supply and venous drainage are from the middle and superior rectal vessels, and the lymphatics drain to pelvic and lumbar nodes. The anal canal inferior to the pectinate line is composed of stratified squamous epithelium, is supplied by branches of the inferior rectal artery and vein (from the pudendal canals), and has a lymphatic drainage to the superficial and deep inguinal nodes. Superior to the pectinate line the bowel is fairly insensitive except to stretching, whereas inferior to the line, touch, pain, heat, and cold are perceived. The superior rectal artery and vein are continuations of the inferior mesenteric vessels. They divide into right and left branches, which descend in the submucosa of the rectum and anal canal down to the anal columns. Superior to the pectinate line they anastomose with the paired middle rectal vessels, and inferior to the line with the paired inferior rectal vessels. Dilation of the veins in the anal columns produces rectal hemorrhoids. When they remain superior to the pectinate line, they are called internal hemorrhoids. When they become large enough to project distal to the line, they are called external hemorrhoids. As the uterus enlarges during pregnancy, the venous return from the pelvis and perineum may be compromised. Anastomoses between the superior and middle rectal veins are sites where the portal and systemic circulations join. The increased venous pressure in this area during pregnancy may result in rectal hemorrhoids. Metastatic tumors superior to the pectinate line may remain undetected for a long time, because the area is moderately insensitive to pain and the lymphatic drainage is to pelvic nodes. Tumors or infections distal to the pectinate line, however, are often readily evident.

The anal canal is closed by the internal and external anal sphincters. The internal sphincter is merely a thickened portion of the circular coat of involuntary muscle surrounding the bowel. The external anal sphincter is under voluntary control.

THE INTERNAL GENITALIA

The internal female genitalia consist of the ovaries, oviducts (uterine, or fallopian, tubes), uterus, and vagina (Figs. 2–9 and 2–10).

The normal adult ovary measures 3 cm × 2 cm × 1.5 cm and weighs about 3 g. It is located on the side wall of the pelvis between the ureter and external iliac vein. The ovary is oriented so that its superior end projects toward the uterine tube and its inferior end toward the uterus. It is held by a short fold of peritoneum, the mesovarium, which is one of the parts of the broad ligament. The suspensory ligament of the ovary is continuous with the mesovarium and connects the tubal end of the gonad to the lateral pelvic wall. The suspensory ligament contains: the ovarian artery, which arises from the aorta just inferior to the renal artery; the ovarian veins, which drain into the inferior vena cava on the right side and into the left renal vein on the left; lymphatic vessels that drain to the lateral aortic and preaortic nodes (because they follow the ovarian veins superiorly); and a plexus of autonomic nerves. The ligament of the ovary extends from the uterine pole to the lateral margin of the uterus. It is about 2.5 cm long and raises a slight fold of peritoneum along the posterior surface of the broad ligament.

In the young nullipara, the ovary is smooth and pink; in elderly multiparas, it is gray and shrunken. Each ovary has a hilum, where the ovarian vessels and lymphatics enter and leave. The lateral surface of the ovary lies against the obturator internus muscle, the umbilical artery, and the obturator vessels and nerve. Its medial surface is covered partially by the lateral end of the uterine tube and by ileum or sigmoid colon.

The oviduct extends from the junction of the body and fundus of the uterus laterally, superiorly, and posteriorly toward the side wall of the pelvis. Each tube is about 11 cm long and may be divided into four parts: the infundibulum, ampulla, isthmus, and interstitial portion. The infundibulum is funnel-shaped and surrounded by fimbriae. One of them, the fimbria ovarica, is longer than the others and attaches to the ovary. The infundibulum contains the abdominal orifice

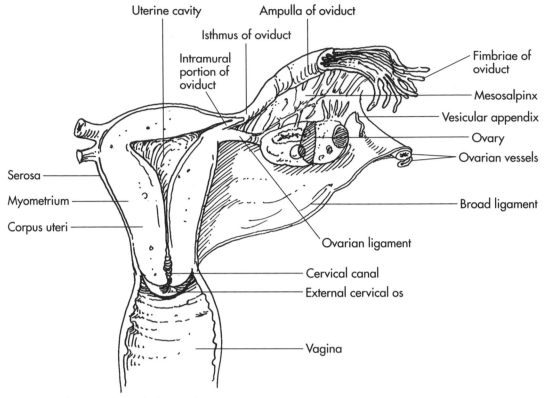

FIG. 2–9. Section through the vagina, uterus, uterine tube, and ovary.

of the uterine tube, which is about 2 to 3 mm in diameter. The ampulla of the uterine tube is long and irregularly dilated. It narrows to a short, straight isthmus, which connects to the uterus at the junction of its body and fundus. The intrauterine (interstitial) part of the uterine tube is about 1 cm long and extends through the myometrium to the uterine cavity. Most of the uterine tube lies in the free edge of the broad ligament, but its infundibulum emerges from it near the side of the pelvis to overlie the medial surface of the ovary. The part of the broad ligament that invests and is immediately adjacent to the uterine tube is called the mesosalpinx. In the male, the peritoneal cavity is a closed sac, but in the female it is open to the outer world via the vagina, uterus, and uterine tubes.

Several embryologic remnants are commonly encountered in the female genital tract. The epoophoron consists of a few minute tubules located in the mesovarium. These tubules course to the duct of the epoophoron, which lies horizontally in the broad ligament. The epoophoron and its duct are embryonic remnants of the mesonephric tubules and duct, respectively. The paroophoron consists of minute tubules lying in the broad ligament adjacent to the uterus. It is a remnant of the mesonephros. Vesicular appendices (hydatids) are small pedunculated cysts found in the broad ligament inferior to the infundibulum of the uterine tube. They form from the upper end of the mesonephric duct.

The uterus is a pear-shaped organ containing a flattened cavity; it lies between the rectum and bladder. It is about 8 cm long, 5 cm at its widest part, and 2.5 cm thick. Its walls are made of smooth muscle. The uterus often deviates from the midline, usually to the right. Its anterior, or vesical, surface is flattened against the bladder, and its posterior, or intestinal, surface is convex. The isthmus of each uterine tube enters the uterus at its widest part, the junction of the body and fundus. Peritoneum covers the

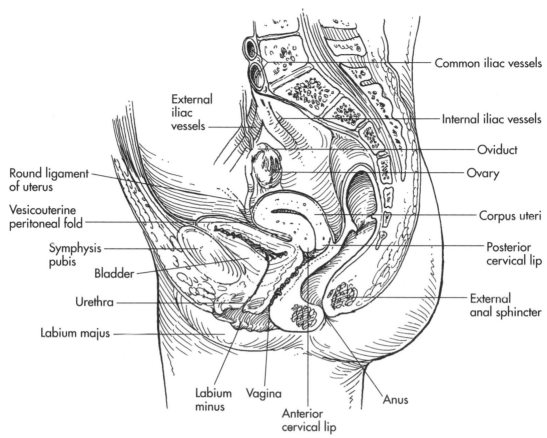

FIG. 2–10. Median sagittal section of female pelvis. The bladder is empty: the uterus and vagina are slightly dilated. (Eycleshymer and Jones.)

fundus and part of the body and continues laterally as the broad ligament, which drapes over the outstretched uterine tubes. The utero-ovarian ligament attaches the ovary to the uterus just inferior to its junction with the uterine tube. The round ligament of the uterus begins anterior to the isthmic portion of the oviduct and extends laterally to the side wall of the pelvis, over the external iliac vessels to the deep inguinal ring, just lateral to the origin of the inferior epigastric artery. From there the ligament continues through the inguinal canal and the abdominolabial meatus to attach to the skin of the labium majus. Just as the utero-ovarian ligament (proper ligament of the ovary) raises a ridge of peritoneum on the posterior surface of the broad ligament, the round ligament raises a similar ridge on its anterior surface.

The cervix of the uterus is about 3 cm long and roughly cylindrical. It projects at a right angle into the vagina near its superior end. The cervical canal extends from the external os about 3 cm to the internal os. It is spindle-shaped, with anterior and posterior ridges, each with lateral branches. These two configurations are called plicae palmatae because of their resemblance to the branches of a palm tree. The cervical canal joins the triangular-shaped cavity of the uterus at the internal os. This triangle is formed by the openings of the two uterine tubes and the internal os of the cervical canal. The anterior and posterior walls of the uterus are apposed to each other. The cavity is lined with endometrium, which is surrounded by the thick, muscular myometrium. The uterus is frequently anteflexed and anteverted. Its body is slightly flexed where the flattened anterior surface lies against the bladder. The uterus lies at right angles to both the vagina and pelvic brim and therefore is anteverted when the bladder is empty. Retroversion occurs naturally when the bladder is full.

The parametrium is the fibroadipose tissue along the sides of the uterus; it supports the vessels and nerves supplying the organ. Because the end of the cervix projects into the vagina, the uterus is said to have intravaginal and supravaginal parts. The uterus is supplied by the uterine and ovarian arteries. The uterine artery, a branch of the internal iliac, courses medially in the cardinal ligament and divides into superior and inferior branches at the junction of the body and cervix. The uterus is innervated by branches of the sympathetic plexus around the arteries that supply it. These nerves arise from ganglia of the sympathetic chain located adjacent to vertebrae T-10 to L-1 and S-2 to S-4. Lymphatic vessels from the cervix travel to nodes alongside the rectum, on the pelvic surface of the sacrum, and associated with the iliac artery. Lymphatic vessels from the corpus of the uterus follow the ovarian vessels to nodes associated with the inferior vena cava and aorta, drain to nodes adjacent to the external iliac artery, and course along the round ligaments of the uterus through the inguinal canal, to the labia majora, and ultimately to the superficial inguinal nodes.

The vagina is a fibromuscular sheath located in the interior part of the pelvis and in the perineum. It extends from the external vaginal orifice in the vestibule through the urogenital diaphragm into the cavity of the pelvis. Its anterior wall is about 7.5 cm long and may be divided into three parts: an inferior third in contact with the urethra, a middle third in contact with the bladder, and a superior third that connects to the anterior part of the cervix. The posterior wall of the vagina is about 9 cm long and may be divided into three parts: the inferior segment contacts the perineal body, which separates it from the anal canal; the middle part is separated from the ampulla of the rectum by a heavy layer of connective tissue known as the rectovaginal septum; and the superior part connects to the posterior wall of the cervix and is covered by peritoneum of the rectouterine pouch. The attachment of the vagina to the anterior, lateral, and posterior walls of the cervix produces a continuous gutter around the cervix. The anterior part of this gutter is shallow and is called the anterior fornix. The posterior fornix is much deeper, and the lateral fornices are intermediate in depth.

The sides of the vagina are supported by endopelvic fascia; fibers from the puborectalis part of the levator ani insert into its side walls. These muscular fibers can act as a constrictor of the vagina. More inferiorly, the vagina passes through the urogenital diaphragm, where it receives some additional support. Finally, the bulbs of the vestibule and the bulbospongiosus muscle help to stabilize its distal portion. The anterior and posterior walls are in contact from a point just inferior to the cervix to the urogenital diaphragm and project into the lumen so that its cross section inferiorly resembles the letter "H." These projections into the lumen are known as anterior and posterior rugal columns; a series of raised ridges, or rugae, project from them laterally. The bulbs of the vestibule and their muscular covering tend to orient the introitus in an anterior-posterior direction. The hymen is a fold of mucous membrane inferior to the urogenital diaphragm at the introitus. After parturition, its remnants are called the carunculae hymenales (myrtiformes). The vagina is supplied by branches of the uterine, vaginal, middle rectal, and internal pudendal arteries and is surrounded by a very extensive venous plexus, which drains into veins of the same names. The vagina receives both sympathetic and parasympathetic nerves from the inferior hypogastric plexus as well as direct branches from the pelvic splanchnic nerves. Stimulation of the parasympathetic nerves produces an engorgement of the extensive perivaginal vascular plexus with subsequent production of vaginal lubricant, which is a serum-like transudate that passes from the vascular plexus through the vaginal wall. The vagina is devoid of glands, and neither those of the cervix nor those of the corpus have anything to do with production of this lubricant. The greater vestibular glands do not contribute to the normal vaginal lubrication.

Support of the pelvic viscera is accomplished by both muscles and connective tissue. The levator ani is particularly important. Its puborectal fibers pull the rectum anteriorly in such a manner that it provides considerable support for the vagina posteriorly. The urinary bladder lies against the vagina posteriorly and the pubic symphysis and levator ani anteriorly and inferiorly. The levator ani inserts into the sides of the vagina and the perineal body, and the urogenital diaphragm provides a floor anteriorly. The connective tissue of the pelvis is arranged loosely around the bladder (vesical fascia) and rectum (rectal fascia) and allows for their easy expansion, but the vesical and vaginal fascias are more closely attached, particularly inferiorly, where they form a vesicovaginal septum. The endopelvic fascia is further organized into pairs of suspensory "ligaments": the pubovesical, the lateral cervical, and the uterosacral ligaments. The pubovesical ligaments extend from the posterior part of the pubis just lateral to the symphysis to the neck of the bladder. The lateral cervical (transverse cervical, or cardinal) ligaments are condensations of endopelvic connective tissue around the uterine, vaginal, and vesical vessels and course from the sides of the pelvis to the junction of the cervix and vagina. Other parts of the ligament connect to the side of the bladder anteriorly and to the side of the rectum posteriorly. The uterosacral ligament is continuous with the lateral cervical ligament and projects from the junction of the body and cervix of the uterus to the middle of the sacrum. Thus, it lies in the rectouterine fold of peritoneum, which forms a boundary for the pararectal fossae. The round ligaments of the uterus provide little support for the uterus. They project anteriorly and laterally across the external iliac vessels to the deep inguinal ring, where they course through the inguinal canals to the labia majora.

PELVIC AND PERINEAL VASCULATURE

The pelvic viscera are supplied by one paired and two unpaired arteries. The unpaired vessels are the median sacral and superior rectal arteries; the paired vessels are the internal iliacs. The median sacral artery is a very small vessel that arises at the level of L-4 from the dorsal wall of the aorta, crosses the body of L-5, and continues in the midline inferiorly on the pelvic surface of the sacrum. The superior rectal artery is a continuation of the inferior mesenteric as it crosses the pelvic brim. The vessel divides

into right and left branches to supply the rectum and anastomose distally with the middle rectal arteries. The aorta branches into the two common iliac arteries at L-4, and they in turn divide into the internal and external iliac arteries. This division takes place about one third of the way along a line drawn from the origin of the common iliac arteries from the aorta to the midinguinal point, where the external iliacs pass into the thigh. The right common iliac artery crosses anterior to the left common iliac vein and lies at first medial and then anterior to the right common iliac vein. Both internal iliac arteries pass into the pelvis medial to the internal iliac veins (Fig. 2–11).

The pattern of branching of the internal iliac arteries is quite variable, but generally each vessel divides into an anterior and posterior division. The anterior division of the internal iliac artery usually has the following branches: the umbilical, superior vesical, obturator, inferior vesical, uterine, vaginal, middle rectal, inferior gluteal, and internal pudendal.

The umbilical arteries are obliterated after birth, but their remnants can be seen extending along the side wall of the pelvis to the anterior abdominal wall. The superior vesical arteries supply the superior and lateral surfaces of the urinary bladder. The obturator artery is deep to all the other vessels; it arises from the internal iliac and hugs the side wall of the pelvis in its course anteriorly to exit through the obturator canal. There usually is an anastomosis between the obturator artery and the inferior epigastric. One or more inferior vesical arteries supply the urinary bladder. The uterine artery descends anterior to the ureter to the base of the broad ligament. It then crosses superior to the ureter near the lateral fornix of the vagina, where it divides into a descending vaginal branch and an ascending uterine branch. The ascending uterine takes a serpentine course up the side of the uterus before turning laterally to follow the uterine tube to anastomose with branches of the ovarian artery. A separate vaginal artery arises from the internal iliac and supplies the distal part of the vagina. It anastomoses with the vaginal branch of the uterine artery. The middle rectal artery is quite variable in size. It anastomoses superiorly with the superior rectal artery, a continuation of the inferior

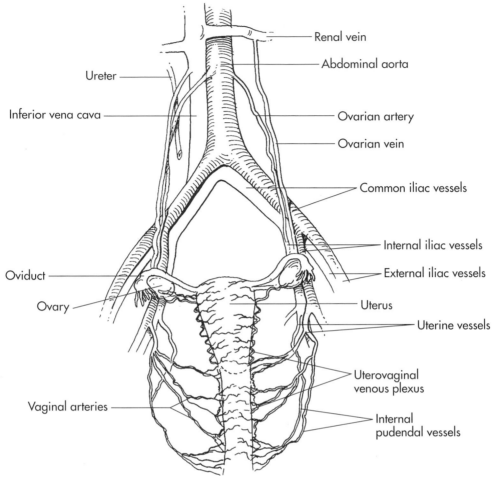

FIG. 2–11. The blood vessels of the female pelvis, showing the chief source of blood supply to the uterus and vagina. (From Eycleshymer and Jones.)

mesenteric; inferiorly it anastomoses with the inferior rectal artery, a branch of the internal pudendal, which supplies the ischiorectal fossa and anal canal inferior to the pelvic diaphragm. The last two branches of the anterior division of the internal iliac are the inferior gluteal and internal pudendal arteries, which leave the pelvis through the greater sciatic foramen inferior to the piriformis muscle. The internal pudendal artery hooks around the ischial spine to enter the pudendal canal inferior to the pelvic diaphragm in the perineum.

The posterior division of the internal iliac artery is smaller and usually has only three branches: the superior gluteal, the iliolumbar, and the lateral sacral. The superior gluteal artery is the largest branch; it passes superior to the piriformis muscle, out of the greater sciatic foramen, and into the gluteal region. The iliolumbar artery courses posterosuperiorly anterior to the ala of the sacrum. It gives rise to the ascending lumbar artery and a branch to the iliac fossa. The lateral sacral artery descends on the pelvic surface of the sacrum just anterior to the roots of the sacral plexus.

The veins of the pelvis are named the same as the arteries and generally follow a similar course but in the opposite direction. The internal iliacs join the external iliacs to form the common iliac veins. The vessels arise from a very extensive, thin-walled basketwork of veins around the urinary bladder, vagina, uterus, and rectum. They are easily torn during surgical manipulation, and the resulting bleeding may be difficult to control. There are important anastomoses between the uterine and vaginal venous plexuses and the superior and inferior rectal veins as well as the lateral sacral veins.

The anastomosis with the superior rectal vein allows venous blood from the pelvis to enter the portal circulation via the inferior mesenteric vein. This connection between the systemic and portal circulations provides a means for cancer in the pelvic organs to metastasize to the liver. The connections between the lateral sacral veins and others in the pelvis are equally important, because the lateral sacral veins anastomose with those of the perivertebral plexus, a valveless system of veins that extends throughout the vertebral canal and connects with the venous sinuses of the brain. These anastomoses provide a route by which cancer may spread from the pelvic viscera directly to the brain without involving other areas of the body.

PELVIC AND PERINEAL INNERVATION

The pelvis is innervated by the lumbar, sacral, and coccygeal plexuses (Fig. 2–12). The anterior rami of L-4 and L-5 join to form the lumbosacral trunk, which crosses the ala of the sacrum to join S-1 on the anterior surface of the piriformis muscle. The lumbosacral trunk is the contribution from the lumbar plexus. The sacral plexus is formed by L-4, L-5, and S-1 to S-4. Arising from the roots of the plexus are the nerve to the piriformis (S-1 and S-2), the pelvic splanchnic nerves (S-2, S-3, and S-4), and the nerves to the levator ani and coccygeus (S-3 and S-4). These nerves are distributed principally to the muscles and organs of the pelvis.

Other branches from the sacral plexus leave the pelvis through the greater sciatic foramen to innervate the lower extremity, the gluteal region, and the perineum: the

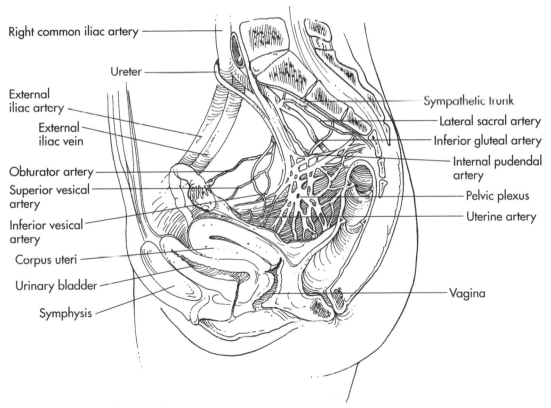

FIG. 2–12. Sagittal section of an adult female pelvis, with the peritoneum and subserous fascia partially dissected away to show the pelvic plexus of autonomic nerves. (Redrawn from Töndury.)

sciatic (L-4, L-5, and S-1, S-2, and S-3), pudendal (S-2, S-3, and S-4), superior gluteal (L-4, L-5, and S-1), inferior gluteal (L-5, S-1, and S-2), nerve to the quadratus femoris (L-4, L-5, and S-1), nerve to the obturator internus (L-5, S-1, and S-2), and the posterior femoral cutaneous nerve (S-1, S-2, and S-3). Finally, there are two cutaneous branches that pass through the coccygeus muscle to innervate the skin around the coccyx: the perforating cutaneous branches of S-2 and S-3 and the perineal branch of S-4.

The pelvic splanchnic and pudendal nerves are particularly important, because they innervate the pelvis and perineum. The pudendal nerve leaves the pelvis through the greater sciatic foramen inferior to the piriformis muscle. It lies medial to the sciatic nerve and hooks around the sacrospinous ligament to enter the pudendal canal in the perineum. It is possible to effect a perineal block by injecting an anesthetic in the vicinity of the perineal nerves as they course around the sacrospinous ligaments. The tip of the ischial spine is palpated through the wall of the vagina and the needle is passed through the vaginal wall and the sacrospinous ligament just medial to the tip of the ischial spine. The internal pudendal vessels course around the ischial spine just lateral to the nerve but are protected by the bone.

The coccygeal plexus is formed by S-4, S-5, and C-1. It gives rise to dorsal and ventral rami, which supply the dorsum of the sacrum and the skin around the coccyx. The organs of the pelvis and perineum receive a rich supply of autonomic nerve fibers from both the sympathetic and parasympathetic nervous systems. The sympathetic fibers arise directly from the sympathetic trunks in the pelvis or indirectly through the superior and inferior hypogastric plexuses. The parasympathetic nerves arise either directly from the pelvic splanchnic nerves or indirectly from the inferior hypogastric plexus.

The abdominal sympathetic trunks give rise to the preaortic (intermesenteric) plexus, which is joined by lumbar splanchnic nerves from L-3 and L-4 and extends inferior to the bifurcation of the aorta as the superior hypogastric plexus. This latter plexus divides into right and left hypogastric nerves, which descend into the pelvis. In the abdomen, the sympathetic trunk lies on the bodies of the lumbar vertebrae. The two trunks pass deep to the common iliac vessels and enter the pelvis, where they lie medial to the sacral foramina. Along their course, four pairs of ganglia can be identified, and the trunks converge on a single ganglion impar just anterior to the coccyx. Gray rami communicantes from the ganglia pass laterally to join sacral and coccygeal nerves, and other visceral branches from these ganglia join the right and left hypogastric nerves and the inferior hypogastric plexus lying on either side of the rectum. The right and left hypogastric nerves (composed of fibers from the preaortic plexus, lumbar splanchnic nerves, and contributions from the sacral sympathetic chain) join the inferior hypogastric plexus, which then becomes a mixture of postganglionic sympathetic fibers and preganglionic parasympathetic fibers from the pelvic splanchnic nerves (S-2, S-3, and S-4). Pelvic splanchnic nerves also send fibers superiorly across the common iliac vessels to the inferior mesenteric artery, where they are distributed to the transverse, descending, and sigmoid portions of the colon. In general, the parasympathetic fibers, which originate from the pelvic splanchnic nerves (S-2, S-3, and S-4) and are distributed either directly or through the inferior hypogastric plexus to the viscera, cause the muscle of the bladder and bowel to contract but their sphincters to relax. They dilate the vessels supplying the erectile tissue of the clitoris and perivaginal plexus and carry sensory fibers for the perception of pain and distention from the bladder and rectum. The sympathetic fibers distributed through the superior and inferior hypogastric plexuses and pudendal nerves as well as those coming directly from the sympathetic ganglia provide motor innervation to the involuntary sphincters of the rectum and bladder and mediate detumescence.

Sensory nerves from the perineum and distal end of the vagina travel with the pudendal (somatic) nerves to S-2, S-3, and S-4. Those from the remainder of the vagina and cervix of the uterus travel with the pelvic splanchnic (parasympathetic) nerves to S-2, S-3, and S-4. The nerves from the body and fundus of the uterus go through the hypogastric plexus and enter the spinal cord at the level of T-11 and T-12. The sensory nerves from the ovaries follow the ovarian arteries, which arise from the aorta just inferior to the renal vessels and enter the spinal cord at the level of T-10.

PELVIC AND PERINEAL LYMPHATICS

The lymphatics of the pelvis and perineum are clinically important but difficult to visualize. The lymphatic vessels from these areas drain into pelvic, abdominal, and inguinal lymph nodes. The pelvic lymph nodes are located either inside the pelvic cavity itself or along the pelvic brim. (Fig. 2–13). Those in the pelvic cavity include nodes associated with the vessels supplying the area, such as the internal iliac, vesical, rectal, lateral sacral, and medial sacral; those in the broad ligament near the cervix; perirectal nodes posterior to the rectum; and others along the course of the superior rectal artery. Along the pelvic brim are found external iliac and common iliac nodes, as well as some that are just superior to the promontory of the sacrum. Many nodes are associated with the abdominal aorta; those receiving drainage from pelvic structures include the inferior mesenteric and the lateral and

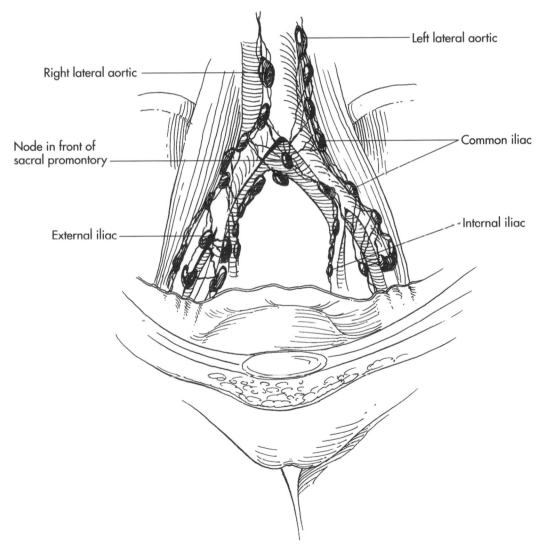

FIG. 2–13. The parietal lymph nodes of the pelvis. (Cunéo and Marcille.)

preaortic nodes that lie between the renal and the common iliac arteries. The inguinal lymph nodes include the superficial nodes that lie just inferior and parallel to the inguinal ligament, and the deep inguinal nodes that lie along the femoral vessels and in the femoral canal.

Lymphatics from the ovary follow the ovarian vessels to the lateral aortic and preaortic nodes in the abdomen. Lymph from the uterus drains into abdominal, pelvic, and inguinal nodes. From the fundus and oviducts (uterine tubes), lymphatics course laterally and follow the ovarian vessels to the lateral aortic and preaortic nodes. From the body of the uterus, they pass via the broad ligament to the external and common iliac nodes, but the areas near the attachments of the round ligaments of the uterus drain to the superficial inguinal nodes. Thus, it is possible for disease in the uterus to manifest itself first in nodes that can be easily palpated just inferior to the inguinal ligament. The vessels from the cervix and superior part of the vagina pass laterally to the external and internal iliac nodes along the course of the uterine and vaginal arteries and posteriorly in the utero-sacral folds to the lateral sacral nodes and those near the promontory (Fig. 2–14).

In general, lymph from the vulva drains to the superficial inguinal nodes, but like that of the anus and anal canal, some of it follows the course of the internal pudendal vessels to the internal iliac nodes. The entire female urethra is drained by the internal iliac nodes. Lymphatics from the glans of the clitoris follow its deep dorsal vein and pass to the deep inguinal nodes.

Lymph from the urinary bladder drains mainly to the pelvic nodes, both the external iliac and internal iliac. Lymphatics from the superior and inferolateral surfaces of the bladder follow the superior vesical vessels to the side wall and up to nodes along the external iliac artery. Some of the lymphatic vessels from the base of the bladder also pass to the external iliac nodes, whereas others

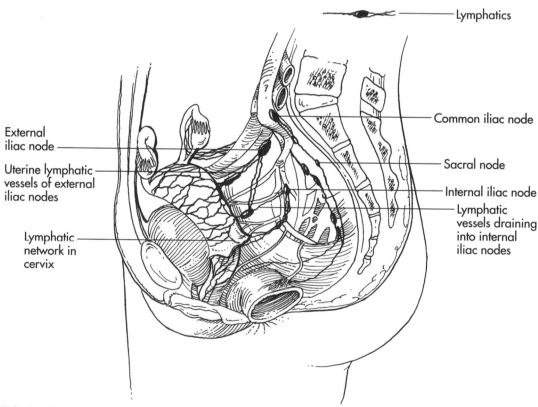

FIG. 2–14. Lymphatic vessels draining the uterus.

drain into the internal iliac nodes or follow the superior surface of the levator ani to the sacral nodes posteriorly.

The rectum drains primarily to the perirectal nodes posteriorly and in turn to the superior rectal and inferior mesenteric nodes. Lymph from the rectum also drains to the lateral and median sacral nodes. The distal portion of the rectum and the part of the anal canal proximal to the pectinate line drain along the middle rectal vessels to the internal iliac nodes. Most of the lymphatics from the anus and the anal canal distal to the pectinate line drain to the superficial inguinal nodes, but some of them follow the inferior rectal vessels to the internal iliac nodes.

PERITONEUM

Peritoneum covers all of the pelvic structures on their superior surfaces to a greater or lesser extent. Peritoneum coats the inside of the abdominal wall inferiorly to the symphysis pubis, from which it is reflected posteriorly over the superior surface of the urinary bladder to a point about 2 cm short of the anterior fornix of the vagina. From there the peritoneum is reflected over the anterior surface of the uterus, creating the vesicouterine pouch. The peritoneum continues over the fundus and posterior surface of the uterus across the posterior fornix of the vagina for about 1 cm before being reflected posteriorly and superiorly to the anterior and lateral surfaces of the rectum. Just as the peritoneal reflection from the superior surface of the urinary bladder to

the anterior surface of the uterus creates the vesicouterine pouch, the reflection from the posterior surface of the uterus and posterior fornix onto the rectum forms the rectouterine pouch. When the bladder is empty, the vesicouterine pouch is nothing more than a transverse slit, but the rectouterine pouch is a sizable excavation in which loops of bowel may lie. The rectouterine pouch is the most dependent part of the peritoneal cavity. It is possible to drain pus and other fluids from this pouch through the posterior fornix of the vagina.

Lateral to the uterus, the peritoneum is draped over the oviducts to form the broad ligaments. The broad ligament comprises the mesovarium, mesosalpinx, and mesometrium. The mesovarium suspends the ovaries from the posterior leaf of the broad ligament. The mesosalpinx is the part superior to the mesovarium that encloses the uterine tubes. The mesometrium is inferior to the mesovarium; its two layers separate to enclose the uterus. A continuation of the broad ligament from the superior pole of the ovary to the side wall of the pelvis is called the suspensory ligament of the ovary. It contains the ovarian vessels, nerves, and lymphatics. Peritoneum from the broad ligaments and lateral walls of the pelvis drapes over the uterosacral ligaments to form the rectouterine folds. The peritoneum then extends into the rectouterine pouch between the uterus and rectum and the pararectal fossae on the sides of the rectum. Between the anterior and posterior folds of the broad ligament along the sides of the uterus is the parametrium.

The development, anatomy, and physiology of the breast are discussed on p. 224.

3
CHAPTER
THE GYNECOLOGIC EXAMINATION

Every gynecologic and obstetric examination should be preceded by a review of systems and a general physical with particular attention to blood pressure, heart, lungs, and eyegrounds. Whenever a patient is examined by a male gynecologist, a female assistant should remain in attendance. The patient should void before pelvic examination except when stress incontinence of urine is to be demonstrated. It is easier to palpate the pelvic organs if the patient's rectum is empty. An outline of the examination of breasts and pelvic organs is given in Table 3–1.

EXAMINATION OF THE BREAST

Careful examination of the breasts routinely should precede gynecologic examination. Inspection and palpation are the basic maneuvers. In certain cases, mammography (roentgenographic examination of the breast) should be employed. Inspection and palpation are performed with the patient in several positions in order to examine each quadrant of the breast with maximal efficiency. First, the patient sits at the edge of the table with her arms extended upward to optimize inspection and palpation of the upper quadrants. She then bends forward with her arms extended outward so that the breasts are dependent. Asymmetry of the breasts is noted in this position. The patient then assumes a recumbent position. She turns first slightly to her right side for examination of the inner quadrants of her right breast and the outer quadrants of her left breast. Alternatively, a small roll may be placed under her left shoulder and chest. She then turns slightly to her left for examination of the inner quadrants of the left breast and the outer quadrants of the right breast. Each portion of the breast is palpated to detect size, consistency, tenderness, and fixation of any masses. Dimpling of the skin or retraction of the nipple and any discrete firm mass require further investigation, including biopsy. The axilla is examined best with the pads of the fingers, which should be inserted while the patient's arms are raised. Palpation is carried out after the patient's arm is brought down against the chest wall with her forearm supported by the examiner. After examination of the axilla, an attempt should be made to palpate supraclavicular nodes. As the physician inspects and palpates the patient's breasts, he or she should teach her systematic self-examination. Additional information concerning the history and physical findings of diseases of the breast is found on page 224.

TABLE 3–1. GYNECOLOGIC EXAMINATION

I. Breasts
  A. Inflammatory lesions
  B. Symmetry
  C. Masses
    1. Cystic or solid
    2. Fixation to overlying skin
    3. Retraction of skin
  D. Discharge from nipple
  E. Tenderness
  F. Lymphadenopathy
    1. Axillary
    2. Supraclavicular
II. Abdomen
  A. Masses and organomegaly
  B. Tenderness
  C. Rigidity
  D. Bowel sounds
  E. Ascites or encapsulated fluid
  F. Scars
III. Pelvic Examination
  A. External genitalia
    1. Congenital anomalies
    2. Hair distribution
    3. Size of clitoris
    4. Inflammation, masses, or lesions of Bartholin's glands, urethra, and Skene's glands
    5. Masses, lesions, and ulcerations of the labia majora, labia minora, perineum, and anus
  B. Vagina
    1. Partial or complete atresia
    2. Transverse or longitudinal septa
    3. Relaxation of walls
    4. Inflammation and atrophy of the mucosa
    5. Masses or nodularity of the vaginal wall
    6. Discharge
  C. Cytologic examination of cervix and vagina (Papanicolaou smear)
  D. Cervix*
    1. Size and shape
    2. Configuration of external os
    3. Pain on motion
    4. Ulcers or masses
    5. Color and consistency
    6. Contact bleeding
  E. Corpus
    1. Size and configuration
    2. Mobility and position
    3. Pain on motion
  F. Adnexa
    1. Masses (size and consistency)
    2. Pain on motion
  G. Rectovaginal
    1. Nodularity of cul-de-sac
    2. Consistency of parametria
    3. Rectal or rectovaginal masses
    4. Rectal bleeding

*Colposcopy is frequently included as part of the routine examination of the cervix. Its use in the diagnosis of cervical abnormalities is described on page 276.

ABDOMINAL EXAMINATION

The abdomen is next examined by inspection, palpation, percussion, and auscultation, with the patient in the recumbent position. Scars, striations, diastasis of the recti, and hernias of the abdominal wall should be noted. Asymmetry of the abdominal contour suggests an abnormal mass. Large myomas are likely to be irregular, whereas a pregnant uterus is normally symmetric. An ovarian cyst may resemble closely a symmetric myoma. On inspection alone, cystic tumors may be indistinguishable from ascites.

Percussion may aid in delimiting the edges of tumors, the height of the urinary bladder, and loops of distended bowel. It may also differentiate the free fluid of ascites from the encapsulated fluid within an ovarian cyst. Paracentesis should not be performed diagnostically because of the risk of rupturing an ovarian cyst that may be malignant or have irritating contents that could initiate a chemical peritonitis.

In the case of ascites, the abdomen is symmetric and there is shifting dullness, dullness in the flanks, and tympany in the anterior abdomen. With an ovarian cyst the upper abdomen is flat, and there is seldom shifting dullness, but there is tympany in the flanks and dullness in the anterior abdomen over the cyst.

Palpation of the upper abdomen should precede that of the lower abdomen and pelvis. In thin women, the lower pole of the kidney normally may be palpated. An attempt should be made to feel the lower edges of the liver and spleen. Tenderness in the costovertebral angles should be noted. The inguinal region should be palpated to detect hernias and lymphadenopathy. Palpation should begin as far away as possible from areas of tenderness. Persistence of spasm after a few moments of gentle depression of the anterior abdominal wall suggests peritoneal irritation. The other major sign of peritonitis is rebound tenderness.

PELVIC EXAMINATION

Pain arising from abdominal viscera should be distinguished from that arising from the abdominal wall. When the cause of pain is visceral, tenderness is elicited when the tensed abdominal wall is palpated. If the tenderness persists when the patient tenses her abdominal muscles by raising her legs or shoulders, the source of pain is more likely to be the abdominal wall itself.

For the pelvic examination proper, the patient's feet are placed in stirrups and her buttocks are brought well over the edge of the table. Her knees should be separated as widely as possible and the examiner positioned comfortably with a well-focused bright light. The external genitalia are examined in the following sequence: clitoris, urethral meatus, Skene's ducts, labia minora and majora including Bartholin's ducts, the perineal body, and the perianal region. Skene's ducts, the urethra, and Bartholin's ducts may be inflamed. In the case of acute gonorrhea, they may produce a purulent discharge. Bartholin's gland is not normally palpable unless involved in a cyst or abscess, and its opening onto the labia is not visible except in the presence of inflammation. The size of the clitoris (especially its width) should be noted and inflammation, atrophy, ulcer, or discharge involving the labia, mons, and perineum recorded. After the labia are separated, the fourchette and hymen should be examined for evidence of tears or scarring. In the virgin, the labia majora are apposed. In the nonvirginal nulliparous woman, various degrees of gaping and scarring are normal. In parous women, these changes are exaggerated. In older women, some degree of labial atrophy is normal. At this point in the examination, the patient is asked to bear down and cough, to see whether she loses urine (stress incontinence). Descent of the anterior vaginal wall, posterior vaginal wall, or cervix represents cystocele, rectocele, and uterine prolapse, respectively.

THE PAPANICOLAOU SMEAR

The systematic examination of the genitalia is now interrupted to obtain a Papanicolaou smear of the vagina and cervix. Because lubricants interfere with preparation of the cytologic smear, the speculum should be inserted without lubrication but moistened with warm water. To minimize discomfort during introduction of the speculum, the perineum should be depressed, avoiding contact with the anterior portion of the vagina and the clitoris. For best results in cytologic diagnosis, bleeding should be minimal and the patient should be instructed to avoid douching and intercourse for the 24 hours preceding examination.

Because the Papanicolaou smear is an integral part of the gynecologic examination, it is described in detail here. Its interpretation in connection with other diagnostic procedures is described on pages 234 and 276.

The most important specimens are obtained from the portio by scraping the squamocolumnar junction with a specially designed spatula and from the endocervical canal by scraping with a spatula or commercially available brush or rubbing with a cotton-tipped applicator. Less valuable for detection of abnormal cells are specimens obtained by aspiration from the vaginal vault or scraping the side walls of the vagina. The smear should be fixed immediately in equal parts of 95% alcohol and ether or dry-fixed with a commercially available spray. The smear must be labeled carefully, preferably by marking the slide itself with a diamond pencil. The smears generally are stained by the Papanicolaou method and examined with the light microscope. Cytologic screening is a most important procedure that should be performed as part of the physical examination of any woman over the age of 18 and in even younger patients who are sexually active. No treatment of a cervical lesion should be attempted before the results of the cytologic screening are available. Electrocauterization, cryosurgical procedures, and use of the laser must be deferred until a diagnosis is obtained by colposcopic examination and appropriate biopsy.

A smear of material pipetted from the posterior fornix includes squamous cells from the vagina and cervix and glandular cells from the endocervix and endometrium. Carcinoma of the cervix is detected best in a smear obtained from around the squamocolumnar junction, whereas a scraping from the lateral vaginal wall was used formerly for hormonal cytodiagnosis until more accurate and specific chemical tests became available. Several "do-it-yourself" kits are available for home use in cancer detection, but there are inherent errors in collection of the specimen. Furthermore, the patient is denied the benefit of a simultaneous examination of breasts and pelvis. The Papanicolaou smear prepared by scraping the squamocolumnar junction and obtaining material from the cervical canal is a good screening method for the detection of cervical carcinoma. Although a single smear may have a false-negative rate as high as 30%, this figure is reduced greatly after three consecutive negative tests, as reported by a competent cytopathologist. Aspiration of cells from the endometrial cavity may improve the rate of detection of carcinoma of the corpus, but definitive diagnosis of this lesion requires adequate histologic sampling of the endometrium.

A stained smear of cells from the vaginal wall may be used to assess the woman's hormonal status as part of the investigation of an endocrine disorder or infertility. The maturation index is the ratio of parabasal to intermediate to superficial cells. For example, a maturation index of 0/20/80 indicates a fair estrogenic effect. The maturation index is normally maximal at the time of ovulation. A maturation index (MI) of 20/75/5, for example, represents a poor estrogenic effect. The karyopyknotic index (KI) is the percentage of superficial cells with deeply pigmented (pyknotic) nuclei. A high karyopyknotic index (greater than 30) is considered to reflect a marked estrogenic effect.

Any suspicious lesion of the cervix should be subjected to biopsy when it is first detected (p. 236). The specimen may be obtained through a single punch of a localized lesion or a large mass. Selection of a site for biopsy is made during colposcopic examination (p. 237). Schiller staining (p. 236) may reveal areas of epithelium that fail to take up iodine and thus may be abnormal. Cone biopsy (p. 243) is never performed as an office procedure. Since the Papanicolaou smear is only a screening procedure, histologic confirmation is required before any treatment is initiated. The management of the abnormal Papanicolaou smear is summarized on page 276.

The squamocolumnar junction is the border between the pink squamous epithelium of the portio and the bright red columnar epithelium of the endocervix. In adolescents, the junction may be far out on the portio, whereas in postmenopausal women, it is likely to be high in the cervical canal. It is important to identify this junction for cytologic sampling because it is the site at which most neoplastic changes in the cervix first occur.

Before removal of the speculum, the color of the cervix is noted. A bluish discoloration may be an indication of pregnancy or a large tumor. The condition of the external os may indicate parity. The nulliparous cervix has a small circular external os, whereas in the parous woman, the os is irregular or transversely lacerated.

The vagina itself is often inspected inadequately because the speculum covers a large part of its surface. Nevertheless, the entire surface of the vagina should be examined carefully under bright light. The color of the mucosa and the condition of the rugae should be noted. Nodularities and ulcers should be described. Any suspicious lesion should be subjected to biopsy.

An attempt should be made to identify the etiologic agent in any profuse vaginal discharge. Organisms that may be identified on initial examination are Gonococcus, Chlamydia, Candida (Monilia), and Trichomonas. Discharge from the urethral meatus, Skene's ducts, Bartholin's ducts, the external cervical os, the anal crypts, and the pharynx may be gram-stained and inoculated on a Thayer-Martin agar plate or another suitable culture medium, to identify gonococci and placed in special culture tubes to identify Chlamydia. Culture is often performed without charge by local health departments.

Hanging-drop smears for trichomonads may be obtained from the urethra, external os, or posterior fornix. The material is suspended in normal saline and examined on a glass slide. The yeast-like organisms that cause candidiasis may be recognized if some of the exudate is suspended in 10% potassium hydroxide or cultured on a medium such as Nickerson's, where they will appear as brown or black colonies within 24 hours.

INTERNAL PELVIC EXAMINATION

The remainder of the internal examination is completed with the patient in the lithotomy position. The patient may help to relax her abdominal wall by taking fast shallow breaths. The uterus and adnexa are palpated between the internal (vaginal) hand and the external (abdominal) hand during the bimanual examination. By depressing the patient's perineum and by resting his elbow on his thigh, the examiner may be able to reach farther into the vagina. The examiner may find it helpful to rest one foot on a low stool. At the beginning of the internal examination, the cervix is located and its size, mobility, and consistency noted. Pain on motion of the cervix should be recorded. The corpus should then be palpated between the abdominal hand, which makes downward pressure on the uterus, and the vaginal hand, which pushes it upward. The size, mobility, consistency, position, and shape of the uterus should be recorded.

Physical diagnosis is rendered difficult when the patient fails to relax, when the examination causes pain, when the patient is obese, and when the bladder or rectum is filled. The normal oviduct (fallopian tube) is rarely palpable even under ideal conditions of examination. Before an attempt is made to ascertain the size and consistency of the ovary, the position and size of the uterus must be known. If an ovarian enlargement is felt, it is most important to describe whether it is cystic or solid, and unilateral or bilateral. Because any solid ovarian mass may represent a malignant tumor, the description of any adnexal lesion must be recorded accurately. The size of a pelvic mass should be noted in centimeters rather than in terms of fruits, vegetables, or eggs of various birds. It is valuable to accompany the description of abnormal findings by a drawing because subsequent management may depend on whether a lesion has regressed, remained the same size, or grown since the last examination.

A normal ovary may be felt in a thin, cooperative patient by even a relatively inexperienced examiner, but even a distinctly enlarged ovary may not be palpable by an expert in an obese or uncooperative patient. If there is any doubt about the presence of an adnexal mass, consultation should be obtained, because any ovarian enlargement is a potentially serious lesion. The average dimensions of the normal adult ovary are $3 \times 2 \times 1.5$ cm, although ovarian size varies considerably during the reproductive period. Any adnexal mass greater in size than the normal ovary should be investigated carefully. The average dimensions of the postmenopausal ovary are $2.0 \times 0.5 \times 0.5$ cm. Any palpable ovary in the postmenopausal woman must be considered abnormal. For accurate diagnosis of an adnexal mass, the pelvic examination occasionally must be performed under anesthesia, especially in children.

RECTOVAGINAL EXAMINATION

The rectovaginal examination should be performed last because it is usually the most uncomfortable, but it should never be omitted from the gynecologic examination. The middle finger is inserted into the rectum and the index finger into the vagina. The tissues of the rectovaginal septum are felt between the two fingers. Moving the fingers laterally from the cervix to the right and left permits systematic palpation of the parametria. The parametria and uterosacral ligaments, which may be involved in inflammatory or neoplastic diseases, are palpable only on rectovaginal examination. Lesions detected on rectovaginal palpation include a high rectocele, an enterocele (p. 211), endometriosis (p. 214), and masses on the posterior uterine wall and in the cul-de-sac and rectovaginal septum. Palpation of the parametria is requisite to clinical staging of carcinoma of the cervix (p. 268).

Occasionally in children and older virgins, the rectal examination is substituted for the vaginal. If the findings are suspicious or inconclusive, examination under anesthesia may be required. During rectal examination, attention is directed to hemorrhoids, fistulas, fissures, anorectal polyps and tumors, and the commonly encountered condylomata acuminata.

Women who have been raped or claim to have been raped may come, often with police escort, for examination and possible treatment. The physician's duty at such time is to record the history as accurately as possible, preferably in the patient's own words, and to record objectively the physical findings, as described on page 359.

OBSTETRIC EXAMINATION

An outline of the physical examination of the obstetric patient is presented in Table 3–2.

TABLE 3–2. OBSTETRIC EXAMINATION

 I. Uterine Size
 II. Consistency and Shape of the Uterus (early in pregnancy)
 III. Presentation and Position of the Fetus
 IV. Size and Movements of the Fetus
 V. Mobility of the Fetal Head
 VI. Consistency, Size, and Engagement of the Head
 VII. Presence of Fetal Heart Tones (by stethoscope or Doptone)
 VIII. Vaginal Examination to Detect Position, Length, Consistency, and Dilatation of the Cervix
 IX. Manual Pelvimetry
 X. Papanicolaou Smear on the First Antepartum Visit If the Patient Has Not Had a Cytologic Examination Within the Last 12 Months
 XI. Sonographic Examination During the First Trimester to Ascertain Developmental Age of the Fetus.*
 XII. Cervical Culture for Gonorrhea and Chlamydia

*Sonography may be repeated later in gestation to assess fetal growth and to detect abnormalities of the fetus or placenta.

II

OBSTETRICS

NORMAL OBSTETRICS

4

CHAPTER

MATERNAL PHYSIOLOGY

DIAGNOSIS OF PREGNANCY

Diagnosis of pregnancy is made on the basis of history, physical signs, and laboratory tests. The history must include an accurate account of the menses, the day of onset of the last normal menstrual period, exposure to pregnancy, and contraception. The signs of pregnancy have traditionally been classified as positive, probable, or presumptive.

The use of serum beta subunit human chorionic gonadotropin (β-hCG) titers and ultrasound has greatly diminished the importance of most of these signs and symptoms as definitive diagnostic indications of pregnancy. Definitive diagnosis of intrauterine pregnancy is now made by a β-hCG concentration greater than 6,500 m.i.u./mL and an intrauterine gestational sac identified by ultrasound. Both are usually present by the sixth week after the last menstrual period. Normal values for concentrations of β-hCG in the serum during the various stages of pregnancy are shown in Figure 4–1. The times of appearance of the various indicators of pregnancy are shown in Table 4–1. Figure 4–1 also shows the corresponding values for the other important trophoblastic polypeptide hormone, human placental lactogen (hPL), or human chorionic somatomammotropin, which is described on p. 56.

The traditional positive signs of pregnancy are not elicited before the second trimester by conventional clinical techniques. They include seeing or feeling fetal movements by the examining physician, hearing and counting the fetal heart rate separately from the maternal pulse, and radiologically delineating the fetus. Fetal movements normally can be felt by the fifth month. The fetal heartbeat can be detected by stethoscope by the eighteenth week and by Doppler ultrasound by the twelfth week. The fetus can be visualized radiologically by the sixteenth week and a gestational sac may be detected sonographically as early as the fifth week (p. 59).

Probable signs of pregnancy include enlargement of the abdomen, enlargement of the uterus, a globular change in shape of the uterus, softening of the cervix and the lower uterine segment (the area between cervix and corpus), irregular painless contractions of the uterus (Braxton Hicks contractions), ballottement of the uterus (repercussion of the fetus after tapping the lower uterine segment), and positive urinary hormonal tests for pregnancy. The hormonal tests, which may be immunologic or biologic, depend essentially on the detection of human chorionic gonadotropin, the level of which is normally highest between the fiftieth and ninetieth days of gestation. Pro-

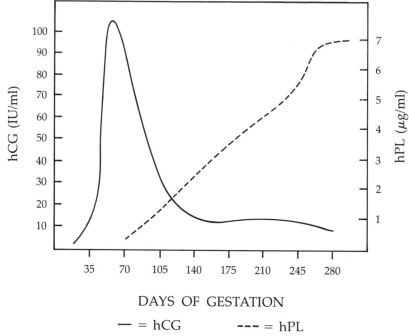

FIG. 4–1. Concentrations of chorionic gonadotropin and placental lactogen in serum during various stages of pregnancy.

gestin-induced withdrawal bleeding is no longer an acceptable technique to rule out pregnancy. Examination of the cervical mucus in pregnancy reveals either a beaded (cellular) or an intact fernlike pattern. An intact fern is not compatible with normal early pregnancy.

Presumptive signs and symptoms of pregnancy include amenorrhea, fullness and tenderness of the breasts, enlargement and darkening of the areola, prominence of sebaceous glands of the areola (Montgomery's tubercles), and secretion of thick yellow fluid (colostrum) from the nipple after the first few months. Additional presumptive symptoms include lassitude, nausea and vomiting (morning sickness), frequency of urination, and quickening (appreciation by the patient of fetal movements after the fourth month). Presumptive physical signs

TABLE 4–1. TIMES OF APPEARANCE OF IMPORTANT INDICATORS OF PREGNANCY

Positive Test or Observation	Interval After Onset of Last Normal Menstrual Period
Serum β-hCG (RIA)	24 Days
Serum β-hCG (ELISA, "Icon")	26 Days
Urine β-hCG (ELISA, "Icon")	28 Days
Softening of the cervix	4-5 Weeks
Intrauterine gestational sac (Ultrasound)	5-6 Weeks
Other urinary pregnancy tests	5-8 Weeks
Softening of the lower uterine segment (Hegar's Sign)	6 Weeks
Fetal cardiac activity (Ultrasound)	6-8 Weeks
Fetal cardiac activity (Doppler)	10-12 Weeks
Perception of fetal movement	16-20 Weeks
Auscultation of fetal cardiac sounds	18 Weeks

include bluish discoloration of the vagina and cervix, increased pigmentation of the skin, and abdominal striae.

The average duration of human pregnancy is 40 weeks (p. 42). To calculate the estimated date of confinement (EDC), count back 3 months from the last menstrual period (LMP) and add 7 days. For example, if the first day of the LMP was March 18, 1992, the EDC is December 25, 1992. These calculations apply to a normal, regular 28-day menstrual cycle. If the cycle is 35 days in length, it is necessary to add 14 rather than 7 days. For example, if the first day of the last LMP was November 1, 1992, the EDC would be August 15, 1993. If the cycle is normally 21 days in length, it is necessary only to count back 3 months without addition of days. For example, if the first day of the LMP was September 30, 1993, the EDC would be June 30, 1994. Recent data suggest that perhaps the length of normal human gestation is several days greater than that calculated by the aforementioned rule.

About 40% of women deliver within 5 days of the EDC and about two thirds within 10 days of the EDC. Because many women experience vaginal bleeding during the first 2 months of pregnancy (p. 97), erroneous calculation of EDC is not uncommon.

Urinary immunologic pregnancy tests have replaced the biologic tests. All are semiquantitative, utilizing an immunologic reaction to human chorionic gonadotropin; the preferable tests are specific for β-hCG (p. 39). Accuracy and sensitivity vary among the individual tests. The "Icon" test is specific, with a sensitivity of 50 m.i.u./ml. It gives a positive reaction as early as 10 days after ovulation and in normal pregnancy is consistently positive by the time of the expected menses. Use of the first voided morning urine increases the concentration of hCG and therefore the effective sensitivity of the test. Other tests available for home use are less specific and less sensitive, but all should give a positive reaction in normal pregnancy within 6 weeks after the last normal menstrual period (4 weeks after ovulation). False-positive reactions are rare, particularly if the test has been repeatedly positive, but a negative reaction does not necessarily indicate the absence of pregnancy. The urinary concentration of hCG

may simply be too low to elicit a positive response. Because concentrations of hCG rise rapidly in early normal pregnancy, a negative test in the presence of a high clinical suspicion of pregnancy should be repeated after 1 week and, if still negative, after a second week. Persistently negative tests, including at least one performed more than 3 weeks after the "missed" period, provide a fairly reliable indication of the absence of normal pregnancy. Most of the newer tests to detect urinary chorionic gonadotropin use an enzyme-linked immunoassay (ELISA) involving monoclonal antihuman chorionic gonadotropin antibody.

The differential diagnosis of pregnancy includes myomas, ovarian cysts, pseudocyesis (false, or spurious, pregnancy), and hematometra (collection of blood within the uterus). None of these conditions is accompanied by a positive test for pregnancy or a gestational sac on sonographic examination. With myomas, there is usually no amenorrhea and the uterus is firmer. With ovarian cysts, the mass may be felt separate from the uterus. Both myomas and ovarian cysts, however, may coexist with pregnancy. With pseudocyesis, a normal sized uterus may be palpated under anesthesia. The signs of false pregnancy may occasionally be reversed under hypnosis.

The definitive sign of fetal death is absence of a fetal heartbeat in real-time sonographic examination. Suggestive signs of fetal death include failure of growth or regression in size of the uterus, regression of mammary changes, and disappearance of fetal heart tones and fetal movements. Radiologic examination is much less commonly performed today. Radiologic signs include collapsed cranial bones, exaggerated curvature of the spine, gas in the heart and great vessels, and failure to demonstrate swallowing of amnionic (amniotic) fluid into which a contrast medium has been injected (amniography).

Some of the physical signs in a first pregnancy are different from those in later pregnancies. In a woman pregnant for the first time, the abdominal wall is tenser, the uterus and breasts are firmer, the labia may be apposed, and tags of hymen and vaginal rugae are more obvious. The primigravid cervix is more likely to be conical and closed, with a regular circular external os.

The vagina of the multipara is wider, the vulva gapes, and the external os is irregular.

PHYSIOLOGIC CHANGES

The average duration of human pregnancy is 40 weeks (280 days) from the first day of the LMP, or 38 weeks (266 days) after ovulation. The growth of the uterus is a response to hormones in the first few months of pregnancy. Thereafter the growth is related to the mechanical effects of the enlarging products of conception. The uterus changes in shape from pyriform in the nonpregnant state to globular in early pregnancy and to ovoid in later pregnancy. It is frequently rotated laterally, more often to the right (dextrorotated). The uterus increases in length from 7 cm in the non-pregnant state to 35 cm at term and from 500 to 1000 times in volume. By the third lunar month of gestation, the top of the uterus reaches the pelvic brim. By the fourth month, it is four fingerbreadths above the symphysis. By the fifth month, the top of the uterus is almost at the level of the umbilicus. By the sixth month, it is slightly above the umbilicus. By the seventh month it is three fingerbreadths above the umbilicus. By the eighth month, it is three fingerbreadths above the level reached in the seventh month. By the ninth month, it is just below the xiphoid, and by the tenth month, it has fallen back to its position in the eighth month. An estimate of fundal height can be made by measuring from pubic symphysis to top of fundus with a tape measure.

The descent of the fetal head into the true pelvis, particularly in the primigravida, often occurs about 2 weeks before term. This phenomenon, which suggests that the fetal head is not too large for the pelvis, is called lightening.

The uterus increases in weight from 60 g in the nonpregnant state to 1000 g at term. Myometrial fibers stretch and hypertrophy but undergo little if any hyperplasia. The myometrial fibers are disposed in figure-of-eight arrangements, which serve as living ligatures to effect hemostasis. Uterine blood flow increases to 600 mL/min at term with a parallel increase in oxygen consumption. Myometrial contractions progress from an irregular and painless (Braxton Hicks) pattern to regular and painful contractions at term. The decidual reaction of the endometrium involves hypertrophy of the endometrial glands and formation of large polygonal stromal cells filled with glycogen and lipid (decidual cells). The basal cells of the cervical epithelium undergo hyperplasia. The cervix increases in vascularity and softens as its glands hypertrophy. It remains occluded by a mucous plug until near the onset of labor. This mucus forms a beaded (cellular) rather than a fernlike pattern when allowed to dry on a glass slide.

A fernlike pattern is a manifestation of estrogenic dominance, which is not characteristic of normal pregnancy. The estrogen is associated with a high content of electrolytes in the mucus, particularly sodium, which is responsible for the fern. As labor approaches, the cervix effaces, thins, and becomes increasingly dilatable near term, probably because estrogens depolymerize the acid mucopolysaccharides that form the ground substance.

The uteroplacental circulation develops as a low-resistance system. Uterine blood flow is only 1 to 2% of cardiac output in the nonpregnant state, whereas at the end of pregnancy it accounts for over 10% of the cardiac output, which itself may be increased almost 50%. Uterine blood flow remains fairly constant, however, throughout the course of gestation when calculated in terms of flow per unit weight to uterus and products of conception. The figure remains close to 10 to 15 mL/100 g of tissue/min. Oxygen consumption is fairly constant at 1 cc/100 g tissue/min. The weight of evidence suggests that the uterine blood flow is not autoregulated. Lack of autoregulation of uterine blood flow is relevant to the use of antihypertensive drugs in pregnant women. The reduction in blood pressure probably decreases uterine blood flow, which is already half or less than half of normal in hypertensive gravidas.

The vagina undergoes an increase in vascularity early in pregnancy, developing a bluish discoloration that may aid in the diagnosis of pregnancy (p. 41). The increased production of lactic acid from glycogen by lactobacilli maintains the acidic pH of the vagina.

The primary change in the ovary is the formation of the corpus luteum of pregnancy, with accompanying cessation of ovulation and menstruation. The ovarian vessels undergo a huge increase in caliber.

The breasts undergo an increased growth in both number and size of ductal and alveolar elements. Development of the ducts is under the control of estrogen and that of the alveoli under the control of progesterone. Additional hormones involved in mammary development include prolactin, growth hormone, insulin, cortisone, and thyroxine. In addition to the general increase in size of breasts, areolae, and sebaceous glands (p. 40), the nipples enlarge and become more deeply pigmented and erectile.

The normal average weight gain in pregnancy is about 20 to 25 pounds. Two pounds are normally gained in the first trimester and about 11 pounds in each of the last two trimesters. The average weight gain in pounds at term is distributed roughly as follows: fetus, 7.5; placenta, 1.0; amniotic fluid, 2.0; uterus, 2.5; breasts, 2.0; blood, 2.5; and interstitial fluid, 5.5.

Many of the physiologic changes in pregnancy begin in the latter half of the menstrual cycle and are maximal, or nearly so, by the sixth week of gestation, including increase in concentration of renin in plasma, reversal of circadian rhythm of day/night renal function, and decrease in plasma osmolality. The net gain in protein amounts to about 1 kg, about half of which is in the products of conception and half in the uterus, breasts, and blood. About 7 liters of water are retained until delivery; about half of this volume is lost at the time of delivery of the fetus, placenta, and amniotic fluid. Additional important metabolic changes include a lowering of glucose tolerance (p. 108), a positive nitrogen balance, and an increase in free fatty acids, phospholipids, and total lipids. The mother ordinarily needs about 800 mg of iron during the course of gestation (500 mg for increased mass of maternal erythrocytes and 300 mg for the fetus and placenta).

Hypochlorhydria and vomiting in pregnancy may interfere with absorption of iron by the mother. The mother stores more calcium than the fetus requires until the last month of pregnancy, when the fetus needs about twice as much as the mother ordinarily can assimilate. The maternal reserves are then taxed and the mother may require additional calcium during lactation.

The increase in blood volume in pregnancy amounts to about 30 to 40% above nonpregnant levels. The maximum is achieved at about 34 weeks of gestation and is maintained throughout pregnancy without a terminal decrease. The elevation of the diaphragm with displacement of the heart to the left creates the false impression of cardiomegaly in normal pregnancy. Increases occur in cardiac rate, stroke volume, and cardiac output. The circulation time is somewhat decreased in the upper portion of the body and increased below the pelvis. Soft systolic apical and pulmonic murmurs are common, but diastolic murmurs indicate disease (p. 111).

The extent of the hemodynamic increases is as follows; erythrocyte mass, 25 to 30%; plasma volume, 40 to 50%; cardiac output, 30 to 40%; uterine blood flow, 1000%; and cardiac rate, 10 to 15 beats/min.

Hematocrit and hemoglobin concentration normally decrease as a result of the hemodilution of pregnancy, reaching their lowest values at about 26 to 28 weeks of gestation. The leukocyte count normally may increase to 15,000 in pregnancy and to 25,000 in labor and the puerperium. There is no morphologic or numeric change in platelets, but increases in fibrinogen, and in Factors VII, VIII, IX, and X are found. Fibrinolytic activity, however, is depressed. An increased erythrocyte sedimentation rate and tendency to thrombosis may result from these changes.

Fibrinogen normally increases about 50% over nonpregnant levels from an average of 300 mg% to about 450 mg%. The decrease in concentration of plasma proteins amounts to about 1 g%. Most of the decrease is in the albumin fraction, with perhaps a slight increase in globulins. As a result, the plasma oncotic pressure and the A/G ratio fall. Among the numerous changes in serum enzymes, the increases in alkaline phosphatase and cystine aminopeptidase are consistent.

The rise in femoral venous pressure is a result of compression of the vena cava by the enlarging uterus. Arterial blood pressure, however, is normally somewhat decreased in the second trimester.

Edema is common in normal pregnancy. About three quarters of all pregnant women have pedal edema that increases while they are erect and regresses while they are recumbent. Many women also have edema, which is normally slight, of the hands and face. The pedal edema, caused mechanically, is attributable to the increase in femoral venous pressure that occurs when the woman in late pregnancy sits, stands, or lies supine. The bulky uterus occludes the vena cava while she is supine and blocks the common iliac veins while she is erect. The generalized nondependent edema is an effect of estrogens; the depolymerization of the ground substance permits increased binding of sodium and water. In the absence of preeclampsia, women with such edema have larger babies, as do those with larger plasma volumes, more total body water, and greater gains in weight.

The arterial blood pressure, especially the diastolic, decreases some time during the first trimester and begins to rise again late in the second. Inasmuch as the cardiac output has increased by 30 to 40% by the end of the first trimester, there must be a remarkable decrease in total peripheral vascular resistance. Suggested explanations for the decrease have invoked progesterone, prostaglandin E_2, and prostacyclin, but they all increase while the blood pressure is rising late in pregnancy.

Glomerular filtration rate (GFR) and renal plasma flow (RPF) both increase about 30 to 50% in normal pregnancy. Glucosuria, sometimes heavy, and aminoaciduria are common in pregnancy; their occurrence and intensity vary sporadically. Proteinuria, however, is abnormal. Increased renal excretion results in decrease in blood urea nitrogen and creatinine. Urinary stasis results from hypomotility and dilation of the ureters and renal pelves, a consequence primarily of the relaxation of smooth muscle by progesterone.

Dilation of the ureter in pregnancy begins before the mechanical effect of the enlarging uterus is brought into play. The ureter in pregnancy is dilated, angulated, and elongated. The trigone of the bladder is elevated and edema of the base of the bladder predisposes to trauma. The combination of trauma, stasis, and increased urinary dextrose and amino acids predisposes to ascending infection of the urinary tract.

Because the average increase of 50% in the filtered load of glucose is presumed to be constant, tubular function must vary for unknown reasons. Experimental expansion of the blood volume is known to inhibit the renal tubular reabsorption of dextrose, sodium, and urate, and probably of other substances, but the hypervolemia of pregnancy does not fluctuate significantly.

The increased GFR and progesterone and the expanded plasma volume tend to increase the excretion of sodium and the retention of potassium. Estrogen and aldosterone tend to retain sodium and increase the excretion of potassium. The net result is retention of both sodium and potassium. For accurate results in pregnancy, the GFR and RPF must be measured in the lateral recumbent rather than the supine position. Paradoxically, however, the supine position reduces the maximal concentrative capacity.

Since tidal volume and respiratory rate increase in pregnancy, minute volume is increased. This hyperventilation may be a result of an increased sensitivity of the maternal respiratory center to carbon dioxide, perhaps as an effect of progesterone. Respiratory alkalosis may occur but is compensated by a decrease in serum bicarbonate with resulting stability of pH of the blood. In nonpregnant subjects, the decrease in bicarbonate is balanced by retention of chloride but, remarkably, that does not occur in early pregnancy. The result is a decrease of about 5 meq/L in both bicarbonate and sodium, matching the decrement of about 10 milliosmolals/kg in plasma. The interrelation is uncertain, for the reduction in osmolality depends upon altered thresholds for thirst and the release of antidiuretic hormone. Injections of progesterone do not have those effects, but chorionic gonadotropin does.

Probably beginning in the luteal phase of the cycle and continuing after conception, progesterone sensitizes the respiratory center to carbon dioxide, leading to increased ventilation, blowing off of carbon dioxide, and reduction in P_{CO_2} in blood from about 38 to 32 mm Hg, with a subsequent trend to alkalosis and compensatory renal excretion of bicarbonate. In nonpregnant subjects, loss of bicarbonate is balanced by retention of chloride and therefore little, if any, reduction in sodium and osmolality. In pregnancy, something other than progesterone seems to prevent the compensatory retention of chloride. The mechanism leading to the remarkable decrease appears to be a decrease in the thresholds for thirst and release of antidiuretic hormone. Injections of progesterone into rats do not have this effect, but injections of human chorionic gonadotropin do to some extent. Furthermore, patients with hydatidiform mole (p. 249) and persistently high levels of chorionic gonadotropin for some time after evacuation have a decreased plasma osmolality that slowly returns to normal as the urinary excretion of hCG abates. In the nonpregnant subject, the plasma osmolality varies so little that the decrease of about 10 osmol is remarkable and in a nonpregnant person would lead to maximal diuresis.

Elevation of the diaphragm lowers the functional residual capacity, but vital capacity and maximum breathing capacity are not altered significantly.

Progesterone causes decreased motility of the gastrointestinal tract and, by inference, delayed absorption and constipation.

Additional changes in the digestive tract include reduction in free HCI, reflux esophagitis (the probable cause of "heartburn"), increased stasis in the gallbladder (possibly leading to formation of stones), and upward displacement of the appendix (possibly interfering with the diagnosis of acute appendicitis in pregnancy). Ptyalism (excessive salivation) and hyperemia of the gums, alterations in appetite, increased size of hemorrhoids, and constipation are commonly encountered in pregnancy.

The hypochlorhydria is especially marked in the first half of pregnancy. For that reason, even severe vomiting seldom results in hypochloremic alkalosis, as it would in nonpregnant women.

General endocrine changes in pregnancy include alterations in secretory and excretory rates, in binding by globulins, and in metabolic interactions, and increase in size and vascularity of the endocrine organs. The most pronounced changes affect the ovary, with persistence of the corpus luteum, cessation of ovulation, and increased and prolonged elaboration of progesterone.

Moderate enlargement of the thyroid gland is accompanied by increases in basal metabolic rate (up to 25%), thyroid-binding globulin (TBG), and thyroxine (T_4). Triiodothyronine (T_3) uptake is decreased and serum cholesterol increased. Free thyroxine levels are essentially unchanged.

Pregnancy and hyperthyroidism share the following: increase in BMR, total T_4, and RAI uptake (which should not be performed during pregnancy); palpitation; tachycardia; perspiration; and emotional lability. Pregnancy and hyperthyroidism differ in the following respects: cholesterol is increased in pregnancy but decreased in hyperthyroidism; TBG is increased in pregnancy but is normal in hyperthyroidism; unbound thyroxine is not increased in pregnancy but is increased in hyperthyroidism; absolute iodine uptake is not increased in pregnancy but is increased in hyperthyroidism; and resin T_3 uptake is decreased in pregnancy but increased in hyperthyroidism.

The pancreas in pregnancy is subjected to a diabetogenic stress. Since islet cell function and secretion of insulin are increased while the antagonism of insulin by placental lactogen (chorionic somatomammotropin) and, much less important, its destruction by placental insulinase increase, the pancreas is taxed in order to produce enough insulin to maintain the hyperinsulinemia of pregnancy (p. 109).

Production of cortisol increases, although much of the steroid is bound by corticosteroid-binding globulin, or transcortin, which is increased in pregnancy. Some increase in free cortisol can be measured, however.

Concentrations of aldosterone, renin substrate, and angiotensin, and both concentration and activity of renin in plasma increase from twofold to tenfold. The change in plasma renin activity is attributable chiefly to changes in plasma renin substrate, the hepatic synthesis of which is influenced by estrogens. The increase in aldosterone protects against the natriuretic and antikaliuretic effects of progesterone. Enlargement of the adrenal cortex involves primarily the zona fasciculata, with the result that glucocorticoids but not 17-ketosteroids are considerably increased. The pituitary gland enlarges and, rarely, may compress the optic chiasma and reduce the visual fields. Parathormone levels are regulated by calcium levels in the blood, which ordinarily do not undergo great change. The concentration of ionized calcium remains almost unchanged but that of total calcium decreases somewhat because of the decrease in the fraction bound to albumin.

Hyperpigmentation in pregnancy involves the areola, vulva, and linea nigra. Facial hyperpigmentation may result in melasma (chloasma), or the mask of pregnancy, which generally regresses post partum. These changes may be the result of an increase in melanocyte-stimulating hormone. Striae on the abdominal wall and breasts are pink during pregnancy, but later may become silvery, providing evidence of prior pregnancy. Vascular spiders and palmar erythema develop as effects of estrogen.

Cutaneous blood flow increases about sevenfold; this effect serves to dissipate the extra heat associated with the changes in basal metabolic rate. Changes in the musculoskeletal system include progressive lumbar lordosis, with increased mobility of the pelvic joints and an anterior displacement of the center of gravity.

The commonly encountered increase in emotional lability is manifested by anxiety, apprehension, identity crises, and changes in libido. Alterations in appetite may include craving for unusual substances not normally considered as food (pica), such as starch and clay. Mild postpartum depression is not uncommon, although frank psychotic reactions reflect a preexisting tendency.

5

CHAPTER

FETOPLACENTAL DEVELOPMENT AND PHYSIOLOGY

GAMETOGENESIS AND FERTILIZATION

Somatic cells divide by mitosis, which results in two daughter cells with the same diploid number of chromosomes as the parent cell. Gametogenesis (ovogenesis, or oogenesis, and spermatogenesis) requires meiosis, or reduction division, during which the chromosomal number is halved to produce haploid gametes. The diploid number is restored during fertilization.

Ovogenesis begins around the middle of the third month of gestation, when primary ovocytes (oocytes) can first be defined. All ovogonia (oogonia) have become primary ovocytes by the seventh month. Ovogenesis begins with the entrance of ovogonia into prophase of the first meiotic division. The lengthy prophase in the female is divided into five phases: leptotene, zygotene, pachytene, diplotene, and diakinesis. During pachytene, the longest phase, pairing of homologous chromosomes and exchange of genetic material occur. At the end of the pachytene phase, ovocytes enter the diplotene phase, in which they remain until they resume maturation or become atretic.

As many as 7 million ovocytes are present in the ovary during the fifth month of fetal development. At birth, only 2 million remain. By the age of 7 years, the number is reduced to between 200,000 and 400,000.

The decline continues throughout life, few ovocytes surviving beyond menopause.

Primordial germ cells migrate from the endoderm of the yolk sac to the gonadal ridge, where they increase in number by mitotic division in the gonadal anlage. Ovogonia are primordial germ cells that have ceased mitosis but have not yet begun to enlarge or entered the meiotic prophase. Upon entering prophase I, ovogonia become primary ovocytes, which when surrounded by a single layer of flattened follicular cells form primary follicles.

In each menstrual cycle between 5 and 20 follicles begin to develop, but normally only one will ovulate. As many layers of follicular, or granulosa, cells are formed, spaces appear between the individual cells. As these spaces coalesce to form an antrum, the antral, or secondary, follicle develops. As the follicle enlarges and ovulation approaches, the mature, or graafian, follicle is formed. During folliculogenesis an acellular layer, the zona pellucida, is deposited around the ovocyte by the granulosa cells.

During the follicular (proliferative) phase of the menstrual cycle, increasing titers of estradiol produced by the developing follicle eventually result in a surge of both FSH and LH from the pituitary. This release of pituitary hormones occurs on about day 14 of the normal cycle. The surge of LH is responsible for ovulation.

Follicle-stimulating hormone is a glycoprotein with a large sialic acid moiety and a half-life of about 2 hours. It is secreted by the basophilic cells of the anterior pituitary and is released by gonadotropin-releasing hormone (GnRH). Negative feedback to estradiol occurs in both the pituitary and the hypothalamus. FSH effects follicular growth to the antral stage by promoting uptake of amino acids and steroid precursors by the follicle. LH, probably through its steroidogenic action, is required for complete follicular maturation.

Luteinizing hormone is a glycoprotein with a small sialic acid moiety and a short half-life of about 30 minutes. It too is secreted by the basophilic cells of the anterior pituitary and is released by GnRH. Negative feedback to progesterone and low levels of estradiol, and positive feedback to high levels of progesterone, as found in the mature graafian follicle, occur. The action of LH is to stimulate steroidogenesis in the ovary.

The portion of the brain with the greatest concentration of GnRH is the hypothalamus, from the septal-preoptic region anteriorly to the premamillary nucleus posteriorly. The cells that form GnRH are found first in the olfactory region of the brain. GnRH fibers originating from the arcuate nucleus and from cell bodies in the anterior hypothalamic region terminate in the median eminence of the hypothalamus near the long portal vessels. Originating in the hypothalamus, these vessels descend along the pituitary stalk to the anterior pituitary gland. GnRH is secreted directly into this specialized vasculature and thus reaches the pituitary gland undiluted by passage through the peripheral circulation. Biologic activity of GnRH requires interaction with a specific membrane receptor on the gonadotrope.

Follicular development requires both FSH and LH. The surge of LH triggers resumption of meiotic activity within the ovocyte. After the LH surge, the ovocyte rapidly completes the first meiotic division, with production of a large secondary ovocyte and a small first polar body. No synthesis of DNA occurs at this point and the secondary ovocyte proceeds immediately to the metaphase of the second meiotic division, which is completed only after fertilization.

After ovulation, the corpus luteum is formed, but luteinization may sometimes occur without ovulation. Luteinization results in two changes in the ovary: an alteration in the biosynthesis of steroids and a proliferation of granulosa cells. In the follicular phase of the menstrual cycle, the follicle synthesizes estrogens from progesterone and androgenic precursors as well as *de novo* from cholesterol. In the luteal phase, the granulosa cells lose the capacity to convert progesterone into androgens. As a result, a large amount of progesterone is released from the ovary. The theca interna, which secretes estrogen during the follicular phase, continues to produce estradiol during the luteal phase. The concentration of progesterone rises from the time of the midcyclic surge of gonadotropin to a peak that occurs about 7 days later. The variability in the length of the normal ovulatory cycle is a function primarily of the length of the follicular phase, for the corpus luteum has a finite life span of about 14 days.

Development of spermatozoa begins with spermatogonia, which comprise Type A and Type B elements. Spermatogonia of Type B grow and divide mitotically to produce primary spermatocytes, which give rise through meiotic division to haploid secondary spermatocytes and then spermatids, half of which carry an X chromosome and half a Y. The process by which spermatids are transformed into spermatozoa is called spermiogenesis. When the spermatozoon achieves its definitive shape, it is released into the seminiferous tubule. Ability of the spermatozoon to fertilize is not achieved until its passage through the epididymis. The biochemical changes that render the spermatozoon capable of fertilization are known as capacitation, which occurs in the uterus, oviduct, or both. Capacitation is stimulated by estrogen and inhibited by progesterone.

Fertilization requires a capacitated spermatozoon, a mature secondary ovocyte, and a milieu in which union of sperm and egg can occur. Fertilization generally occurs in the ampulla of the oviduct.

The secondary ovocyte presents three barriers to spermatozoa: the mass of cumulus cells, the zona pellucida, and the vitelline membrane. In the process of penetration, spermatozoa undergo the acrosome reaction. This reaction involves fusion of the plasma membrane of the spermatozoon with the outer acrosomal membrane, vesiculation of both membranes, and finally their disappearance. The result is the release of several enzymes. The two most important are hyaluronidase, which disperses the cells of the cumulus and allows spermatozoa to reach the zona pellucida; and acrosin, a proteinase that lyses a path for the spermatozoon through the zona pellucida. In addition, acid phosphatase and neuraminidase are released. After penetration of the ovocyte by a spermatozoon, the Golgi apparatus of the ovocyte disintegrates into small membrane-bound cortical granules, which migrate to a position immediately beneath the vitelline membrane. Release of material from the granules into the perivitelline space effects a block to polyspermy.

After fusion of the membranes of spermatozoon and ovum to form the zygote, meiosis resumes and the second polar body is extruded. The haploid sets of chromosomes from spermatozoon and ovum are quickly surrounded by pronuclear membranes to form the male and female pronuclei. Fertilization is completed when the pronuclei move to the center of the zygote, the pronuclear membranes disintegrate, and the maternal and paternal chromosomes are aligned on the metaphase plate of the first cleavage division. In the human being, the two-cell stage is not attained until at least 24 to 36 hours after fertilization.

After ovulation, the ovocyte normally remains capable of being fertilized for not longer than 12 hours. Although it may be penetrated at a later stage, it will probably degenerate before implantation. Breakdown of the metaphase II spindle may result in trisomy (a condition of three homologous chromosomes resulting from nondisjunction) or failure of extrusion of the second polar body (triploidy). During aging of the ovocyte, cortical granules move toward the center of the ovocyte, where they are no longer in a position to block polyspermy.

EARLY DEVELOPMENT OF THE FETUS

For the first 24 hours after fertilization, the zygote remains in the one-cell stage. The two-cell stage begins 24 hours after fertilization and ends 12 hours later. The four-cell stage lasts from hour 36 to hour 48; the eight-cell stage lasts from hour 48 to hour 72; and the 16-cell stage lasts from hour 72 to hour 96. The zygote enters the uterine cavity as a solid ball of cells, the morula, between three and five days after fertilization. In the uterus the morula is transformed into a fluid-filled blastocyst, which consists of an outer covering of trophoblast and a small inner cell mass (embryo-forming cells). The zona pellucida is lost at this stage and the blastocyst then implants on approximately day 6 with the embryonic pole in contact with the endometrium. During the second week the bilaminar embryo is formed and during the third week the trilaminar embryo develops. The embryonic period comprises the second through the eighth weeks and the fetal period the remainder of gestation (third through tenth lunar months). Organogenesis is completed by 16 weeks or earlier.

By day 16, the trilaminar embryonic disc comprises ectoderm, endoderm, and mesoderm. At about day 20, the paraxial mesoderm begins to divide into paired cuboidal bodies called somites, the primordia of the axial skeleton and associated musculature. Each column of paraxial mesoderm is continuous laterally with the intermediate mesoderm, the primordia of the urogenital system (p. 324). Laterally, the intermediate mesoderm thins and becomes continuous with the lateral mesoderm, the primordia of the body wall and the wall of the primitive gut.

The most significant event in the establishment of general form of the developing body occurs during the embryonic period, namely, the process of folding, which transforms the flat, ovoid trilaminar disc into a cylindrical embryo (Fig. 5–1). This folding in both longitudinal and transverse planes is caused by rapid growth in the region of the neural tube, a slower rate of growth at the periphery of the embryonic disc, and a slight constriction in the region of the future umbilical cord.

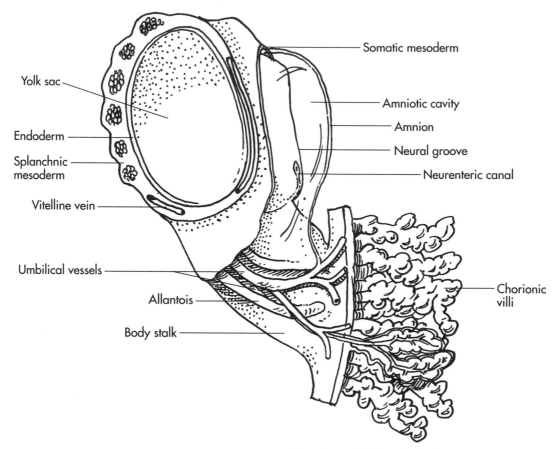

Yolk sac

Endoderm

Splanchnic
mesoderm

Vitelline vein

Umbilical vessels

Allantois

Body stalk

Somatic mesoderm

Amniotic cavity

Amnion

Neural groove

Neurenteric canal

Chorionic
villi

FIG. 5–1. Model of human embryo 1.3 mm. long. (After Eternod, Actes helv. Sci nat. Zurich, 1896.)

DEVELOPMENT OF THE PLACENTA AND FETAL MEMBRANES

The human placenta is basically a chorioallantoic structure, for although a vesicular allantois is lacking, the precociously developed allantoic mesenchyme, which later forms the umbilical cord, gives rise in situ to the allantoic vessels that vascularize the chorion. Because maternal blood is in direct contact with trophoblast-covered villi, the human placenta is classified as hemochorial. Because only one layer of trophoblast (the syncytium) is continuous throughout pregnancy, the human placenta is considered hemomonochorial.

The yolk sac, or umbilical vesicle into which it develops, is prominent at the beginning of pregnancy. The embryo is at first a flattened disc, situated between the cavities of amnion and yolk sac. As the embryo grows, it bulges into the amnionic cavity, and the dorsal part of the yolk sac is incorporated into the body of the embryo to form the gut. The yolk sac may occasionally be recognized even in the mature placenta as a crumpled vascular sac between amnion and chorion (Figs. 5–2 to 5–4).

The allantois may project into the base of the body stalk. Its mesoderm normally contains two arteries and one vein. The right umbilical vein disappears early, leaving only the original left vein.

The amnion forms around the eighth day of development by cavitation. Distention of its sac brings the amnion into contact with the internal surface of the chorion. Apposition of the mesoblasts of chorion and amnion occurs between the fourth and fifth months of gestation with the result that the extraembryonic coelom is obliterated.

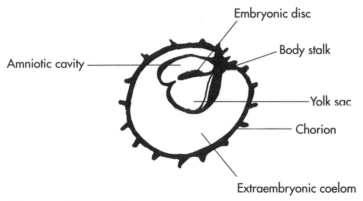

FIG. 5–2. Diagram illustrating early formation of allantois and differentiation of body stalk.

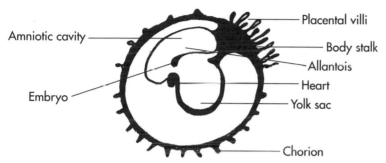

FIG. 5–3. Diagram showing later stage of allantoic development with commencing constriction of the yolk sac.

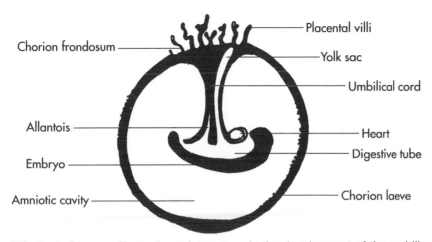

FIG. 5–4. Diagram illustrating a later stage in the development of the umbilical cord.

The changes that culminate in the transformation of the endometrium to decidua are not complete until several days after implantation (nidation). Directly beneath the site of implantation is the decidua basalis. Surrounding the ovum and separating it from the rest of the uterine cavity, in the early months of gestation, is the decidua capsularis, which forms as a result of deep, or interstitial, implantation, with the endometrium relining the uterus over the site of the implanted blastocyst. The remainder of the pregnant uterus is lined by decidua parietalis.

The human blastocyst is completely embedded in the endometrium by day 11 or 12 after fertilization. The greater part of the chorion, in contact with the decidua capsularis, loses its villi between the third and fourth months of gestation and forms the smooth chorion, or chorion laeve. The villi on the side of the chorion toward the decidua basalis enlarge and become elaborately branched to form the chorion frondosum. By the third month the decidua capsularis degenerates and the chorion laeve comes into contact with the parietal decidua of the opposite wall of the uterus. The human placenta is thus of dual origin, comprising fetal (chorion frondosum) and maternal (decidua basalis) elements.

Once the cytotrophoblast has penetrated the deepest layer of decidua, continued growth of normal placenta cannot be accomplished by further trophoblastic invasion. Increased thickness of the placenta must therefore be the result of growth in length and size of the villi of the chorion frondosum, with accompanying expansion of the intervillous space. Until the end of the fourth month, the placenta grows in thickness and circumference; thereafter, there is no appreciable increase in thickness, but growth in circumference continues almost throughout pregnancy.

The earliest form of nutrition is derived from endometrial secretion; later, maternal blood is the source. During and after implantation, there appear within the syncytiotrophoblast numerous vacuoles, the coalescence of which creates lacunae, which merge to form the intervillous space. Maternal venous sinuses are tapped early, but until day 14 or 15, no arterial blood enters the intervillous space. By day 17, the chorionic villi are vascularized, but until villous

and fetal vessels are connected and the fetal cardiac pulsations are initiated (in the second month), no true circulation can be described.

Villi may first be distinguished on or about day 12. The period between days 9 and 20 is characterized by intense growth and differentiation of the chorion. The trophoblastic trabeculae develop a cellular core as a result of multiplication of cytotrophoblastic elements. These highly modified trabeculae may then be designated primary villi. The villous stems later develop mesodermal cores, which convert primary into secondary villi. Vascularization of the secondary villi transforms them into tertiary villi, the principal organs of exchange in the human placenta. Proliferation of cellular trophoblast at the tips of the villi forms the cytotrophoblastic cell columns, which are not invaded by mesenchyme but are anchored to the decidua at the basal plate.

As the placental villi mature, several morphologic changes render them more efficient in maternofetal transfer. The early villi are less finely branched (Fig. 5–5),

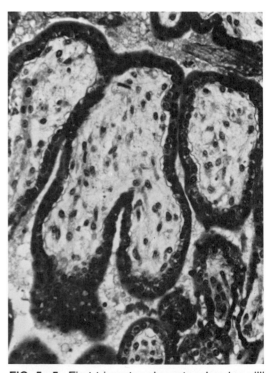

FIG. 5–5. First-trimester placenta, showing villi with well defined syncytial and cytotrophoblastic layers.

have a smaller surface-to-volume ratio, and are less well vascularized than are the terminal villi of the mature placenta (Fig. 5–6). In the early villi, a prominent layer of cytotrophoblast (Langhans cells) is evident (Fig. 5–7), whereas in the mature villi, the trophoblastic covering is thinner, with capillaries more numerous and closer to the surface (Fig. 5–8). Although the Langhans layer thins and becomes discontinuous as pregnancy advances, it never disappears completely from the normal human placenta. Electron microscopy shows that the syncytium is the differentiated form of trophoblast, whereas the Langhans layer, to which mitotic activity is confined (Fig. 5–9), comprises the less well differentiated cells that are the source of syncytiotrophoblast.

Some changes that accompany maturation of the placenta cannot be interpreted as indications of increased efficiency of placental transfer. They include thickening of basement membranes of endothelium and trophoblast, obliteration of villous capillaries, fibrosis of placental connective tissue, and deposition of calcium. A knot of syncytium in one part of the villus may accom-

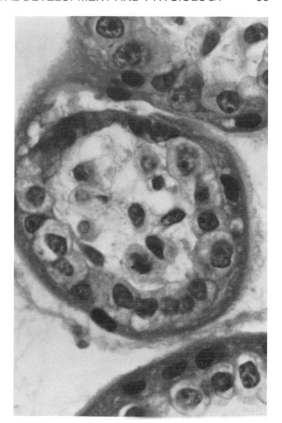

FIG. 5–7. High-power view of first-trimester placenta, showing details of trophoblast.

pany intimate approximation of endothelial and trophoblastic membranes to form a very thin vasculosyncytial membrane in another part.

FETOPLACENTAL PHYSIOLOGY

The fetus derives all of its nutrition from the mother through the placenta, which serves as a fetal kidney, liver, lung, and endocrine organ. The unusual dual circulation of the placenta allows effective fetomaternal exchange. Maternal blood enters the basal plate of the placenta, whence it is driven by the maternal systolic blood pressure toward the chorionic plate. As the blood falls back toward the basal plate, exchange takes place. The deoxygenated blood then returns to the uterine veins through the basal plate.

The unique features of the placenta include its extracorporeal location, its limited life span, its multiplicity of functions, and its apparent escape from immunologic rejec-

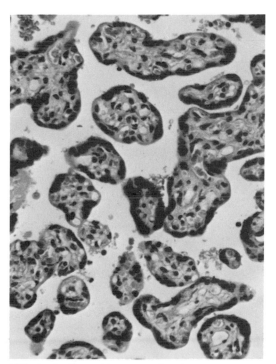

FIG. 5–6. Term placenta, showing mature, well vascularized villi.

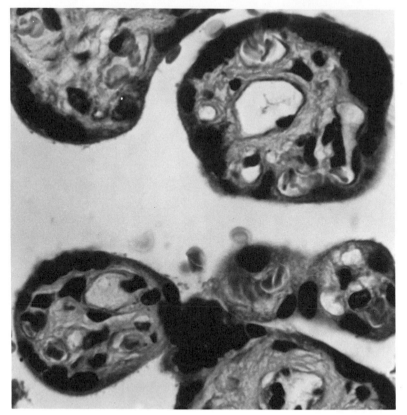

FIG. 5–8. High-power view of term placenta, showing well vascularized terminal villi.

tion. The retention of fetal (placental) tissue within the mother for a period of time far exceeding that of allograft rejection depends primarily on the special properties of the trophoblast. An absence or a deficiency of trophoblastic histocompatibility antigens, presence of extracellular sialomucin coatings of the trophoblast, and perhaps effects of progesterone and immunologic enhancement have been considered principal factors in retention of the foreign tissue.

Two maternal proteins, uteroglobin and transglutaminase, have been shown to protect the mammalian embryo from immunologic rejection during early pregnancy. Additional factors that have been invoked to explain retention of allogeneic fetoplacental tissue include: anatomic separation of maternal and fetal circulations; afferent blockade of the immunologic reflex arc by decidua; inactivation of maternal immunologic effector agents by trophoblast; production by the fetus of immunosuppressive agents such as alpha-fetoprotein; and pro-

duction by the mother of immunoregulatory agents that confer protection upon the fetoplacental unit. It has been suggested recently that the increases during pregnancy in decidual interleukin-1β and human leukocyte antigen HLA-DR$_\alpha$ may be involved in maternal recognition of the placenta and that transforming growth factor-β may regulate the local maternal immune response and thus prevent recognition of the fetus.

PLACENTAL HORMONES

The trophoblast produces both protein and steroid hormones. The complete proteins are assembled by the trophoblastic syncytium; synthesis of the steroids involves participation by the mother and fetus as well as the syncytium. The level of human chorionic gonadotropin (hCG) is elevated abruptly in early pregnancy, reaching a peak at about 80 days and gradually declining to a level that remains low throughout pregnancy. The production of hCG by the tro-

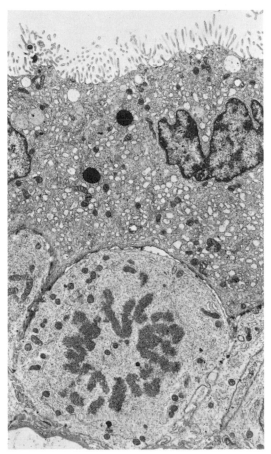

FIG. 5–9. Electron micrograph of placenta from six weeks' gestation, showing well differentiated syncytium with microvillous border and Langhans cells (cytotrophoblast), one of which displays a prominent mitotic figure.

phoblast is the basis for hormonal pregnancy tests (p. 41).

Chorionic gonadotropin is a glycoprotein with a large sialic acid moiety, which gives it a long half-life of 6 to 24 hours. This hormone has primarily LH-like properties on bioassay, with a very small amount of FSH-like activity. It substitutes for pituitary gonadotropins in maintaining steroidogenesis in the corpus luteum of pregnancy. Cellular gonadotropin is produced by a variety of human tissues but appears to be glycosylated to its physiologic form only by placenta.

Chorionic gonadotropin reaches a peak of 100,000 to 300,000 IU/liter of maternal urine by the end of the second month of pregnancy. By the fourth month, the level is down to 25,000 to 50,000 IU/liter. A low level is maintained to term. Between 45 minutes and 6 days after expulsion of the placenta, hCG normally disappears from the urine.

Human chorionic gonadotropin is a dimeric glycoprotein produced by the trophoblast during normal and pathologic pregnancies and rarely in certain disorders unassociated with pregnancy. The dimer consists of an α chain with 92 amino acids and a β chain with 145 amino acids. The α and β chains are linked by noncovalent hydrogen bonding. The α chain of hCG is virtually identical with that in all three of the pituitary glycoprotein hormones: follicle-stimulating hormone (FSH), luteinizing hormone (LH), and thyroid-stimulating hormone (TSH). The β chain, however, is distinct among the four hormones and appears to be under different genetic control from that of the α chain. Intact hCG is produced very early in pregnancy by the human trophoblast and may be measured in maternal serum by monoclonal antibody techniques as early as 9 days after conception, that is, several days before the missed menses. The free subunits, although present in much lower concentrations, may be measured by 16 to 20 days after conception. Throughout normal pregnancy, the concentration of intact dimeric hCG far exceeds that of either the α or the β subunit. The value for the dimer ranges from 2000 to 10,000 ng/mL or 10,000 to 50,000 mIU/mL, whereas that of the β subunit usually ranges from 20 to 100 ng/mL. The ratios of these subunits to the intact hormone vary from early to late pregnancy and from normal to pathologic pregnancies.

The ratios of the subunits to each other and to the intact dimer have been used in the study of trophoblastic disease (hydatidiform mole and gestational trophoblastic neoplasia) (Chapter 39) and chromosomally abnormal fetuses (Chapter 12). The free β subunit is elevated significantly in gestational trophoblastic disease. Recent studies suggest that the measurements of the subunits, the intact dimer, and their ratios may be useful in the early detection of trisomy 18 and trisomy 21.

The currently employed so-called β subunit assays actually measure intact hCG (sometimes together with the comparatively insignificant quantities of free β subunit). A monoclonal antibody has been generated against a specific site on the bound β chain and this site may or may not be recognized on the free β chain because of differences in the tertiary structure of the free and bound chains. Thus, current "β subunit" kits measure either the dimer or the dimer together with the free β subunit but not the free β subunit alone. At the present writing, controversy persists regarding the specific cells of origin, in the normal and pathologic trophoblast, of the subunits of hCG.

The other important protein hormone is human placental lactogen (hPL), also named human chorionic somatomammotropin (hCS), which undergoes a gradual increase from 6 weeks' gestation to term. It is diabetogenic and shares certain physiologic and chemical properties with human growth hormone.

Placental lactogen is a polypeptide with both prolactin-like and growth-hormone-like activities. It may substitute for prolactin in supporting ovarian function in early pregnancy and may promote development of the breast, inasmuch as growth hormone is necessary for expression of the effects of estrogen and progesterone on mammary tissue.

The plasma level of hPL reaches a maximum of between 5 and 15 μg/mL near term. The level of this hormone may be an index of placental function. Levels below 4 μg/mL after the thirtieth week of gestation have been associated in some but not all studies with poor perinatal outcome.

The placenta has been shown to produce a gonadotropin hormone-releasing hormone that is immunologically identical with that of the hypothalamus. It may be produced by the cytotrophoblast to act on the syncytium in paracrine fashion. The trophoblast also may secrete inhibin, a glycoprotein hormone, which appears to inhibit the secretion of GnRH and of hCG.

Progesterone is synthesized by the placenta from maternal precursors. The concentration of this steroid, which is essential for the maintenance of pregnancy, gradually increases in the plasma to term. The main estrogen excreted in pregnancy is estriol. Its production requires a supply of androgens by the fetal adrenal cortex and metabolic participation by the fetal liver and placenta.

Its production rises throughout pregnancy with a sharp increase at 28 weeks. Defective function of the fetal adrenal or liver or of the placenta may lead to low levels of estriol in the maternal urine or plasma. A decrease in the level of maternal estriol may result from administration of steroids and certain antibiotics. Measurement of estriol was formerly thought to be an indicator of fetal well-being. Because of high variability and low sensitivity, however, estriol is not measured frequently today for this purpose.

The principal metabolite of progesterone in pregnancy is pregnanediol, which reaches a maximum at about 32 weeks' gestation. It is not a reliable index of placental function. At the fourteenth week of pregnancy, the maternal excretion of urinary estrogen is 1 mg/day. At term, the level is normally 30 mg/day, about 90% of which is estriol (E_3).

Maternal cholesterol is converted to pregnenolone by the placenta. This compound is then converted to dehydroisoandrosterone sulfate (DHAS) by the fetal adrenal. DHAS is then hydroxylated at the 16-position in the fetal liver. This is the rate-limiting reaction. The 16-alpha-OH-DHA is converted to estriol in the placenta. It is conjugated to a glucosiduronate or a sulfate and is excreted as E_3G or E_3S in the maternal urine. (Fig. 5–10). The placenta does not synthesize corticosteroids. TSH-like activity has also been identified in the placenta. The placenta is somewhat permeable to thyroxine but not to TSH, parathormone, posterior pituitary extract, or insulin.

PLACENTAL TRANSFER

Placental transfer in either direction may be active or passive. The rate of transfer depends principally on the following factors: the rates of maternal and fetal blood flows, the respective concentrations of substances in the maternal and fetal plasmas (concentration gradients), the area and thickness of the placental membrane, the molecular weight and electrical charge of the compound, the physical properties of the barrier, the biochemical mechanisms for active transfer, and the metabolism by the placenta itself.

Since most drugs administered to the mother—including antibiotics and anesthetics, as well as gases, nutrients, many

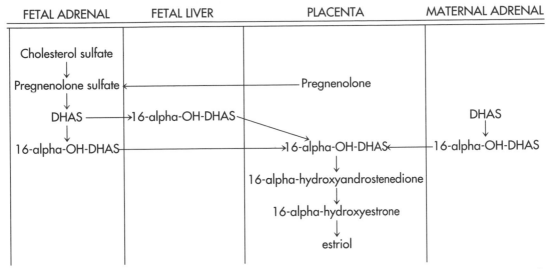

FETAL ADRENAL   FETAL LIVER   PLACENTA   MATERNAL ADRENAL

FIG. 5–10. Participation of fetal adrenal, fetal liver, placenta, and maternal adrenal in the synthesis of estriol.

hormones, and some immunoglobulins— cross the placenta, everything prescribed for the mother during pregnancy must be considered in terms of effects on the fetus as well. A few agents, such as succinylcholine, d-tubocurarine, and heparin, however, cross very slightly or not at all. Other substances are concentrated preferentially in the fetal circulation.

The fetus meets its requirements for iron even in the presence of maternal anemia. It maintains oxygenation of its blood by several mechanisms. First, fetal erythrocytes have a higher affinity for oxygen than do maternal erythrocytes. The higher hemoglobin level of the newborn resembles that seen in the adult at high altitude. Fetal blood has a greater oxygen capacity, but has a lower saturation and a higher hematocrit than does adult blood. Accumulation of iron in the fetal liver occurs mainly in the third trimester.

Placental transfer occurs as a result of several mechanisms. Respiratory gases and some electrolytes are transferred by simple diffusion. Sodium is probably transferred actively, with chloride then diffusing to maintain electrostatic balance. Carbohydrates are transferred by facilitated diffusion, and amino acids and some vitamins by active transport. Ascorbic acid, for example, is concentrated on the fetal side. Differential rates of transfer of stereoisomers, such as D-

and L-histidine, are evidence of enzyme-mediated carrier mechanisms. In general, the greater the degree of lipid solubility and the smaller the molecular weight, the greater is the rate of transfer. Certain molecules of high molecular weight, however, such as some of the immunoglobulins, cross the placenta, whereas others of equal molecular weight do not. In general, uncharged particles are transferred more readily. Macromolecules may be transported across the placenta by pinocytosis. Water is transferred by bulk flow in response to small hydrostatic or osmotic pressure gradients. Breaks in placental villi lead to leakage of fetal erythrocytes into the maternal circulation and possible Rh-isoimmunization in certain circumstances (p. 126). Some viruses such as rubella may cross the placenta and produce fetal disease (p. 113).

IgG crosses the placenta, whereas IgM and IgA do not. Passive immunity to some diseases may be conferred on the fetus as a result of the transfer of these antibodies. In addition, the fetus may produce some of its own antibodies after midpregnancy.

The fetus receives most of its nitrogen as amino acids and synthesizes its own protein. Although the placenta transfers phospholipids, which are subsequently degraded, most of the fetal lipid is synthesized by the fetus itself. Similarly, the fetus synthesizes its own nucleic acids. Glucose is readily transferred in both directions, but the maternal level is usually higher than the fetal. The levels of calcium and phosphorus, however, are higher on the fetal side.

FETAL DEVELOPMENT

A fetus reaches term at 40 weeks. It is considered mature at 37 weeks' gestation. If the birth weight is under 2500 g, the fetus is considered to be of "low birth weight." Viability is often considered to begin at 500 g, which corresponds roughly to midpregnancy.

The fetal internal iliac arteries continue extraabdominally as umbilical arteries, which carry deoxygenated blood to the placenta. The umbilical vein carries relatively well-oxygenated blood from the placenta back to the fetus. Various shunts of oxygenated blood characterize the fetal circulation. Some blood from the umbilical vein is shunted through the ductus venosus to avoid the liver, the only organ to receive undiluted freshly oxygenated blood. The upper half of the fetal body receives more oxygen than does the lower half. The foramen ovale shunts blood to the left side of the heart to supply the head. The ductus arteriosus shunts much of the pulmonary arterial flow to the aorta, thus bypassing the lungs.

At birth, the lungs expand as the infant draws its first breath. As blood begins to flow through the pulmonary vessels, the ductus venosus, foramen ovale, and ductus arteriosus undergo functional closure (Fig. 5–11).

The high cardiac output of the fetus and the high hemoglobin content and better oxygen dissociation of fetal hemoglobin compensate for the relatively poor oxygen content of fetal blood. The fetal heart rate of 135/min drops to about 110/min in the newborn.

By the third month of fetal life, the genitalia are sufficiently differentiated to allow diagnosis of sex. By the second trimester, the liver has replaced the placenta as

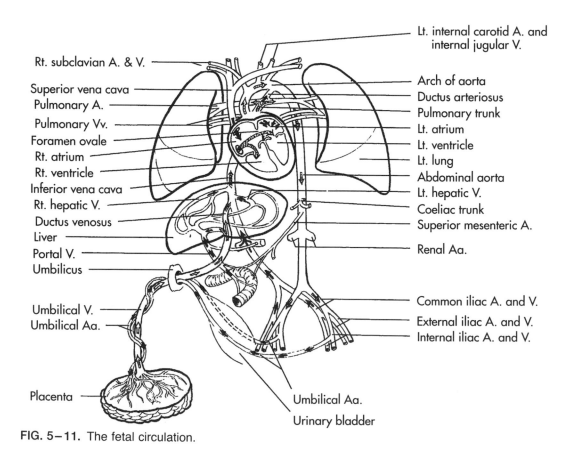

FIG. 5–11. The fetal circulation.

the principal organ for storage of carbohydrate.

The growth of the fetus by weight and length is as follows:

Gestational Week	Length (cm) (Crown-heel)	Weight (g)
8	3	1
12	10	18
16	18	100
20	25	300
24	32	600
28	37	1,000
32	42	1,700
36	47	2,500
40	50	3,200 or more

The composition of the amniotic (amnionic) fluid is determined in part by metabolic products of the fetus. The fluid is at first isotonic with maternal serum and is later diluted by hypotonic fetal urine. The volume of fluid increases to a maximum of slightly over 1000 mL at about 35 weeks and gradually decreases to between 500 and 800 mL at term. Examination of the amniotic fluid can be used to assess fetal well-being and maturity. The cells and fluid are examined to detect sex of the fetus and many metabolic and chromosomal abnormalities (Chapter 12).

Severe diminution in the volume of amniotic fluid (oligohydramnios) is associated with a poor prognosis if it occurs during the second trimester. If oligohydramnios does not occur until the third trimester, however, it may respond to therapy by infusion of fluid into the amnionic cavity. Causes of severe oligohydramnios include chromosomal anomalies such as triploidy and genitourinary disorders such as bilateral obstruction of the urethrovesical junctions, posterior urethral valves, and renal agenesis. A marked decrease in amniotic fluid may also occur with restriction of intrauterine growth (Chapter 26).

Fetal maturity may be assessed by a variety of clinical and laboratory methods. An accurate knowledge of the date of onset of the last menstrual period, auscultation of the fetal heart by standard fetoscope by 20 weeks, and several early measurements of the size of the uterus (before 16 weeks) are the best means of assessing gestational age and fetal maturity by history and physical examination. Ultrasonic detection of the onset of fetal cardiac activity at 5 to 7 weeks and measurements of crown-rump length between 7 and 14 weeks and of biparietal diameter and femoral length between 16 and 30 weeks also provide accurate assessments of gestational age. Ultrasonic measurements of crown-rump length have proved most accurate, with an error of ± 3 to 5 days. In each case, serial measurements are always more accurate than a single measurement. Assessment of gestational age during the third trimester is considerably less accurate than during the first or second trimester. A biparietal diameter of 9.0 cm or more or a femoral length of 7.1 cm or more usually indicates a fetus that weighs at least 2500 grams. Serial measurements of fundal height in centimeters above the symphysis (with a tape measure) provide another simple means of assessing fetal growth. Radiologic examination of the fetus for assessment of gestational age is contraindicated. Sonographic assessment of gestational age is illustrated in Table 5–1 and Figures 5–12 through 5–15. Sonography is discussed further in Chapter 26.

Placentas may be graded from 0 (least mature) through I and II to III (most mature). A grade III placenta has a chorionic plate with indentations extending to the basal layer, a placental mass divided into compartments with echo-free areas, and a basal layer with dense, almost confluent echogenic areas.

Several chemical studies of the amniotic fluid have proved fairly reliable in ascertaining fetal age. The most important chemical indices of fetal maturity are the phospholipids in the amniotic fluid. The lecithin/sphingomyelin ratio is approximately 1.0 at

TABLE 5–1. SONOGRAPHIC CRITERIA FOR DATING GESTATIONAL LENGTH

First Trimester

1. Gestational sac
2. Crown to rump length (CR)
3. Biparietal diameter (BPD) after 9 weeks

Second Trimester

1. Biparietal diameter
2. Transverse cerebellar diameter
3. Outer orbital diameter
4. Abdominal circumference (AC)
5. Femoral length (FL)
6. Fetal foot length

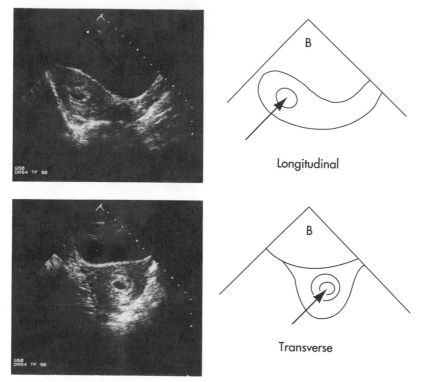

FIG. 5–12. Transverse and longitudinal sonograms of a five to six weeks' intrauterine gestation. A 1 cm sac with an echogenic rim is seen within the uterus but no fetus is yet visible. Sac (arrow) and bladder (B) are shown. The early sac of an intrauterine gestation may be confused with a decidual reaction or "pseudosac" that is associated with ectopic pregnancy.

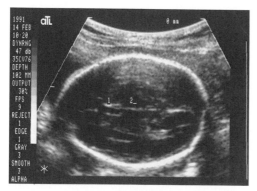

FIG. 5–13. Axial scan of fetal head showing biparietal diameter of 70 mm at 28 weeks' gestation. 1 = Cavum septi pellucidi (CSP); 2 = Thalamus. This method, although frequently employed, is somewhat less accurate than the crown-rump length. Accuracy of both methods, however, varies with gestational age. For the biparietal diameter (BPD), accuracy at 16 weeks is ±1 week; near term it is ±3 weeks.

the thirty-fifth week. An L/S ratio of about 2.0 indicates pulmonary maturity and little likelihood of respiratory distress syndrome (Fig. 5–16). A lower ratio, however, does not necessarily indicate the likely development of respiratory distress syndrome. Measurement of phosphatidyl glycerol (PG) is also a very useful means of assessing pulmonary maturity, especially in diabetic pregnancies. In mature fetuses, the ratio of PG to the other phospholipids in the amniotic fluid is increased. A "shake test" (foam stability test) is a rough guide to the presence of surface-active substances.

Several additional chemical tests are less commonly employed today. The concentration of creatinine, for example, should be 2 mg% or more after the thirty-seventh week of gestation. In the normal term fetus the bilirubin concentration should be negligible. In the mature fetus the osmolality, which is measured by depression of the freezing

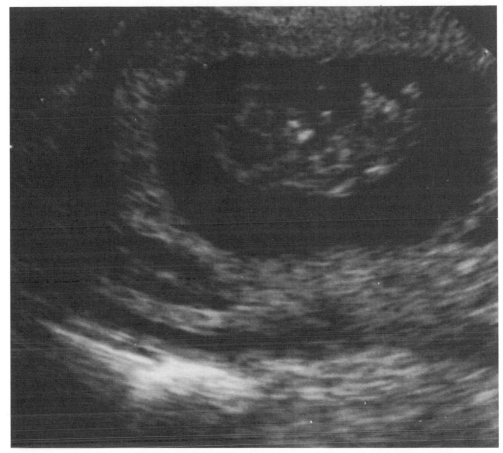

FIG. 5–14. Sonogram showing the crown-rump length (32 mm) of the fetus at 10 weeks' gestation. The head is identified by the intracerebral echoes. Crown-rump measurements are the most accurate means of assessing gestational age between 7 and 13 weeks of gestation.

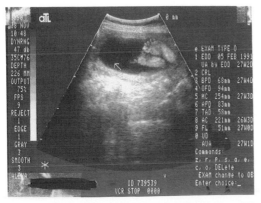

FIG. 5–15. Ultrasonic view of fetal foot at 27 weeks' gestation as seen in plantar view.

point and reflects predominantly the concentration of sodium, should be less than 250 milliosmoles.

Measurement of the optical density of the amniotic fluid at 650 nm is another rapid, inexpensive test of fetal pulmonary maturity.

Further use of ultrasound in conjunction with amniocentesis is discussed in the sections dealing with prenatal diagnosis of genetic and metabolic disorders (Chapter 12) and the sections on abnormalities of fetal growth (Chapter 26).

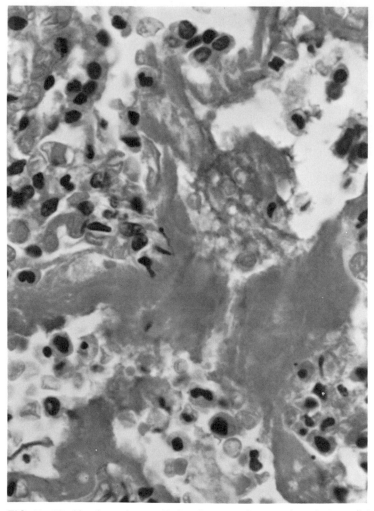

FIG. 5−16. Newborn lung with hyaline membranes (respiratory distress syndrome).

6
CHAPTER
ANTEPARTUM CARE

EDUCATION

A major purpose of antepartum care is education of the patient about pregnancy, labor, and delivery. Pregnancy should be explained as a physiologic process rather than an illness. The antepartum period is a good time to practice preventive medicine, since ideally the patient is under a physician's supervision for at least half a year. During this time, dental care may be obtained, an adequate diet planned, and advice about sexual activity and contraception given.

Diet should be well-balanced to include meat, eggs, fresh fruits and vegetables, and a total daily intake of 2500 calories. Iron should be prescribed with meals (p. 116). Prenatal vitamins may be given routinely, although a well-balanced diet with iron supplementation is usually adequate for a healthy woman. The pregnant patient must be urged to discontinue smoking cigarettes and drinking alcoholic beverages for at least the duration of the gestation and to avoid illicit drugs permanently (p. 64).

The patient should be told that bathing is permissible, especially since bath water does not enter the vagina, and that coitus may be continued, if desired, so long as there are no abnormalities of pregnancy and it causes no discomfort. Normal physical activity should be permitted to the point of fatigue. The patient should be encouraged to walk about a half mile a day and to continue work as long as she is physically and emotionally comfortable. Short-distance travel is associated with no increased risk, but long trips may be hazardous during the third trimester, especially if opportunities for ambulation and recumbency are limited.

Vigorous exercise during pregnancy is contraindicated in the following circumstances: history of three or more spontaneous abortions, ruptured membranes, premature labor, plural gestation, incompetent cervix, bleeding, and cardiac disease.

Classes for both parents are valuable to allay fear of labor and delivery. The patient should be informed that any drug taken during pregnancy may affect the fetus (Table 6–1) and that maternal infectious diseases may affect the fetus and neonate (Table 6–2). The obstetrician must therefore be consulted before the patient undergoes any diagnostic investigation or treatment. In general, no drug or treatment, including over-the-counter preparations, should be given to the pregnant woman unless the benefits clearly outweigh the risks to mother and fetus. The mother should receive no immunizations with live virus during pregnancy. Vaccines with killed organisms and tetanus toxoid may be administered during pregnancy.

TABLE 6–1. EFFECTS OF MATERNAL DRUGS ON THE FETUS AND NEWBORN

Maternal Drug	Effect
Alcohol	Deficiencies in growth; mental retardation; facial anomalies
Amethopterin	Anomalies; abortion
Ammonium chloride	Acidosis
Androgens	Masculinization
Cephalothin	Positive direct Coombs' test
Chlorambucil	Anomalies; abortion
Chloramphenicol	"Gray baby syndrome"
Cocaine	Congenital anomalies; abruptio placentae
Coumadin	Fetal death; hemorrhage; osseous deformities
Diethylstilbestrol	Vaginal adenosis; uterine anomalies
Diphenylhydantoin (Phenytoin)	Dysmorphic facies; cardiac defects; abnormal genitalia
Diuretics	Imbalance of electrolytes
Heroin	Neonatal death or convulsions
Hexamethonium	Neonatal ileus
Iodine-containing preparations	Abnormal development of thyroid
Isoretinoin	Abortion; multiple fetal defects
Lead	Abortion; stillbirth
Methimazole	Goiter; mental retardation
Morphine	Neonatal death or convulsions
Novobiocin	Hyperbilirubinemia
Phenobarbital	Neonatal bleeding
Potassium iodide	Goiter; mental retardation
Progestins	Masculinization; possible cardiovascular anomalies
Propylthiouracil	Goiter; mental retardation
Reserpine	Nasal congestion and drowsiness
Salicylates (excess)	Neonatal bleeding
Streptomycin	Damage to acoustic nerve
Sulfonamides	Kernicterus
Tetracyclines	Discoloration of teeth; inhibition of osseous growth
Thalidomide	Phocomelia
Thiazides	Thrombocytopenia
Tobacco (cigarettes)	Low-birth-weight babies
Trimethadione	Craniofacial and cardiac anomalies
Valproic acid	Neural tube defects
Vitamin K analogues (excess)	Hyperbilirubinemia

During the antepartum visits, the various methods of analgesia and anesthesia should be discussed and the patient informed about the available kinds of contraception. She should be given the opportunity to decide whether she prefers breast feeding or a bottle and to discuss circumcision of a male infant. She should also be encouraged to select possible names for the baby. The patient must be taught to recognize uterine contractions, or "hardening" of the uterus, and the feeling of pelvic pressure that is associated with premature labor. She should also be taught to recognize the onset of labor, that is, the regular, painful, progressive contractions, and to report any "bloody show" (blood-tinged mucous discharge from the vagina that accompanies dilation of the cervix during the first stage of labor) or rupture of the membranes (definite or suspected). The patient should be instructed to take no food after the onset of labor. It is important that she be taught to report any of the danger signs of pregnancy, including vaginal bleeding, abdominal pain, nondependent edema, blurred vision, head-

TABLE 6–2. EFFECTS OF MATERNAL INFECTIONS AND RADIATION ON THE FETUS AND NEWBORN

Maternal Insult	Effect
Cytomegalovirus	Microcephaly; retardation of somatic growth; cerebral damage; hearing loss
Rubella	Cataracts; deafness; cardiac lesions; expanded syndrome including effects on all organs
Syphilis	Fetal death with hydrops (severe); abnormalities of skin, teeth, and bones (mild form)
Toxoplasmosis	Chorioretinitis; hydrocephalus; calcification in CNS; and possible effects on all organs
Varicella-zoster	Intrauterine and persistent postnatal disease; possible effects on all organs, including scarring of skin and muscular atrophy
X-Radiation	Microcephaly; mental retardation

ache, or any significant change in well-being.

The daily diet should contain 150 g of carbohydrate, 100 g of fat, and 85 g of protein. Six to 8 glasses of fluid including a quart of milk a day are desirable. The diet should specifically contain adequate amounts of calcium, iron, vitamin A, thiamine, riboflavin, niacin, folic acid, and vitamins C and D. The sodium content of carbonated beverages and beer and the caloric content of alcohol must be considered in planning the diet. Consumption of alcohol should be discontinued during pregnancy p. 65. If specific dietary problems arise, a professional dietician should be consulted.

A maternity girdle and low-heeled walking shoes may add to the patient's comfort. No hand-bulb syringes must be used for douching because of the danger of air embolism, and the douche bag should be held not more than two feet above the level of the hips to avoid undue pressure. Coitus may be continued unless premature labor, rupture of the membranes, vaginal bleeding, or infection supervenes. Cunnilingus during pregnancy may introduce air into the vagina and cause fatal air embolism.

DRUGS IN PREGNANCY

The use of alcohol, tobacco, and illicit drugs has become a problem of increasing impor-

tance in obstetrics. Between 70 and 90% of Americans between the ages of 15 and 40 have used mood-altering drugs, and about half of them are women of reproductive age. Many women are not aware that they are pregnant when they use drugs and thus may expose their fetuses at the time most likely to cause congenital malformations, that is, within 58 days after conception. Furthermore, many women who use illicit drugs during pregnancy do not admit to doing so and thus deprive themselves of the opportunity to discuss the effects with their obstetricians.

Pregnant women who are substance abusers require prenatal care beyond what is sufficient for the normal pregnancy. Substance abusers are at increased risk of sexually transmitted diseases, hepatitis, bacterial endocarditis, and poor nutrition. They therefore require screening for syphilis, gonorrhea, chlamydial infection, hepatitis, and the human immunodeficiency virus (AIDS). Women who use drugs parenterally are at greatest risk. Although few illicit drugs cause easily identifiable fetal malformations, substance abuse during pregnancy is an indication for fetal evaluation, which may include high-resolution ultrasound, maternal serum alpha-fetoprotein screening, and fetal echocardiography. Because users of illicit drugs seldom abuse only one drug, the potential for adverse effects is magnified.

Almost all substances that are acquired illegally are contaminated. For example, in the extraction of cocaine base from coca, leaded gasoline is used as a solvent, with the potential danger of lead poisoning. Marijuana may contain dangerous vegetable contaminants, which may cause serious morbidity or even mortality. Marijuana may be contaminated, furthermore, with the herbicide paraquat and the pesticide chlordane. Warfarin, which has been used to "cut" heroin, is associated with a well-described embryopathy.

Alcohol, a commonly used central nervous system depressant, is consumed socially by as many as 70% of Americans. Problem drinking, which may be considered equivalent to alcoholism by some students of the subject, implies 8 or more ounces of 80 proof alcohol a day. That amount of ethanol is found in eight cocktails, eight glasses of wine (6 ounces each), or eight cans or bottles of beer (12 ounces each). Women who drink alcohol during pregnancy are putting their fetuses at risk of the fetal alcohol syndrome, which comprises deficiencies of prenatal and postnatal growth, mental retardation, behavioral disturbances, and midfacial hypoplasia. Congenital cardiac defects and anomalies of the brain are also common. The syndrome affects 30 to 40% of the newborns of alcoholic women. The full-blown syndrome usually affects the children of mothers who drink more than 3 ounces of alcohol a day throughout their pregnancies. Consumption of smaller amounts of alcohol may be associated with less severe manifestations, called collectively "fetal alcohol effects." No recommendation can be made regarding a safe level of drinking, and the effects of episodic drinking have not been defined clearly. Consumption of alcohol during pregnancy is the most commonly identified nongenetic cause of mental retardation.

Cigarette smoke contains a large number of noxious chemicals, but nicotine and carbon monoxide are the most important from an obstetric viewpoint. The rates of prematurity, spontaneous abortion, and low birth weight are all increased in mothers who smoke tobacco. Abruptio placentae is more common in mothers who smoke, but the rate of congenital anomalies does not seem to be increased.

Marijuana is usually smoked or eaten as a recreational drug. The active ingredient is tetrahydrocannabinol (THC). The rate of major anomalies in infants of mothers who smoke marijuana during pregnancy does not appear to be increased over the background risk.

The amphetamines are drugs that are prescribed for narcolepsy and as stimulants of the central nervous system and depressants of appetite. The major problems that arise from their use during pregnancy are related to the impurities in the illicitly obtained drugs. Their use does not seem to be related to an increase in congenital anomalies.

Cocaine is a local anesthetic derived from the leaves of *Erythroxylon coca*. It is a vasoconstrictor, a central nervous system stimulant, and one of the most widely abused drugs in the United States and elsewhere. Abruptio placentae is one of the more serious complications of pregnancy in women who use this drug. Premature separation of the placenta is thought to result from the vasoconstrictive and hypertensive effects of cocaine. Similarly, congenital anomalies in infants exposed to cocaine in utero are attributed to vascular disruption. They include intestinal atresia, limb reduction anomalies, disruptive brain anomalies, congenital cardiac defects, "prune belly" syndrome, and anomalies of the urinary tract. Additional adverse effects of cocaine on pregnancy include an increased rate of low birth-weight infants and possibly an increased risk of sudden infant death syndrome (SIDS).

Barbiturates are used regularly as hypnotics, sedatives, and anticonvulsants. Although these drugs on occasion are used illicitly, they do not appear to cause an increase in congenital anomalies in the infants exposed to them.

Diazepam (Valium) is a benzodiazepine widely used as a mild tranquilizer, muscle relaxant, anticonvulsant, and preanesthetic medication. The data regarding the relation of use of diazepam during pregnancy to embryopathy are inconsistent. The risk of cleft lip or palate in the offspring of women who use the drug during pregnancy does not seem to be greater than the background risk.

Codeine is commonly found in many antitussive preparations. It is a narcotic analgesic that is widely used, but it does not seem to be associated with an increased risk of congenital anomalies in the offspring of users. Heroin, another opiate, is abused throughout the world. The studies of the effects of this drug during pregnancy are complicated by maternal use of other drugs at the same time. The rate of congenital anomalies in the offspring of heroin users is not increased above background values, but fetal growth restriction and perinatal death occur more commonly. Postnatal growth, however, appears to be normal in most cases. Neonates exposed in utero to heroin commonly manifest signs of withdrawal, including tremors, irritability, sneezing, vomiting, fever, diarrhea, and seizures.

Methadone is used principally as maintenance therapy for heroin addiction. Although there is no increased rate of congenital anomalies above background values, withdrawal syndrome and low birth weight occur much more frequently in the neonates of mothers who use the drug than in those of controls.

ANTEPARTUM VISITS

An important aspect of antepartum care is identification of the high-risk pregnancy. First, a history of medical, surgical, or obstetric complications in prior pregnancies must be elicited. Risk is increased in patients of low socioeconomic status and possibly unwed mothers, in whom the effects of environment and heredity are often difficult to separate. Extremes of age (under 15 and over 40) are associated with more obstetric complications. Obesity, addiction or habituation to drugs, and intake of ethanol are all associated with an increased rate of complications. Heavy smoking by the mother leads to lighter but not necessarily premature infants. High parity itself, moreover, is associated with a significantly increased rate of obstetric complications.

In obtaining the obstetric history the doctor should inquire specifically about diabetes mellitus, preeclampsia-eclampsia, tuberculosis, rheumatic fever, cardiac disease, hypertensive and renal disease, syphilis, rubella, pelvic operations, transfusions, hereditary diseases, and a familial history of twins. History of the menses and prior pregnancies should be recorded in detail.

The most common complication leading to serious perinatal morbidity and mortality in the United States today is preterm labor. A major factor associated with preterm labor is a prior preterm birth (p. 140).

Many findings obtained on examination of the mother give clues to high-risk pregnancy. The more important include: abnormal growth of the uterus (suggesting plural gestation, hydramnios, and hydatidiform mole), dead fetus, contracted pelvis, abnormal presentation, and large or abnormal fetuses. Fetal indications of a high-risk pregnancy include restriction of growth and abnormal cardiac sounds.

Laboratory tests used to detect possible complications of pregnancy include: serologic test for syphilis; examination of urine for glucose and protein; urine culture (particularly with a history of urologic infection); hemoglobin and hematocrit; Papanicolaou smear; and a glucose tolerance test in the presence of glycosuria, a history suggestive of diabetes, or a history of prior newborns weighing greater than 9 pounds. It is advisable to perform a single measurement of plasma glucose after an oral glucose load at about the twenty-sixth week of gestation. If this value is elevated, a full 3-hour glucose tolerance test is performed. Cultures for gonorrhea and chlamydia should be obtained from urethra, cervix, and anus. Fetal disease may be anticipated by identifying the mother's blood group (ABO) and Rh-type. In cases of Rh-negative mothers, antibody titers are indicated (p. 126).

Antepartum visits should be made monthly during the first 6 months, every 2 weeks from the twenty-eighth to the thirty-sixth week of gestation, and weekly during the last month. The patient should consult the obstetrician as early in pregnancy as possible. Advantages include early assessment of gestational age and careful surveillance during the period of early fetal growth. In the first few months of pregnancy, the fetus is most susceptible to the effects of ingested drugs and environmental factors such as radiation.

Accurate records must be kept in an effort to optimize maternal and fetal well-being. The patient must be encouraged to ask questions during her visits and the obstetrician must answer them factually and completely. Several suitable books are readily available to provide further information to the patient.

At each antepartum visit the blood pressure, weight, and urinary protein should be checked, primarily to detect preeclampsia (p. 120). The normal midtrimester drop in blood pressure should be recognized. Weight gain is normally kept to about 25 to 30 pounds, but in the absence of fluid retention a greater weight gain in itself is not harmful to the outcome of the pregnancy. In no case should the patient be placed on a program of weight reduction, and "diet pills" of all varieties are contraindicated in pregnancy. In cases of suspected recent exposure to rubella, antibody titers should be obtained. (p. 114).

The height of the fundus should be measured at each visit and the fetal heart tones recorded (by stethoscope or Doptone). The presence of plural gestation or abnormalities of presentation should be noted as soon as they are suspected. In the third trimester it is appropriate to repeat the hemoglobin, the serologic test for syphilis, and the gonococcal and chlamydial cultures. A pelvic examination including Papanicolaou smear is performed at the initial visit, but it may be easier to perform manual pelvimetry later in pregnancy when the pelvic tissues are more relaxed. Frequent vaginal examinations are helpful in identifying early cervical dilation in patients who are at risk for preterm delivery.

Manual pelvimetry should include an estimate of the diagonal conjugate (the distance from the promontory of the sacrum to the inferior border of the pubic symphysis), which is normally about 12.5 cm. The true conjugate is the distance from the promontory of the sacrum to the superior border of the symphysis. It cannot be measured manually, but is estimated by subtracting between 1 and 2 cm from the diagonal conjugate, depending on the height and inclination of the symphysis, to give a figure of about 11 cm. The intertuberous diameter (the distance between the inner aspects of the ischial tuberosities) is the transverse diameter of the outlet and is generally about 11 cm. If the diagonal conjugate is below 11.5 cm, further study is often indicated (p. 73).

Other pelvic features of obstetric importance are the shape of the pubic arch, the width of the sacrosciatic notch, the prominence of the ischial spines, the shape of the forepelvis, the convergence of the side walls, and the thickness of the bones. Because x-ray pelvimetry exposes mother and fetus to ionizing radiation and because appropriate clinical management is usually possible without it, the technique is employed only for unusual, specific indications today.

COMMON COMPLAINTS

In discussing common complaints with the patient, it is important to distinguish physiologic alterations of pregnancy from disease and to discourage the use of drugs whenever possible. Lassitude, urinary frequency without dysuria, ptyalism, tingling of the breasts, palpitation, tachypnea, and occasional syncope ordinarily require no special therapy. Backache may be relieved by supportive garments and a firm mattress. Constipation may be treated with mild laxatives, a high intake of fluids, and a diet high in bulk. Varicosities may require supportive stockings and elevation of the legs. Leukorrhea, hemorrhoids, and heartburn occasionally require symptomatic therapy. Painful uterine contractions must be distinguished by continued observation from true progressive labor (p. 73). Any severe abdominal pain requires ruling out appendicitis, cholecystitis, partial abruption of the placenta, and urinary tract infection.

Pica, which may interfere with a regular diet, should be recognized and discouraged. Emotional lability, as opposed to a true psychiatric disturbance, usually responds well to simple support and reassurance.

Hyperemesis gravidarum is an exaggeration of nausea and vomiting of pregnancy, with systemic effects such as acetonuria and substantial weight loss. It is best treated with multiple small feedings high in carbohydrates and sometimes antiemetics.

Hyperemesis gravidarum appears to be less common today than formerly and is no longer considered a form of preeclampsia. Etiologic factors may include elevated levels of gonadotropins and steroids, delayed gastric emptying, and emotional predisposition. It is most common between the second and fourth months of pregnancy. The important components of therapy include maintenance of fluid and electrolyte balance, correction of other diseases, and avoidance of obnoxious odors. Other causes of nausea and vomiting must be ruled out, including viral hepatitis and ulcers. Hyperemesis gravidarum is often associated with immature personalities but is apparently not increased in unwed mothers. Psychologic support is important and antiemetic agents such as cyclizine, meclizine, and dicyclomine have been useful and have not proved to be teratogenic. Despite its value, the drug Bendectin was taken off the market by its manufacturer for reasons of product liability. Drastic and punitive measures have no place in the management of hyperemesis, and abortion is rarely indicated.

7

CHAPTER

INTRAPARTUM CARE

LABOR

Labor is divided into three stages. The first stage begins with the onset of true labor and ends with full dilation of the cervix (10 cm). The second stage begins with full dilation of the cervix and ends with birth of the fetus. The third stage begins with birth of the fetus and ends with the expulsion or extraction of the placenta and membranes.

Labor is characterized by progressive dilation and effacement of the cervix, which accompany regular painful uterine contractions normally associated with descent of the presenting part (that part of the fetus that is lowest in the pelvis). The presenting part is the part of the fetus that is palpated by the examining finger on vaginal examination, for example, occiput, sacrum, or acromion. Dilation of the cervix is the enlargement of the external cervical os caused by the upward retraction of the myometrial fibers during labor. Effacement of the cervix is accomplished when the cervix is completely retracted, the cervicovaginal angle has disappeared, and only the external os remains to be dilated.

During the course of pregnancy, painless irregular uterine contractions (Braxton Hicks contractions) increase in intensity and regularity and eventually become true labor pains. The contractions of true labor begin in the lumbar region at intervals of 20 to 30 minutes. At the onset of labor, the mucous plug is expelled from the cervical canal.

Normal uterine contractions are characterized by fundal dominance (contractions that are strongest in the top of the uterus and weakest in the bottom) and symmetry (contractions that arise simultaneously from both cornual areas). The intensity of normal uterine contractions increases progressively, so that at the height of a contraction the intrauterine pressure rises to between 40 and 60 mm Hg and the myometrium can be indented only with strong digital pressure. Uterine contractions with an intensity of less than 15 mm Hg are ineffective. The tonus of the uterus is the pressure between contractions, when the myometrium can be indented with only moderate digital pressure. Tonus is normally less than 25 mm Hg. The frequency of uterine contractions gradually increases to about one every 2 to 3 minutes and the duration to between 45 and 60 seconds at the end of labor.

The upper segment of the uterus is the thick contractile portion; the lower segment is thin and passive. A retraction ring may divide the two.

The first stage of labor is concerned with overcoming cervical resistance and the second stage with the passage of the fetus through the birth canal. Although the lengths of the stages of labor may normally vary within fairly wide limits, the first stage lasts about 6 to 8 hours in the multipara and 10 to 14 hours in the primigravida. The second stage usually does not last longer than 2 hours. The third stage usually lasts about 15 to 30 minutes and should be terminated after 1 hour at the latest.

The three main factors determining the course of labor are the powers (uterine contractions), the passages (bony pelvis and maternal soft tissues), and the passenger (size and position of the fetus). Progress in labor is determined by the gradual descent of the presenting part, or change in station (the location of the presenting part in the birth canal). Designation of station as "+" or "−" refers to the level in cm below (+) or above (−) the ischial spines. Station 0 is attained when the presenting part has reached the level of the ischial spines. Station +2, for example, is attained when the presenting part is 2 cm below the spines. When the occiput is at station 0, the vertex is said to be engaged clinically. Engagement occurs when the fetal biparietal diameter has passed the plane of the pelvic inlet.

Presentation, or lie, is the relation of the long axis of the fetus to the long axis of the mother. It may be either longitudinal or transverse. With a longitudinal lie, the presenting part is either the head (cephalic) or the breech. With a transverse lie, the shoulder is the presenting part. Cephalic presentations are classified according to the relation of the head to the body of the fetus. When the head is fully flexed and the chin contacts the thorax, the occiput, or vertex, presents. When the neck is fully extended and the occiput contacts the back, a face presentation results, with the chin, or mentum, the presenting part. Intermediate conditions include the sinciput, in which the large fontanelle presents, and the partially extended head, in which the brow presents. Sinciput and brow presentations usually convert spontaneously to vertex or face presentations by flexion or extension, respectively, during the course of labor.

Position is the relation of a designated point on the presenting part of the fetus to the right or left side of the maternal pelvis. Thus, there are two positions, right and left. Each position is divided into three varieties: anterior, transverse, and posterior. These six varieties are designated by letters, as in the following examples. If the occiput is in the left anterior portion of the maternal pelvis, it is designated LOA. If the chin (mentum) is in the right posterior portion of the maternal pelvis, it is designated RMP. If the breech (sacrum) is in the left transverse portion of the maternal pelvis, it is designated LST.

Labor is divided into latent and active phases. The latent phase is the time between the onset of regular contractions and appreciable cervical dilation. During this phase, the cervix effaces but dilates only slightly. The active phase extends from the end of the latent phase to the end of the first stage of labor. The events of labor normally occur in an orderly sequence at accelerating rates. Variations from this pattern may indicate impending abnormalities (p. 132).

The latent phase in a primigravida lasts about 8.5 hours and ends when the cervical dilation is about 2.5 cm. The accelerated phase lasts about 2 hours and occurs while the cervix dilates from 2.5 to 4 cm. The phase of maximal slope lasts about 2 hours and occurs while the cervix is dilating from 4 to 9 cm. The phase of deceleration lasts about 2 hours and occurs during the last centimeter of dilation of the cervix. In the second stage, intrauterine pressures in excess of 100 mg Hg may result from bearing down. The total length of labor in the multigravida is normally several hours shorter than in the primigravida.

During labor, the fetal head may be in various degrees of flexion or extension (habitus or attitude). A fully flexed vertex occurs in about 95% of all deliveries. The fetal head may undergo certain changes in shape to accommodate to the configuration of the maternal pelvis. Molding is a change in shape of the fetal head in labor that is brought about by the forces of labor, the resistance of the bony pelvis, and the loose connections between the bones of the fetal skull. The head may also undergo lateral flexion (asynclitism). Synclitism exists when the fetal head presents with the sagittal suture midway between the maternal symphysis pubis and the sacral promontory. In anterior asynclitism, the sagittal suture approaches the sacral promontory and the anterior parietal bone of the fetus is the most dependent portion of the head in the birth canal. In posterior asynclitism, the sagittal suture approaches the symphysis pubis and the posterior parietal bone is most dependent.

During long labor, a caput succedaneum may be formed. In the process, the portion of the fetal scalp immediately over the cervical os becomes edematous and may prevent the differentiation of sutures and fontanelles by the examiner. Molding, asynclitism, deflexion, and caput may all lead to an erroneous diagnosis of station, since the head feels lower than it actually is.

Throughout labor, the fetal status must be monitored by the recording of heart rate by stethoscopic auscultation or electronic methods. The maternal status must be monitored by the recording of vital signs every 30 to 60 minutes, urinary output, and the quality and frequency of uterine contractions. Fetal position should be ascertained by abdominal and vaginal examination. When the fetal position or presentation is in doubt, consultation is mandatory. Failure of progress of labor for 2 hours and detection of a small pelvis or a fetal abnormality also require consultation. The method of pain control, analgesia and anesthesia, may affect the progress of labor and the status of the fetus (p. 82).

If no vaginal bleeding is detected, vaginal examination should be performed to ascertain station, cervical dilation, and effacement. The vaginal examinations must be repeated under aseptic conditions at appropriate intervals. During the first stage, the patient may have an enema, but the perineal preparation need not include shaving of pubic hair. A large-bore intravenous needle should be inserted, especially if there is increased likelihood of excessive loss of blood. The patient should take nothing by mouth after the onset of labor. The bladder should not be catheterized unless the patient cannot void or a difficult delivery or cesarean section is expected. During the second stage, as the patient begins to bear down, maternal vital signs and fetal heart rate are monitored more frequently. The multipara is often transported to the delivery room when the cervix is 7 to 8 cm dilated, and the primigravida at full dilation, depending on the rapidity of labor.

The normal mechanism of labor in a vertex involves: engagement, descent, flexion, internal rotation, extension, external rotation, and expulsion. When the fetal head has negotiated the pelvic outlet and its largest diameter is encircled by the vulvar ring, crowning is said to take place. After the head is born, the shoulders are delivered, followed more or less rapidly by the remainder of the body.

Diagnosis of presentation and position is made by abdominal palpation, vaginal examination, auscultation of the location of the fetal heart, and sonography. The breech feels softer than the head, and the back feels larger, smoother, and firmer than the small parts, which are nodular and irregular. If the cephalic prominence is felt on the same side as the small parts, the head is flexed. If the cephalic prominence is on the same side as the back, the head is extended.

The cause of the onset of labor is basically unknown, but important factors may include: release of the progesterone block of myometrial activity, changing relations of oxytocin and oxytocinase, and fetal endocrine activity. The enzymatic release of arachidonic acid, a precursor of prostaglandins, is important in the initiation of parturition. The increased synthesis of prostaglandin E_2 in the amnion may be stimulated by a substance in fetal urine. Thus, the fetus may play a major role in determining the onset of labor. Oxytocin may stimulate uterine contractions by acting both directly on the myometrium and indirectly on the production of decidual prostaglandin.

Extensive data derived from animal experimentation suggest that prostaglandins are the final links in the chain leading to the onset of uterine contractions. In sheep there is a striking increase in the production of cortisol by the fetal adrenal gland 1 to 2 days before the onset of parturition. This increase is followed by a decrease in the production of progesterone by the placenta and an increase in that of estrogen, with the result that the production of prostaglandins is enhanced significantly. In the human being, the relations among fetal cortisol, estrogen, and progesterone are not proven, although data suggest that in women also the production of prostaglandin and the ratio of estrogen to progesterone may be critical in the initiation of labor. It is known that interleukin-1β stimulates formation of prostaglandin in several tissues, including amnion, endometrium, and myometrium. It has been suggested therefore that interleukin-1β (IL-1β) is the intermediate modulator of parturition, acting to stimulate hydrolysis of glycerophospholipids, release of arachidonic acid, formation of prostaglandins, and synthesis of platelet-activating factor (PAF) by uterine and extraembryonic fetal tissues.

The principal problem in diagnosis of labor is its differentiation from false labor, which unlike true labor is unaccompanied by progressive dilation of the cervix or increasingly forceful contractions. It can be differentiated from the latent phase of labor with certainty only on retrospective evaluation. The hazards of false labor include maternal exhaustion, apprehension, and premature intervention by the obstetrician.

The typical obstetric inlet has an anteroposterior diameter of 11.5 cm and a transverse diameter of 13 cm. The plane of least pelvic dimensions in the midpelvis has an anteroposterior diameter of 12 cm and a transverse diameter of 10.5 cm. If the inlet and midpelvis are adequate, it is unlikely that the outlet will cause difficulty in delivery. The normal biparietal diameter of the term fetus is about 9.25 cm and the bitemporal about 8.0 cm. When there is difficulty in engagement in the transverse diameter, the bitemporal diameter is often substituted for the biparietal diameter and extension is the result. In normal circumstances, flexion results in making the suboccipitobregmatic (9.5 cm) rather than the occipitofrontal (11.5 cm) the engaging diameter.

The anterior fontanelle (bregma) is the diamond-shaped junction of the parietal and frontal bones. The posterior fontanelle is the triangular junction of the two parietal bones and the occipital bone (Fig. 7–1).

X-ray pelvimetry, although used frequently before the advent of obstetric sonography, has been largely replaced by a trial of labor with electronic fetal monitoring.

If the membranes rupture during the first stage of labor, the size of the uterine cavity decreases and the pressure of the head directly on the lower uterine segment may improve the efficiency of labor. Immediately after rupture of the membranes, the fetal heart should be auscultated and a vaginal examination should be done to detect pro-

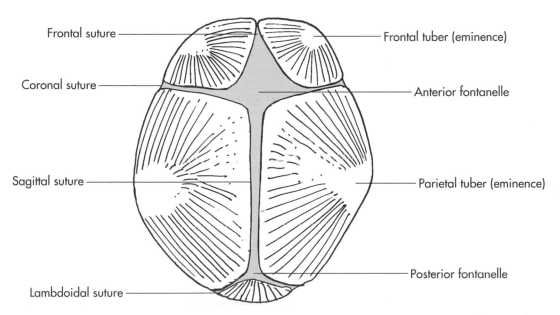

FIG. 7–1. Skull at birth, showing frontal and occipital fontanelles. The greatest width of the skull at this stage is at the level of the parietal tubers.

lapse of the umbilical cord. If the origin of the fluid is in doubt, nitrazine paper may be used to detect the alkaline pH that is characteristic of amniotic fluid but not urine. Microscopic examination may be employed to detect fetal epithelial cells, globules of fat, and hair, which are normally released into the amniotic fluid. Ferning is also characteristic of amniotic fluid but not urine. If the patient with ruptured membranes bears down (Valsalva), fluid may be seen escaping from the cervix.

Fetal monitoring during labor is greatly improved by adding electronic surveillance to clinical methods. In the first stage of labor, the fetal heart rate may drop during contractions but it rises again to between 120 and 160/min between contractions. Occasionally detection of tachycardia, bradycardia, or irregularity of the fetal heart rate by stethoscope calls attention to the need for more precise electronic monitoring. The combination of abnormalities of the fetal heart rate and passage of meconium is serious. Auscultation of the fetal heart should be even more frequent during the second stage.

Several patterns emerge when simultaneous electronic monitoring of the fetal heart rate and uterine contractions is carried out. In normal tracings, beat-to-beat variability is found. When deceleration of the fetal heart rate occurs immediately after the onset of uterine contractions, the pattern known as early deceleration results (Fig. 7–2A). This pattern should suggest compression of the fetal head and is not an ominous sign. Bradycardia occurring late after the onset of uterine contractions is called late deceleration (Fig. 7–2B). This pattern usually indicates uteroplacental insufficiency. A variable onset of deceleration with respect to the uterine contraction often indicates compression of the umbilical cord (Fig. 7–2C).

Late decelerations may be caused by placental insufficiency, maternal hypotension, or excessive uterine activity resulting from administration of oxytocin. If correction of maternal hypotension and discontinuation of the oxytocin do not correct the pattern, prompt delivery may be indicated. Variable deceleration is often corrected by repositioning of the mother and administration of oxygen. If these factors do not reverse the pattern, operative delivery may be required to avoid the hazards of prolonged compression of the cord. Analysis of the pH of blood from the fetal scalp is helpful in deciding the management. Acidosis (pH of less than 7.20) suggests a more serious degree of fetal compromise necessitating delivery (Fig. 7–3).

Whether to use electronic fetal monitoring in all labors is still controversial. The technique is indicated, however, in all high-risk pregnancies including, but not limited to: meconium-stained amnionic fluid, restriction in intrauterine growth, oligohydramnios, preterm or postterm gestation, antepartum medical complications, the use of oxytocin in labor, and abnormalities of the fetal cardiac rate identified by other methods. Inasmuch as a low-risk pregnancy may become high-risk intrapartum, electronic monitoring should always be available. If intermittent cardiac auscultation is used instead of electronic monitoring, it must be done at least every 30 minutes during the first stage of labor and at least every 15 minutes during the second stage; in both stages it should be performed for a period of 30 seconds after the uterine contraction.

Maternal assessment of fetal activity is a simple but valuable method of monitoring the fetal condition. So-called fetal kick counts are recorded by the mother as an indication of fetal activity. Several large clinical studies have demonstrated the efficacy of this method of maternal assessment in the prevention of unexplained fetal death.

The contraction stress test (CST), also known as the oxytocin challenge test (OCT), has been used extensively for antepartum fetal surveillance. The response of the fetus at risk of uteroplacental insufficiency to uterine contractions is the basis of this test, for it is known that such contractions reduce blood flow to the intervillous space. Uterine contractions may be evoked by administration of oxytocin with an infusion pump or by stimulation of the maternal nipple. If stimulation of the nipple produces sufficient uterine activity, infusion of intravenous oxytocin may be avoided. In a negative test (Fig. 7–4), no late decelerations occur with adequate contractions (three in 10 minutes, each lasting 40 to 60 seconds). The actual pressure exerted during each contraction

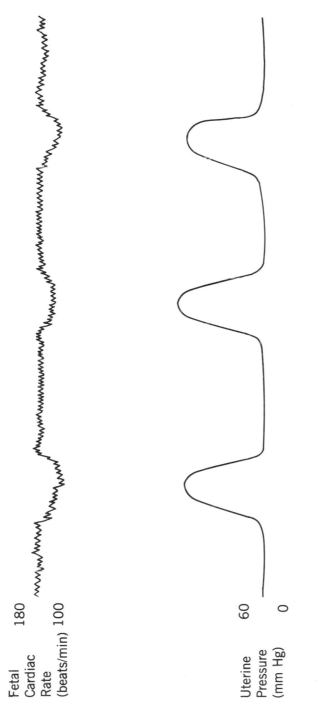

Fetal
Cardiac
Rate
(beats/min)

180

100

Uterine
Pressure
(mm Hg)

60

0

Diagrammatic Representation of
Early Deceleration (Compression of Fetal Head)

FIG. 7–2. A. Early deceleration, showing uniform pattern with onset and end of deceleration synchronous with onset and end of uterine contraction. Pattern is related to pressure on fetal head.

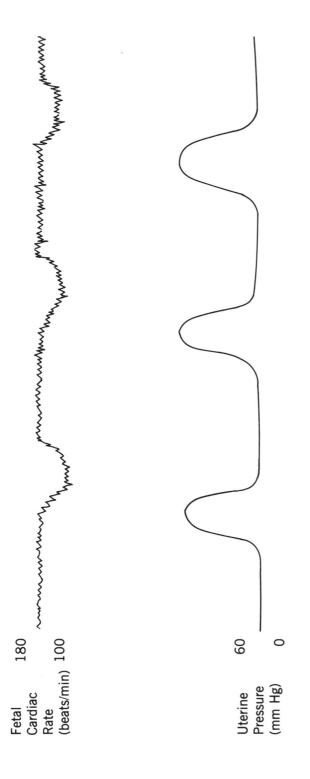

Diagrammatic Representation of
Late Deceleration (Uteroplacental Insufficiency)

FIG. 7–2. (continued) B. Late deceleration, showing uniform pattern with onset after beginning of uterine contraction and recovery after end of uterine contraction. Pattern is related to uteroplacental ischemia.

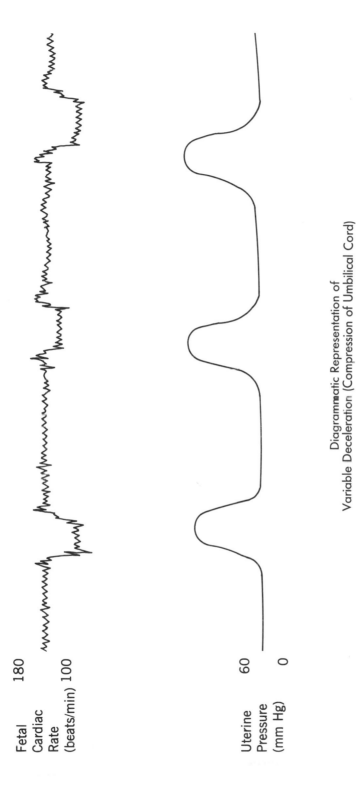

Diagrammatic Representation of
Variable Deceleration (Compression of Umbilical Cord)

FIG. 7–2. *(continued)* C. Variable deceleration, showing irregular pattern with onset and end of deceleration bearing no consistent relation to onset and end of contraction. Pattern may be related to compression of cord.

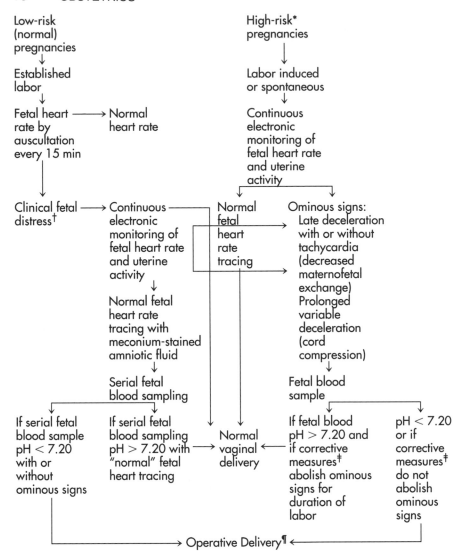

FIG. 7–3. Management of fetal distress

*For example: diabetes, chronic hypertension, preeclampsia, premature labor, and third-trimester bleeding.

†Auscultated fetal heart rate >160 or <120/min or meconium staining of amniotic fluid.

‡Change in maternal position to alleviate maternal hypotension or compression of the umbilical cord. Decrease or discontinuation of intravenous oxytocin to alleviate uterine hyperactivity.

¶Anticipate birth of depressed newborn and have available obstetric or pediatric personnel skilled in direct resuscitation.

usually is not known because an external monitor is used in the test. In a positive test (Fig. 7–5) late decelerations occur at the same level of stress and persist with the majority of contractions. Fifty percent of these tests have been shown to be falsely positive, but the rate of false negativity is much lower. The contraction stress test requires at least an hour of monitoring. Usual contraindications to the test include premature labor, ruptured membranes, prior classical cesarean section, plural gestation, and placenta previa.

The nonstress test is currently the most widely used technique of antepartum fetal evaluation. It depends on the response of the fetal cardiac rate to fetal activity, uterine contractions, or stimulation (for example,

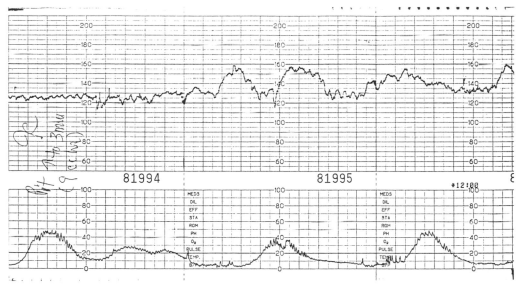

FIG. 7–4. Negative contraction stress test.

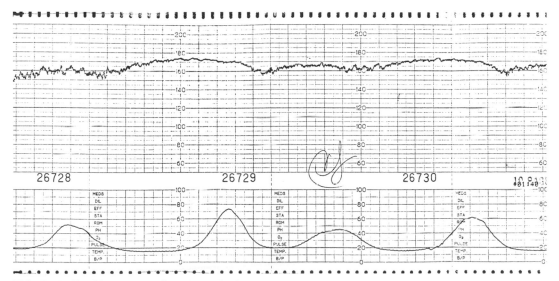

FIG. 7–5. Positive contraction stress test.

acoustic). Its advantages are capability of performance in an outpatient setting, short duration of testing, lack of necessity for drugs, and virtual absence of contraindications. The test is considered reactive when at least two accelerations of the fetal heart rate of an amplitude of 15 beats or more per minute and a duration of 15 seconds occur during 20 minutes of monitoring (Fig. 7–6). With a reactive pattern, the baseline rate is normally between 120 and 150 beats per minute and the baseline variability is 15 beats or more per minute. The test is not useful before the twenty-eighth week of gestation because the mature fetal response is not present until then.

In both stressed and nonstressed monitoring, the prediction of fetal compromise is less certain than the confirmation of fetal well-being. These tests must be used in conjunction with indices of fetal maturity and other relevant clinical data in deciding the need for delivery.

Fetal well-being may be assessed by the so-called biophysical profile, which includes the nonstress test and measurements of fetal breathing movements, gross fetal movements, fetal tone, and volume of amniotic fluid. The biophysical profile uses real-time ultrasonography to perform, in essence, a physical examination of the fetus and to evaluate the integrity of its central nervous system. Each of the five variables receives a score of 0 (abnormal) or 2 (normal). A normal fetus has, in addition to a reactive nonstress test, the following responses: at least one episode of fetal breathing of at least 30 seconds' duration within a period of 30 minutes; at least three discrete fetal movements within the 30-minute period; upper and lower extremities in full flexion, trunk in flexion and head flexed on chest, and

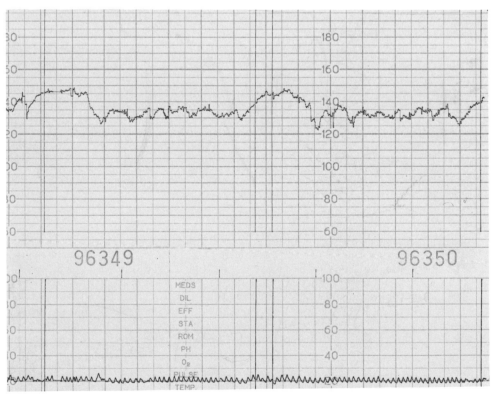

FIG. 7–6. Reactive nonstress test (NST). The dark vertical lines indicate the mother's perception of fetal movement.

extension of extremities or spine with return to flexion (good fetal tone); and qualitative assessment of the volume of amniotic fluid. Normally the fluid is present throughout the uterine cavity, with the largest pocket of fluid greater than 2 cm in two perpendicular planes. Fetuses with scores of 10 are at low risk of chronic hypoxia, whereas those with scores below 6 are at risk. The amniotic fluid index (AFI) is calculated by adding the vertical dimensions of the largest pockets of amniotic fluid after dividing the maternal abdomen into four quadrants. A normal value is between 6 and 10 cm. The pockets must be free of fetal parts or umbilical cord.

Amnioscopy is a technique for evaluation of the color and turbidity of the amniotic fluid by means of transcervical examination through an endoscope. Meconium staining is associated with a lower Apgar score and a higher perinatal mortality. It is used more often in countries other than the United States and is valuable principally in conjunction with other tests of fetal well-being.

Most fetuses engage in the occiput transverse position and deliver as occipitoanteriors. In a typical labor, the head is born by extension over the perineum, followed by restitution to the oblique and another 45° of external rotation back to the transverse position. The patient should be instructed not to bear down before the second stage.

Delivery is most safely accomplished spontaneously or by low forceps extraction. Excessive or premature administration of anesthesia results in the need for more difficult forceps deliveries.

The head should be delivered between contractions. During spontaneous delivery the obstetrician should cover the patient's anus with a towel and apply upward pressure on the chin through the perineum. The obstetrician's other hand should be used to control the egress of the head by gentle pressure on the occiput. As soon as the head is delivered, loops of cord should be removed from the infant's neck. Delivery of the shoulders should be delayed until they are in the anteroposterior diameter of the outlet. One shoulder should be delivered at a time. The rest of the body ordinarily follows with ease. In normal circumstances, the newborn should be suspended by its feet below the level of the placenta to allow transfusion of placental blood.

The third stage of labor comprises separation and expulsion of the placenta. Its successful spontaneous termination depends primarily on uterine activity. After the placenta separates, the shape of the uterus changes from discoid to globular and the top of the uterus is felt at a somewhat higher level. At the same time there is a gush of blood and a lengthening of the cord, which yields when slight traction is applied. Uterine bleeding after expulsion is controlled by occlusion of blood vessels by sustained uterine contraction.

The placenta should be routinely inspected for completeness and the birth canal should be examined for injuries. A missing placental cotyledon or a torn vessel on the chorionic surface indicates retention of a placental fragment within the uterus.

The vital signs of the mother and the uterine tone should be monitored for at least one hour post partum (the period sometimes called the fourth stage). The patient should remain in the recovery room for 2 to 3 hours before being returned to her room.

The average blood loss during normal vaginal delivery without episiotomy is at least 300 mL. The blood loss is often greater than it appears without accurate measurement. Loss of blood of 500 mL or more is considered postpartum hemorrhage.

The placenta should be delivered as soon as possible after it has separated, with care taken to remove all the membranes as well. In the presence of excessive bleeding or after 30 minutes in the third stage, it is wisest to remove the placenta manually under appropriate anesthesia. No traction should be applied to the cord until the placenta has separated. Premature or forceful traction may result in inversion of the uterus, a serious accident that may lead to shock and may require hysterectomy.

Many regimens for the administration of oxytocic agents after delivery of the fetus are employed. One satisfactory method is the addition of 10 units of oxytocin to the intravenous infusion. The oxytocin should not be given in a single intravenous push. To avoid trapping of the placenta, it is wisest to defer the administration of oxytocin until after the completion of the third stage, although some obstetricians use it at the time of delivery of the shoulders. Derivatives of ergot are used less often now immediately post partum and should be avoided in the presence of hypertension or preeclampsia.

When uterine atony is anticipated, as in cases of overdistension of the uterus (plural gestation, macrosomia, hydramnios), grand multiparity, prolonged labor, and prior infusion of magnesium sulfate or oxytocin, it is best to keep the oxytocin infusion running for several hours after the third stage.

OBSTETRIC ANESTHESIA

The problems of obstetric anesthesia differ from those of anesthesia in general because of the altered maternal physiologic functions in pregnancy, the presence of the fetus (which is particularly sensitive to anesthetic agents), alterations in maternal homeostasis resulting from anesthesia, and often the emergency during which obstetric anesthesia must be administered. In particular, the changes in maternal respiratory and cardiovascular function tend to enhance the speed of induction of inhalation anesthesia because of a decrease in functional residual capacity and an increase in sensitivity to inhalation agents. The diminished volumes of spinal canal and epidural spaces necessitate smaller amounts of local anesthetic agents to achieve a similar level of anesthesia; furthermore, there is the effect of the diminished venous return, which results from the compression of the inferior vena cava by the gravid uterus (supine hypotensive syndrome). The drop in peripheral resistance and the venous dilation secondary to sympathetic blockade resulting from major regional anesthesia, in combination with compression of the inferior vena cava, may cause life-threatening hypotension. Finally, all general and local anesthetic agents, barbiturates, tranquilizers, and narcotics cross the placenta. Most relaxants of skeletal muscle (curare, pancuronium, and succinylcholine), however, cross the placenta poorly or not at all because they are highly charged. Analgesia may be achieved during labor and delivery by means of narcotics and other types of analgesic agents, regional blocks, or general anesthetics.

General anesthesia must be avoided when the patient's stomach is full, unless intubation can be carried out promptly. Analgesia (such as 100 mg of meperidine) should be withheld until labor is clearly established, and regional blocks should not be performed until the cervix is at least 4 to 5 cm dilated. The choice of anesthetic agent depends on the availability of the technique and the skills of the personnel. It should be tailored to the type of delivery and the desires of the patient whenever possible. For example, a low forceps or a normal spontaneous delivery of a multipara can often be effected by analgesia and a pudendal block. A forceps delivery of a primigravida, however, may often be managed best by lumbar epidural, caudal, or low subarachnoid (saddle) block. Deliveries that require extensive intrauterine manipulations should be conducted with maximal uterine relaxation, such as is provided by halothane.

Analgesia during labor is most often accomplished by means of narcotic agents. These drugs rapidly cross the placental barrier and may depress the fetus' respiratory center. The intravenous and intramuscular routes of administration are both acceptable. Narcotics are often used in combination with tranquilizers because of a possible synergistic effect. Barbiturates are not analgesic but reduce anxiety. Tranquilizers alone are often helpful early in the first stage of labor when anxiety rather than pain is the principal problem. Use of these drugs, particularly diazepam may, however, result in depressed newborns. Scopolamine in large doses and in combination with narcotics causes amnesia, but also excitation, which may be difficult to control. Inhalation anesthetic agents such as nitrous oxide and methoxyflurane may be used in subanesthetic concentrations to obtund painful sensations during labor and delivery. Inhalation analgesia may be used in conjunction with narcotics. The patient must be carefully watched and protected from unnecessarily deep anesthetic levels. The major inhalation agent used in the United States today for analgesia is 50% nitrous oxide and oxygen delivered on demand.

Anesthesia remains a major cause of maternal mortality in the United States (p. 149), where general anesthesia is still widely used to achieve relief of pain during delivery. General anesthesia, however, is responsible for most of the deaths attributable to anesthesia; 50% are attributed to aspiration of gastric contents. This form of anesthesia must be approached with the greatest care if the patient has eaten within 6 hours of the onset of labor. Even if 6 hours have elapsed, however, the stomach is not necessarily empty. All patients in labor must therefore be considered to have full stomachs. Aspiration of gastric contents is often fatal. General anesthesia should not be used except in unusual circumstances for control of pain in vaginal delivery. Of all maternal deaths related to anesthesia, half are associated with failed intubation and aspiration under general anesthesia. The risk of failed intubation is greater in pregnant than in nonpregnant patients.

All inhalation agents, with the exception of nitrous oxide, depress the myometrium and can abolish uterine contractions. Halothane is a popular halogenated agent that is highly effective for inducing uterine relaxation. Equivalent doses of enflurane and isoflurane produce the same degree of uterine relaxation.

The purpose of regional anesthesia is to block sensations arising from the cervix, uterus, and perineum. The pain pathways during the first stage of labor involve visceral afferent nerve fibers that arise from the uterus and cervix and enter the spinal cord at T 10 to L-1. The pains of the second stage of labor arise from somatic afferent receptors and fibers in the vulva and perineum and travel by way of the inferior hemorrhoidal nerve, the labial nerve, and the dorsal nerve of the clitoris (which join to form the pudendal nerves) and enter the spinal cord at S-2 to S-4. The sacral nerves are larger and therefore more difficult to block.

Paracervical blocks administered in the vaginal fornices block pain impulses at the level of the uterine plexus. Lumbar epidural and caudal blocks interrupt pain sensations in the epidural space before the nerve's entrance into the spinal canal. Subarachnoid anesthesia blocks the nerves in the spinal canal where they bathe directly in the cerebrospinal fluid. Pudendal blocks interrupt only pain sensations arising from the perineum and vulva and are useful only in the second stage of labor. Paracervical anesthesia does not block the sacral segments and therefore does not relieve pain arising from the perineum. Spinal, lumbar epidural, and caudal blocks may be used to interrupt painful sensations from the uterus, cervix, and perineum. Because paracervical anesthesia is frequently associated with fetal bradycardia, it is not popular in modern obstetrics. The bradycardia results from vasoconstriction of the uterine artery or high uptake of anesthetic agent by the fetus because of increased absorption by the uterine artery. Paracervical and pudendal blocks are peripheral nerve blocks, which affect only the specific nerves in the immediate area. Epidural, caudal, and spinal blocks are central and less specific, blocking more than the local nerves.

Toxic reactions to local anesthetics are most often related to overdosage. This result can occur after careless use of any of the aforementioned techniques, although least frequently with spinal anesthesia. Toxic reactions in obstetric anesthesia are most frequently the result of intravascular injection of a dose intended for epidural administration. Toxicity may result also from rapid absorption of a proper dose or administration of an excessive dose of medication. Toxic effects include stimulation of the central nervous system (confusion, vertigo, tinnitus, twitching, or convulsions), cardiovascular collapse, or both. Allergic reactions are uncommon. Treatment is as follows: maintenance of the airway, oxygen, intravenous anticonvulsants such as diazepam to counter stimulation of the central nervous system, intravenous fluids, and cardiac massage or defibrillation for cardiovascular collapse. Hypotension can occur after any major block that results in sympathetic blockade. Therapeutic measures must be taken immediately if hypotension develops. The steps include lifting the uterus off the inferior vena cava or placing the patient on her left side; rapidly hydrating the patient with 1 liter of a balanced salt solution; and administering vasopressors intravenously if the prior measures do not return the pressure to normal levels. Since the drop in blood pressure must be quickly noted and treated, major regional blocks must be preceded by: the application of a blood pressure cuff that is to be left in place, constant monitoring of vital signs, and the establishment of a dependable means of intravenous medication (intravenous cannulas or catheters).

Less local anesthetic is required to achieve a given level of anesthesia in late pregnancy than in the nonpregnant state. Hypotension resulting from regional blocks must be treated to maintain a maternal systolic pressure of at least 100 mm Hg if the pregnant patient was normotensive before the anesthesia. If the patient was hypertensive, the blood pressure should be maintained not lower than 20% below baseline. Lower pressures may impair perfusion of the intervillous space and result in fetal hypoxia, hypercarbia, and acidosis.

Complications resulting from major regional blocks such as spinals and epidurals include overdosage or inadvertent intravenous injection, with respiratory depression or arrest and convulsions; chemical and septic meningitis; constrictive arachnoiditis; and postpuncture headaches. The complications are generally preventable. The most common complication is inadvertent puncture of the dura during placement of an epidural catheter, with resulting high spinal anesthesia.

Anesthetic techniques suitable for labor and vaginal delivery differ from those for cesarean section. Techniques for the laboring parturient include nonpharmacologic methods (e.g., Lamaze), intravenous medications such as Demerol and Vistaril, infiltration of peripheral nerves, (pudendal and paracervical), central blocks (epidural, caudal, and spinal), and inhalation analgesia (50% nitrous oxide in oxygen). For cesarean section, however, the two appropriate techniques are regional (spinal or epidural) and general anesthesia with intubation.

Regional anesthesia is preferred over other forms of anesthesia because the complications arising from these methods are preventable or treatable. Regional anesthesia generally avoids the major risks of failed intubation and aspiration by the mother. Spinal, caudal, and lumbar epidural anesthesia are contraindicated, however, if: the patient is hypovolemic or suffers from a complication that is accompanied by blood loss; the patient is hypotensive; the skin is infected at the site of puncture; there is an active neurologic disorder; the patient is receiving anticoagulants; the patient refuses the procedure; and the physician lacks the experience or adequate equipment for administration, monitoring, and resuscitation.

The need for highly skilled physicians to administer major regional blocks or general anesthesia has not been met. The safest, easiest way of achieving pain relief during parturition thus appears to be the careful administration of small doses of narcotics and tranquilizers during labor, followed by a pudendal block and subanesthetic concentrations of general anesthetic agents for delivery.

General anesthetic agents in obstetrics may be employed for three purposes: in subanesthetic concentrations for analgesia; general anesthesia of a degree sufficient for delivery or cesarean section; and as myometrial relaxants for intrauterine manipulations such as breech extraction or version and extraction, replacement of an inverted uterus, relaxation of tetanic contractions, and removal of a retained placenta. A well performed regional block may be used for many of these purposes as well. Because of the danger of aspiration of gastric contents, endotracheal intubation is always indicated when general anesthesia is administered. Endotracheal intubation can be performed with the patient awake after topical anesthesia of the pharynx or with the patient asleep after the rapid administration of a fast-acting barbiturate, followed immediately by a muscle relaxant. Cricoid pressure should be maintained to compress the esophagus and prevent regurgitation. Pressure should be maintained until the endotracheal tube cuff has been inflated and the airway protected. When a patient is at high risk for aspiration, the larynx is not anesthetized because even when awake, the patient may aspirate. Intubation of the patient while she is awake is usually performed only when difficulty with the airway is anticipated.

Aspiration of gastric contents can cause death by two different mechanisms. First, obstruction of the airway renders the capillary-alveolar gas exchange impossible. Second, if the pH of the gastric juice is below 2.5, contact with the respiratory tree often results in bronchospasm, pulmonary edema, and death. If the patient survives the immediate injury, severe atelectasis and chemical pneumonitis may ensue. The treatment consists in quickly clearing the airway by suction, administering 100% oxygen by means of an endotracheal tube, treating the bronchospasm with bronchodilators, and early use of mechanical ventilation with positive end expiratory pressure (PEEP).

Ordinarily, chemical pneumonitis requires aspiration of at least 25 mL of fluid with a pH below 2.5. If fluid is aspirated it reaches the periphery of the lung within 15 to 18 seconds. Lavage with bicarbonate may worsen the damage. Steroids have not proved useful and broad-spectrum antibiotics are no longer recommended because of the risk of superinfection. When fever and leukocytosis suggest infection, the offending organism should be identified and treated according to sensitivity. The only intervention that seems to improve outcome is PEEP, to increase functional residual capacity and prevent closure of the airway. In the event of major aspiration, bronchoscopy should be employed (to remove any solid objects that may be obstructing the airway) followed by PEEP.

The first and most important factor in the prevention of aspiration pneumonitis is the awareness that every parturient is at high risk. It has been recommended that patients receive nonparticulate oral antacids throughout labor. Although these drugs do not protect against aspiration of solid material, they probably lower the risk of damage to the lung by acidic fluids.

The use of vasopressors for the treatment of hypotension secondary to major regional blocks is based on their ability to increase venous return by activating adrenergic receptors and therefore causing a rise in peripheral resistance and venous constriction. Furthermore, they can increase venous return by activating β-adrenergic receptors and cause an increase in cardiac inotropism and chronotropism. Some vasopressors do both. In obstetrics the use of α-adrenergic stimulants such as methoxamine or phenylephrine is contraindicated because the rise in maternal blood pressure is accompanied by uterine arterial vasoconstriction, diminished perfusion of the intervillous space, and resulting aggravation of fetal distress. Agents that have mainly β-adrenergic receptor-activating effects are preferred. The principal agent is ephedrine. In preeclampsia-eclampsia, vasopressors must be used in smaller doses because of the increased adrenergic receptor sensitivity. Derivatives of ergot must not be used before or after the administration of vasopressors. There is a synergistic effect of these two types of medications that may lead to lethal hypertension.

The rate at which an inhalation agent will affect a fetus is difficult to predict because it is dependent upon many variables involving the mother, placenta, and fetus. An intravenous anesthetic agent such as thiopental,

however, rapidly reaches the fetus. Thiopental has a low molecular weight and is nonionized to a high degree at a physiologic pH. Transfer across the placenta therefore depends primarily on the maternofetal concentration gradient, in accordance with the Fick equation for diffusible substances. After an injection of thiopental, equilibrium between mother and fetus is reached in less than two minutes. Thereafter the fetus continues to accumulate thiopental. As the concentration of thiopental in the mother diminishes, however, as a result of redistribution to various spaces, so does that in the fetus. The concentration in the umbilical vein is always higher than in the umbilical artery. It is therefore impossible to deliver the baby before equilibrium is reached. The anesthesiologist should not hurry the obstetrician, but the obstetrician should work with careful speed. Despite the rapid placental transfer of thiopental, this agent in conjunction with nitrous oxide, oxygen, and succinylcholine is preferred when general anesthesia is chosen.

When spinal anesthesia is to be administered, it is important to be proficient in the use of 25-gauge or 26-gauge spinal needles. The incidence of postpuncture headaches is related directly to the size of the rent made in the dura in the course of the administration of a spinal block. Special needles with a pencil tip and a hole on the side have been used successfully to reduce the occurrence of spinal headache. These needles separate the dura rather than cut the fibers. During administration of an epidural block, a small test dose must be given to ascertain whether the subarachnoid space has been entered inadvertently. The accidental subarachnoid injection of the usual doses of local anesthetics used for epidural anesthesia may result in a very high or total spinal block, which may cause respiratory arrest. Resuscitation equipment and drugs must be on hand at all times.

Popular local anesthetics for use in obstetrics comprise two classes of chemicals: esters and amides. All local anesthetics have an aromatic ring and a carbon chain with an amino group. The ester anesthetics link the two moieties with a $-COO$ group, whereas the amides are linked with a $-NHCO$ group. Currently used local anesthetics include esters (2-chloroprocaine and tetracaine) and amides (lidocaine and bupivacaine).

TABLE 7–1. LOCAL ANESTHETICS USED COMMONLY IN OBSTETRICS

	Onset of Action	Duration	Biologic Half-Life	Maximal Dose
2-Chloroprocaine	Fast	Short (30–60 min)	30–60 min	20–22 mg/kg
Lidocaine	Intermediate	Intermediate (60–120 min)	1–2 hr	4 mg/kg
Bupivacaine	Slow	Long (120–300 min)	3 hr	1.5–2.5 mg/kg

Prilocaine is not used much in the United States for obstetric anesthesia. Use of tetracaine is restricted primarily to spinal anesthesia because of its high potential for toxicity. The small doses used for spinal anesthesia eliminate that problem. Lidocaine has been in use for a long time and is probably the safest member of its chemical group. Contrary to earlier reports, it does not appear to have an adverse effect on neurobehavioral scores of the newborns. Bupivacaine is the drug of choice for laboring patients because of its differential blocking capabilities, with sensory block much greater than motor. The 0.075% dosage is not to be used in pregnant women because this high concentration has been associated with several deaths as a result of cardiotoxicity from inadvertent intravenous injections. Pregnant women appear to be more sensitive to this amide than are nonpregnant patients. A drug soon to be released, ropivacaine, has a structure and a mode of action similar to those of bupivacaine. It is said to have less cardiotoxicity than has bupivacaine.

Chloroprocaine, an ester, is an excellent drug with a rapid onset of action, but it has been implicated in cases of neurotoxicity when inadvertently injected into the subarachnoid space. The problem may have been related to the low pH and the bisulfite that was used as a preservative. The new formulations of this drug do not contain bisulfite.

Esters are degraded by plasma cholinesterases. The byproduct of their metabolism is para-aminobenzoic acid (PABA), the substance used in sunscreens. Because some patients have allergic reactions to PABA, the use of these esters is contraindicated in them. The half-life of the ester chloroprocaine is very short. Amides are broken down in the liver and have a longer half-life of about 2 to 3 hours. Local anesthetics are weak bases. The more acidic the environment, the more highly ionized the local anesthetic becomes. For transfer across the placenta to the fetus, the local anesthetic must be nonionized. If the mother's acid-base balance is normal but the fetus is distressed and acidotic, the local anesthetics cross the placenta, are ionized in the acidic medium of the fetus, and create a "sink" because there is no concentration gradient for equilibrium of the nonionized form. This phenomenon is called "ion trapping." To prevent toxic accumulation of local anesthetics in a distressed acidotic fetus, amide local anesthetics should be avoided and an ester such as 2-chloroprocaine should be used. The ester is hydrolyzed rapidly in the mother's blood and accumulation by the distressed fetus is thus prevented. Table 7–1 compares three local anesthetics that are in common use.

8
CHAPTER
CARE OF THE NEWBORN

IMMEDIATE CARE OF THE NEONATE

As soon as the head is delivered, the infant's nose and throat should be aspirated with a bulb syringe to clear the airway. Particularly when the fetus has been stressed, it is necessary to take these measures to prevent aspiration of amnionic fluid (Fig. 8–1). After delivery, the infant should be held with the head dependent above the obstetrician's lap but below the level of the mother's perineum to facilitate transfusion of placental blood. The cord of a normal infant, who is not likely to require exchange transfusion, should be allowed to stop pulsating before it is clamped. Double clamping is best performed about 4 cm from the umbilicus. The infant should be kept warm and dry before transfer to the nursery. Handling of the newborn, particularly if premature, should be minimized. The newborn's eyes should be treated with erythromycin ointment or silver nitrate (1% solution) to prevent ophthalmia. Penicillin and tetracycline have also been used widely.

The Apgar score should be recorded at 1 minute and 5 minutes after birth to permit objective transfer of information among obstetrician, anesthesiologist, and pediatrician (Table 8–1). Apgar scores of 0 to 3 denote a severely depressed infant; scores of 4 to 6 suggest a fair general condition; and scores of 7 or above indicate a good condition. All newborns with scores of 0 to 3 and many with scores of 4 to 6 need resuscitation.

The newborn's footprints should be obtained and identification bracelets applied as soon after delivery as possible.

The pediatrician should be forewarned of any complications during pregnancy, labor, or delivery and informed about any drugs that the mother may have taken. If the baby is jaundiced soon after birth, it may require an exchange transfusion. In such a case, the umbilical cord should be left long and a pediatric consultation obtained immediately.

The placenta should be examined carefully to see whether it is intact and to detect gross lesions. A cross section of the cord should be inspected to detect the absence of one umbilical artery, an anomaly that is found in 1% of infants and may be associated with other congenital malformations. Placentas that are grossly abnormal and those associated with an actual or potentially poor perinatal outcome should be examined microscopically as well.

RESUSCITATION

The delivery room must have immediately available at all times equipment for resuscitation, including endotracheal tubes and

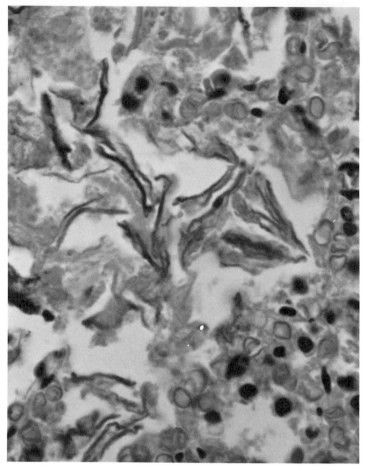

FIG. 8-1. Newborn lung with aspirated amniotic fluid containing numerous squamous cells seen on end.

laryngoscopes, umbilical vein catheters, oxygen, and suction devices.

A newborn may be incapable of maintaining normal respiration for several reasons including: intrauterine depression or inadequate placental exchange, prematurity, congenital anomalies, drugs administered to the mother, trauma during labor or delivery, and anemia secondary to blood group incompatibility.

TABLE 8-1. APGAR SCORE

Sign	0	1	2
Cardiac rate	Absent	Slow (Below 100)	Over 100
Respiratory effort	Absent	Weak cry; hypoventilation	Good effort; strong cry
Muscular tone	Limp	Some flexion of extremities	Active motion; extremities well flexed
Reflex irritability (Response to stimulation) of skin of feet	No response	Some motion (Grimace)	Crying and active
Color	Blue, pale	Body pink; extremities blue	Completely pink

Intrauterine hypoxia may result from maternal disorders such as diabetes, hypertension, hypotension, preeclampsia, and renal disease. Additional factors include premature separation of the placenta, compression of the umbilical cord, and tetanic uterine contractions. Prematurity is associated with incomplete development of the lung and inadequate production of surfactant, leading to alveolar instability and predisposition to respiratory distress syndrome. Narcotics, barbiturates, and all anesthetic agents administered to the mother may depress the fetal central nervous and cardiovascular systems.

The medical team responsible for neonatal resuscitation should include at least two persons, one to manage the airway and the other to monitor the cardiac rate. The equipment required for resuscitation should be checked regularly and kept in a state of continual readiness. The initial steps in resuscitation of the newborn include drying him and keeping him warm, preferably under a source of radiant heat. Next the nose and oropharynx should be suctioned. At this point, the infant's condition should be assessed and recorded, as with the Apgar score. The most important criteria of neonatal status are the respiratory effort and the cardiac rate. Once the infant begins to breathe on his own, attention is turned to the cardiac rate. Stimulation should be provided by rubbing the baby's back with a dry towel and blowing oxygen on him. Once a normal cardiac rate is achieved, attention is turned to his color. If the cardiac rate is below 60 beats per minute, the medical attendant should begin immediate ventilation with a bag and a soft mask that fits snugly around the infant's nose and mouth. Response to ventilation is indicated by improvement in cardiac rate and color. Most neonates can be resuscitated efficiently with a bag and mask, but if there is no response, intubation should be accomplished without delay. Cardiac massage and drugs are needed only infrequently, but if appropriate ventilation does not produce the desired response, the next steps are cardiac massage and epinephrine. Placement of an umbilical catheter provides a route for administration of other drugs and volume expanders. The sequelae of inadequately resuscitated newborns may be cerebral edema, hemorrhage, seizures, cardiogenic shock, persistent fetal circulation, acute tubular necrosis, hepatic failure, necrotizing enterocolitis, and hypoglycemia.

CIRCUMCISION

Circumcision is performed in a sizable majority of newborn males in the United States. Although in 1971 the American Academy of Pediatrics stated that there were no strictly medical indications for routine neonatal circumcision, cultural and personal preferences have maintained the popularity of the procedure in the United States. Among the stated advantages are prevention of penile carcinoma and facilitation of penile hygiene. Alleged additional benefits include prevention of phimosis and paraphimosis and the avoidance of pain, risks, costs, and psychologic effects of late circumcision. New studies supporting the medical benefits of neonatal circumcision appeared between 1990 and 1992. They include a significant decrease in infections of the urinary tract in circumcised as compared with uncircumcised children and young men and conclude that a risk:benefit analysis justifies the procedure. Studies linking circumcision to a decrease in sexually transmitted diseases including chancroid, syphilis, human papillomavirus, herpes simplex type 2, and the human immunodeficiency virus are highly suggestive but inconclusive. Furthermore, an increased incidence of cervical cancer has been found in the sexual partners of uncircumcised men infected with the human papillomavirus. Good technique and instruments minimize the risks, which, although uncommon (0.2 to 0.6%), include hemorrhage and infection. The procedure should be deferred in premature or sick infants and those with a bleeding tendency or a penile anomaly such as hypospadias. The operation should not be performed immediately after delivery but at least 24 hours later, or until the infant has been observed to remain well. The American College of Obstetricians and Gynecologists refers to the decision about neonatal circumcision as a "personal choice." Because it is usually an elective procedure, an informed written consent must be obtained.

9
CHAPTER
POSTPARTUM CARE

PUERPERIUM

The puerperium is the period of time, usually about 6 weeks, from delivery until the genital tract returns to the normal nonpregnant condition. After an uncomplicated spontaneous delivery, the multiparous patient may often be discharged as early as 24 hours postpartum. Primigravidas and many patients with episiotomies are more likely to remain in the hospital somewhat longer post partum. In all cases, the patient should be allowed to ambulate and to use the bathroom as soon after delivery as she can comfortably do so. She should be encouraged to empty her bladder at least every 8 hours to avoid overdistention, which may predispose to infection. A mild cathartic may be prescribed after 48 hours if the patient has not moved her bowels. Codeine (0.06 g) and aspirin (0.6 g) may be prescribed for afterpains. These pains are more common in the multipara but usually subside by 48 hours post partum. The perineum should be kept clean during the puerperium. Painful episiotomy sites or lacerations may be treated symptomatically with sitz baths and a heat lamp. If the lochia (vaginal discharge during the puerperium) are particularly bloody, methergine (methylergonovine maleate) may be prescribed in 6 doses of 0.2 mg at 4-hour intervals.

Postpartum chills are common but not necessarily indicative of infection. The temperature should be recorded every 6 hours for the first 24 hours at least. A slight elevation (rarely over 100.4° F, or 38° C) is common after a difficult labor or delivery, but it usually falls to normal within 24 hours. A sustained elevation or a rising temperature suggests infection (p. 147).

In certain situations in which Rh-isoimmunization is thought to have been initiated, anti-D globulin (RhoGAM) should be given shortly after delivery (p. 126). Since the patient may ovulate very soon after delivery, contraceptive advice should be given while she is still in the hospital and repeated at the time of the postpartum checkup. Coitus is best avoided until all discomfort has subsided and all wounds have healed.

The postpartum examination usually takes place between 4 and 6 weeks after delivery. At that time, the physical examination should include measurement of the blood pressure and hematocrit; examination of the breasts, abdomen, and pelvis; and a Papanicolaou smear if it has not been done in the preceding 6 months.

LACTATION

Colostrum is secreted for about 2 days after delivery, at which time lactation begins. The mammary ducts usually fill with milk between the second and fifth days post partum

(Fig. 9–1). Suckling and the administration of oxytocin stimulate the let-down of milk. The milk attains a stable composition after the first month. If the mother does not intend to breast-feed the baby, lactation may be suppressed by drugs early in the puerperium. Bromocriptine has been effective in suppressing lactation but it requires prolonged use and is expensive. Steroidal estrogens and testosterone are not recommended because of their possible relation to thromboembolism. When no drugs are used, painful engorgement of the breasts normally disappears within 36 to 48 hours. Symptomatic relief of engorgement is pro-vided by supportive binders, ice bags, fluids by mouth, and analgesics. The obstetrician must be aware that many drugs administered to the nursing mother may be transferred to the newborn in the milk.

Prolactin (LTH, lactogenic hormone, mammotropic hormone) is required for lactogenesis (initiation of the secretion of milk) and galactopoiesis (continuation of secretion of milk). The hormone also serves to maintain the cholesterol precursors in the ovary for the secretion of steroids.

Prolactin is a polypeptide similar in structure to growth hormone. It is secreted by acidophils of the hypophysis. Its release is

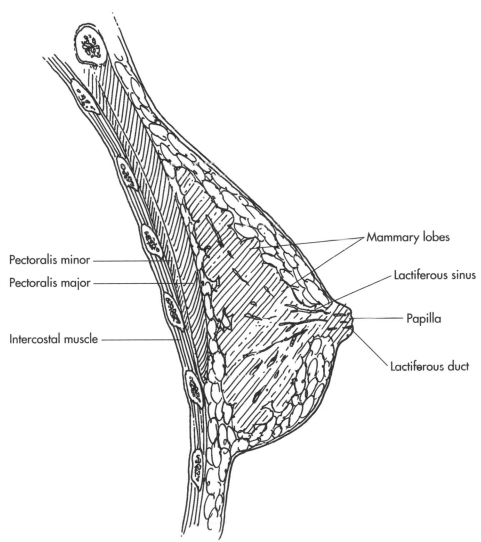

FIG. 9–1. Sagittal section through lactating mammary gland. (Eycleshymer and Jones.)

Pectoralis minor

Pectoralis major

Intercostal muscle

Mammary lobes

Lactiferous sinus

Papilla

Lactiferous duct

promoted by thyrotropin-releasing hormone (TRH) and inhibited by a prolactin-inhibiting factor (PIF) of the hypothalamus, which may be simply dopamine. The prolactin-inhibiting factor and GnRH are generally released and repressed together. Thus, when LH and FSH are secreted, prolactin is inhibited. An exception occurs during the midcycle gonadotropic surge, when there is also marked release of prolactin, presumably an action of TRH. During lactation and occasionally in women receiving phenothiazine tranquilizers, both PIF and GnRH are repressed, with resulting anovulation. Lactation may be induced via the central nervous system from stimulation of the breast or psychologic factors associated with nursing.

RETURN TO NORMAL

By the tenth postpartum day, the uterus has descended into the pelvis, that is, has regressed to the size of a 3 months' gestation. During the puerperium, the weight of the uterus decreases from 1000 to 100 g. In this process, known as involution, individual myometrial cells decrease in size. The endometrial lining is usually restored after several weeks as the placental site regresses. Involution of the placental site is normally complete by 6 weeks postpartum. Interference with this process may result in late postpartum hemorrhage (p. 148). The lochia gradually change from red (lochia rubra) to pinkish or yellowish (lochia serosa) to whitish (lochia alba) as the proportions of erythrocytes, leukocytes, and decidual debris change. Lochial discharge normally continues for 4 to 8 weeks postpartum.

The first normal menstrual period usually occurs between 4 and 8 weeks postpartum and is often heavy. Although the first ovulation usually occurs about 4 to 6 weeks postpartum, the patient may ovulate as early as the second or third day postpartum. Lactation may delay or suppress menstruation, but does not in itself provide sufficient contraception.

During the puerperium, a diuresis resulting in a loss of about 5 pounds takes place between the second and fifth postpartum days. The loss of fluid may be even greater in preeclampsia (p. 120).

Leukocytosis immediately after labor may rise to as high as 30,000. The hemoglobin and hematocrit may vary somewhat during the postpartum period, but normally do not fall below the values before delivery unless the blood loss has been considerable. At 1 week postpartum, the blood volume is normally back to the level before pregnancy.

ABNORMAL OBSTETRICS

10
CHAPTER
ECTOPIC PREGNANCY

Pregnancy in any location other than the body of the uterus is considered ectopic. The vast majority of ectopic pregnancies occur in the oviduct (Fig. 10–1). The diagnosis must be considered in any patient of reproductive age with menstrual irregularity, vaginal spotting, or abdominal pain. Diagnosis of ectopic pregnancy, ruptured or unruptured, is made by the finding of elevated concentrations of β-hCG in the serum (generally greater than 6,500 miu/mL) and the absence of an intrauterine gestational sac on sonographic examination (86% positive predictive value). The finding of a gestational sac in an extrauterine location is also indicative of ectopic pregnancy, but most often it is not recognized by ultrasound. If the β-hCG concentrations are lower than 6500 miu/mL, the measurement should be repeated in approximately 2 days. The levels of β-hCG in the serum should exceed 6500 miu/mL and a gestational sac should be visible by 6 weeks if the pregnancy is intrauterine and viable. At about 6 weeks' gestation, pregnancies showing an increase in serum hCG of less than 66% in 48 hours are likely to be ectopic, or intrauterine gestations with a high probability of subsequent abortion. With transvaginal ultrasound a gestational sac should be visible within the uterus with levels of hCG as low as 1500 to 2500 miu/mL.

Ectopic pregnancies have been increasing at a steady rate in the United States during the last decade and now account for about 2% of all pregnancies. About 5% of maternal mortality in the first trimester of gestation may be related to ectopic pregnancy, and this serious complication accounts for 6 to 10% of maternal mortality in general.

Ectopic pregnancy may be caused by any factor that retards the passage of the fertilized egg (zygote) from ovary to endometrium, for example, prior salpingitis or prior tubal surgical procedures, such as elective tubal sterilization and attempts at surgical reversal. About 7.5% of ectopic pregnancies occur after tubal sterilization, and of all pregnancies occurring after failed tubal sterilization, about 75% are ectopic. The most common antecedent factor in ectopic pregnancy remains prior salpingitis.

Rupture, which usually occurs at about 8 to 10 weeks' gestation, may be heralded by severe abdominal pain, clinical tenderness, syncope, a drop in hematocrit, and shock. Hemoperitoneum often causes pain referred to the shoulder and is frequently diagnosed by culdocentesis, although false-negative and false-positive taps may occur. Ultrasound is usually effective in identifying hemoperitoneum, but laparoscopy may be required for this purpose.

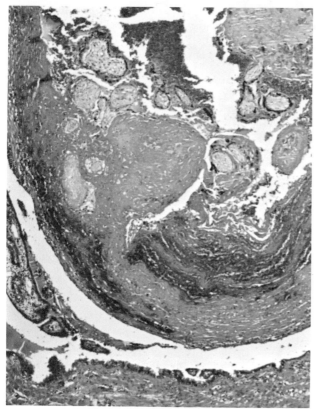

FIG. 10–1. Ectopic pregnancy, showing chorionic villi involving wall of oviduct.

DIFFERENTIAL DIAGNOSIS

The differential diagnosis, which is that of the acute abdomen in a woman of reproductive years, includes appendicitis, pelvic inflammatory disease, rupture of a follicle or corpus luteum cyst, and even threatened abortion. The primary treatment is surgical, with replacement of fluids and blood as soon as possible. If the patient desires future pregnancy, the tube is not severely damaged, and bleeding can be controlled, simple removal of the products of conception through a linear salpingotomy may be performed. In other situations, partial or total salpingectomy may be the preferred procedure.

PATHOLOGY

Tubal gestation appears to have tripled in frequency in the last 15 years, now occurring at the rate of about 20 per 1000 reported pregnancies. Any factor that inter-feres with the function of the fimbriae or causes strictures or adhesions of the tubal wall may predispose to ectopic pregnancy. The intrauterine device and surgical procedures on the oviduct have been important factors, but prior tubal infection remains the most common cause. The uterus usually grows at a normal rate for about 6 to 8 weeks and a decidual reaction (without trophoblastic tissue) is commonly found in the endometrium. The Arias-Stella reaction, which comprises endometrial epithelial atypia and vacuolated cytoplasm, is not pathognomonic of oviductal pregnancy but may be found whenever there is functioning trophoblastic tissue anywhere in the body (Fig. 10–2).

CLINICAL COURSE

The termination of the gestation depends largely on the location. Pregnancies in the ampulla (78%), particularly the distal portion, frequently abort with minimal signs.

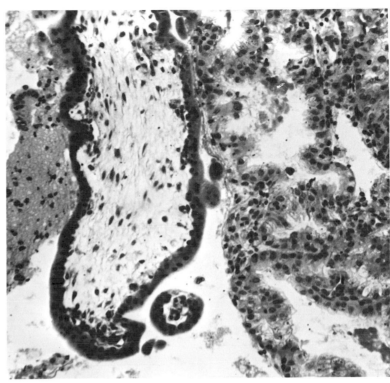

FIG. 10–2. Tissue obtained by curettage from first-trimester pregnancy, showing early villus and Arias-Stella reaction in the adjacent endometrial epithelium.

Pregnancies in the isthmus (12%) usually rupture into the peritoneal cavity or between the leaves of the broad ligament. Rupture of a pregnancy in the interstitial portion of the tube (2%) may be followed rapidly by massive hemoperitoneum and severe shock. Such patients may die before reaching the hospital. Rupture is sometimes precipitated by a Valsalva maneuver, as with straining at stool.

The clinical picture of ectopic pregnancy usually includes a normal temperature and a normal or only moderately elevated white count. The classic triad of amenorrhea, vaginal bleeding, and pain occurs in only 25% of cases. An adnexal mass may be present or absent. None of the individual signs occurs in more than 75% of cases and the accuracy of purely clinical diagnosis does not exceed 80%.

TREATMENT

Conservative (laparotomy or laparoscopy) surgical treatment (expression of the pregnancy from the tube or removal of the products of conception through a linear salpingotomy) should be attempted in a woman who wishes to retain her potential for childbearing. Control of bleeding can often be achieved with pressure, cautery, or fine suture. If hemostasis is not complete, a partial salpingectomy must be performed. Total salpingectomy is performed only when the tube is severely damaged or the patient has no desire for further fertility. Linear salpingotomy is followed by a subsequent rate of intrauterine pregnancy of 76%, as opposed to 44% after unilateral salpingectomy. Oophorectomy should not be performed if the ovary is normal. Hysterectomy is indicated only for cornual pregnancy with severe damage to the uterus. If the uterus is not badly damaged and the patient desires further fertility, hysterectomy should not be performed because pregnancy is still possible after salpingectomy by means of embryo transfer. The use of intravenous methotrexate in conservative management of ectopic pregnancy is not yet standard practice and requires strict adherence to current protocols.

NONOVIDUCTAL ECTOPIC PREGNANCY

Primary abdominal and ovarian pregnancies are rare. Most are secondary to tubal gestation. An abdominal pregnancy is characterized by easy palpation of the fetal parts, abnormal presentations (often transverse lie), and radiologic evidence of a fetus that appears to be overlying the maternal vertebral column. Although the fetus may be carried to term, it is usually removed abdominally as soon as it is diagnosed. The placenta should be left in place unless it can be removed easily without endangering the adjacent maternal structures. The fetus in cases of abdominal pregnancy may die and calcify to form a lithopedion. Ovarian pregnancy almost always requires oophorectomy. The rare cervical pregnancy usually requires hysterectomy to control hemorrhage, although gentle curettement and ligation of the internal iliac arteries occasionally have been successful.

11
CHAPTER

SPONTANEOUS ABORTION AND OBSTETRIC-GYNECOLOGIC SHOCK

The most common causes of vaginal bleeding in women in the reproductive age group are related to complications of pregnancy. Abortion is the termination of pregnancy before fetal viability, or when the fetus weighs less than 500 g. Abortion may be spontaneous (occurring through natural causes) or induced (by mechanical or medicinal means). Most spontaneous abortions occur in the second or third month of gestation. Induced abortion may be medically indicated or elective. Local laws rather than medical grounds determine whether an abortion is legal or criminal.

Spontaneous abortions occur in more than 10% of all pregnancies. The true rate is probably closer to 20%, for many of the earliest abortions are not recognized by the patient. The cause of spontaneous abortion is unknown in the majority of cases, although blighted ova and other less profound fetal genetic abnormalities (proved by chromosomal analysis) may be detected in a significant proportion of conceptuses. Local and systemic maternal disorders and environmental factors may all be operative. Maternal diseases include acute and chronic infections (such as those caused by Toxoplasma, *Listeria monocytogenes,* and T-mycoplasmas), chronic wasting diseases, and endocrinopathies (particularly thyroid and prolactin dysfunction). Local factors include anomalies of the reproductive tract, myomas, or incompetence of the cervix. External environmental factors include trauma, radiation, and cytotoxic drugs. Immunologic factors are not well defined. Such problems should be referred to specialized centers.

THREATENED ABORTION

Threatened abortion is diagnosed on the basis of any vaginal bleeding in the first 20 weeks of pregnancy. Only half of all cases of threatened abortion will progress to abortion regardless of treatment. Diagnosis requires a gynecologic examination to rule out other causes of vaginal bleeding, such as cervical polyps and neoplasms as well as injuries to the lower genital tract. With threatened abortion, the uterine bleeding may be accompanied by cramps and backache, the uterine size is consistent with the menstrual history, and the cervix is not dilated. Especially if the pain accompanying uterine bleeding is severe, other complications of pregnancy must be ruled out, such as ectopic pregnancy and hemorrhagic corpus luteum.

TREATMENT OF ABORTION

Treatment of threatened abortion is conservative, namely, mild sedation and a few days of bedrest. Longer periods are not justified, for abortion cannot be forestalled by further bedrest. There is no drug therapy of proven effectiveness, including progesterone. When the cramping and bleeding are accompanied by dilatation of the cervix, the abortion becomes imminent, and when the membranes rupture, the abortion is considered inevitable. When part of the product of conception is passed, the condition is termed incomplete abortion. In patients with imminent and inevitable abortions, the usual course of action is to complete the abortion. Usually a portion of the placenta is retained and the incompletely emptied uterus continues to bleed. Hemorrhage may be slight or sufficient to produce shock. Abortion is usually preceded by fetal death, and histologic examination generally reveals necrosis and hemorrhage in the decidua. The most effective treatment of incomplete abortion is curettage (suction or sharp), with oxytocin employed in the larger uteri (10 to 12 weeks' size or larger). An intravenous infusion should be started; in the presence of moderate or severe bleeding, blood should be crossmatched and available. Complications (more common before the laws governing induced abortion were liberalized) include sepsis and shock (p. 101). Septic abortion is a major cause of maternal mortality in the United States.

In cases of complete abortion, the entire product of conception is passed. Bleeding is usually minimal and no treatment ordinarily is required.

MISSED ABORTION

In cases of missed abortion, the fetus dies but is retained in utero for more than 2 months. Diagnosis is made on the basis of regression of the signs of pregnancy or absence of fetal cardiac motion on sonographic examination followed by lack of spontaneous abortion. The uterus should be evacuated as soon as the fetus is known to be dead. Early missed abortion may often be managed by intravenous oxytocin followed by curettage. Later abortions may require stimulation of uterine contractions by prostaglandin.

HABITUAL ABORTION

Habitual abortion is defined as three or more consecutive spontaneous abortions. Known causes include uterine anomalies, incompetence of the cervix, inadequate corpus luteum (in which case supplementation with progesterone may be efficacious), hypothyroidism, vascular and renal maternal diseases, and immunologic incompatibilities (or perhaps excessive similarities) between the parents.

Since half of all threatened abortions fail to progress to frank abortion, any treatment will have a 50% chance of success. Progestin therapy has not been proved effective in the usual spontaneous abortion; it may, furthermore, cause retention of the products of conception and possible masculinization of the genitalia of the female fetus. One quarter to one half of all abortuses have chromosomal anomalies such as autosomal trisomy (50%), monosomy X (25%), polyploidy (20%), and others (5%).

An unusual complication of a missed abortion is hypofibrinogenemia, which ordinarily does not occur until 5 weeks or more after fetal death.

Late abortions occurring in the second trimester may be caused by placental abnormalities and maternal diseases such as chronic hypertension. Syphilis may be a cause of late abortion (after the fourth month). Late abortions usually have no discernible cause; they resemble premature deliveries rather than early abortions in the relatively slight bleeding and the moderately severe pain.

INCOMPETENT OS

The incompetent os (technically incompetent cervical canal) is a cause of habitual midtrimester abortion that is not common but is amenable to surgical treatment. It is diagnosed by a history of signs and symptoms that appear in a sequence different from that of the usual incomplete abortion. In the case of incompetent os, the painless, bloodless dilatation of the cervix is followed by rupture of the membranes and then abortion. The pregnancy may be saved by the timely placement of a suture around the internal os (cerclage). If the pregnancy is carried to term, a cesarean section may be performed or the suture may be cut.

INDUCED ABORTION

Induced abortions, particularly those performed illegally, may be complicated by hemorrhage, sepsis, acute renal failure, and bacteremic shock. Treatment includes massive antibiotics, scrupulous regulation of fluids and electrolytes to tide the patient over the oliguric phase, and removal of necrotic foci that may be a source of toxins. Nephrotoxic antibiotics must be employed with great caution in patients with impaired renal function. Roentgenograms of the abdomen should be obtained to rule out a foreign body in the peritoneal cavity or free gas under the diaphragm, both of which indicate perforation of the uterus. Endotoxic shock complicating abortion leads to a high maternal mortality.

Abortion may be induced legally for medical (for example, cardiac, renal, and psychiatric) indications or electively, according to local statutes. Medical indications may be maternal (to preserve the life or health of the mother) or fetal (to prevent abnormalities, as with rubella, or genetic defects, as indicated by amniocentesis.) Techniques, with indications and contraindications for each, are discussed in Chapter 30.

Very early abortions (before 6 weeks) and late abortions (after the sixteenth to twentieth weeks) may be complete. The common abortion (between the eighth and twelfth weeks), however, is usually incomplete, requiring a curettage. In spontaneous abortion many of the villi may show hydropic change, which should not be confused with hydatidiform mole (Chapter 39).

Trauma is not a common etiologic factor in abortion. To prove a traumatic cause, it must be shown that bleeding and abortion occur shortly after the trauma and that there is no abnormality of the conceptus. Habitual abortion requires careful investigation. In addition to a thorough history and physical examination, a minimal investigation includes a chest film, complete blood count, serologic test for syphilis, indices of thyroid function, glucose tolerance test, hystero-gram, measurement of basal body temperature, endometrial biopsy, and progesterone assay.

SEPTIC ABORTION

Septic abortion usually results from instrumental or chemical interference. Uterine perforation, bacterial shock, and hemolysis may be associated. The prominent pathogens were formerly streptococci and staphylococci, which produced bacteremia. The principal offenders now are gram-negative bacilli (*E. coli* and related organisms), which may produce endotoxic shock, with hypotension, oliguria, occasionally disseminated intravascular coagulation, and adult respiratory distress syndrome. Septic abortion caused by pathogenic clostridia may produce, in addition, hemolysis and jaundice. The treatment comprises massive antibiotics and attempts to maintain renal function, normal blood pressure, and tissue oxygenation. The patient may present with a foul purulent discharge, a boggy tender uterus, and temperature spikes. Prompt curettage to remove necrotic foci is indicated, except in the presence of extrauterine spread (parametritis). The following paragraphs outline the physiology and management of obstetric-gynecologic shock.

OBSTETRIC-GYNECOLOGIC SHOCK

Fundamentally, shock involves tissue oxygenation that is inadequate to meet cellular metabolic demands. Cells that are so affected eventually die as a result of progressive inability to meet metabolic needs through anaerobic glycolysis. Shock is thus not definable in terms of blood pressure or an emotional state. In fact, many patients with profound shock maintain a normal or even high blood pressure, a finding that often results in delayed intervention. It might seem that the simple restoration of tissue perfusion would avoid the adverse consequences of shock, and that is usually the case if treatment is initiated immediately. The treatment is complex, however, because tissue perfusion involves a delicate relationship between intravascular volume, intravascular capacitance, cardiac output, peripheral arteriovenous (A-V) shunts, blood oxygen content, and cellular function.

Shock may be categorized into four types: hypovolemic, cardiogenic, septic, and neurogenic. Although pure hypovolemic shock (hemorrhagic shock in a trauma patient) and pure cardiogenic shock (pump failure in acute myocardial infarction) may occur, most patients with systemic hypoperfusion suffer from two or more types that occur simultaneously. The hemodynamic characteristics of the different types of shock are described in Table 11–1. Obstetric and gynecologic patients suffer most frequently from septic shock or the combination of septic shock and hypovolemia. Only rarely does cardiogenic shock contribute significantly to shock in the obstetric-gynecologic patient. Neurogenic shock occurs acutely after injury to the spinal cord. It results from mechanical disruption of sympathetic efferent fibers. There is loss of sympathetic tone and markedly increased peripheral venous and arterial capacitance. Except for the unusual patient with injury to the cervical or thoracic spinal cord, this form of shock is not seen in obstetric-gynecologic practice.

Pure hypovolemic shock is seen in patients with acute hemorrhage, as in postpartum hemorrhage or ruptured ectopic pregnancy. The immediate response to loss of 25% or more of the circulating blood volume in the nonpregnant patient is activation of the sympathetic nervous system with vasoconstriction and resulting increased peripheral vascular resistance (Table 11–1). To maintain circulation to the vital organs (heart, brain, and kidneys), blood is shunted away from organs of lesser immediate priority (skin, gut, and skeletal muscle). Initially, such a state of shock is manifested by sweating (sympathetic nervous system stimulation), cool and pale skin, gastrointestinal

ileus, and weakness. Because of a reduction in stroke volume, systolic blood pressure is reduced. The net effect is a reduction in the pulse pressure because diastolic pressure is maintained by sympathetic reflexes. The heart compensates for the reduced stroke volume by tachycardia, which is also mediated through the sympathetic nervous system. If hemorrhage progresses to 40% of normal blood volume, even vital organs sustain inadequate perfusion, and mental confusion and oliguria occur. The effects of prolonged hypovolemic shock are tissue-specific. For example, prolonged hypoperfusion of the skin leads to decubitus ulcers. Ischemia of the gut leads to breakdown of the mucosal barrier and entry of luminal microbes into the portal venous and lymphatic tributaries, with resulting systemic sepsis. This process of "bacterial translocation" leads to progressive gram-negative septic shock, a precursor of the "multiple organ failure" syndrome. Renal ischemia for as short a time as 45 to 60 minutes can result in acute tubular necrosis with renal failure. Mucosal ischemia, rather than hypersecretion of acid, appears to be the primary inciting factor in the development of stress ulceration of the stomach. As the capacity of the tachycardia to compensate for a reduced stroke volume is exceeded, cardiac output drops with resulting tissue hypoperfusion. The treatment involves simple replacement of volume when shock is hypovolemic in origin. When loss of intravascular volume is obvious, as in hemorrhagic shock, rapid administration of isotonic crystalloid and blood, when indicated by a reduced oxygen-carrying capacity, effects adequate tissue perfusion. In such circumstances, a clear sensorium and adequate urinary output reflect effective intervention. Unfortunately, losses of fluid are often much less evident, as in the case of

TABLE 11–1. HEMODYNAMIC CHANGES ASSOCIATED WITH SHOCK

	Hypovolemic	Septic	Cardiogenic	Neurogenic
Pulse	↑	↑	↑	↓
Blood pressure	↓	↑ ↓	↑ ↓	↓
Intravascular volume	↓	↓ (untreated)	↑	↔
Central venous pressure	↓	↓ (untreated)	↑	↓
Cardiac output	↓	↑ (treated)	↓	↑
Systemic vascular resistance	↑	↓ (treated)	↑	↓

postoperative third-space loss of fluid after extensive retroperitoneal dissection in oncologic surgery. In such circumstances, invasive hemodynamic monitoring with measurement of central venous pressure and, on occasion, pulmonary arterial catheterization for recording left-heart filling pressures are necessary. These measures are indicated also when a patient fails to respond to fluid therapy in the face of obvious fluid loss. Documenting an adequately replaced intravascular volume is essential. Although delayed resuscitation of a hypovolemic patient may appear successful on the basis of restoration of adequate vital signs, the patient usually succumbs to a progressive organ failure syndrome secondary to irreversible cellular oxygen debt.

Septic shock is a much more insidious precursor of the "multiple organ failure" syndrome and usually causes a hypovolemic state and therefore a combined clinical picture. The untreated patient in septic shock manifests signs similar to those occurring in pure hypovolemic shock, including tachycardia, hypotension, and increased systemic vascular resistance (see Table 11–1). As isotonic fluid replacement is initiated and right-heart filling pressures are restored, however, the hemodynamic picture becomes hyperdynamic, with a striking rise in cardiac output and a drop in systemic vascular resistance. The drop in peripheral vascular tone in septic shock appears to be caused by the activation of a number of mediators, including metabolites of arachidonic acid (prostaglandins and leukotrienes), cytokines (interleukins and tumor necrosis factor), complement pathway components, and acute phase reactants. The hemodynamic consequences of gram-negative sepsis were thought previously to be secondary to the direct effects of endotoxin. It now appears, however, that endotoxin and other activators of the septic hemodynamic response act indirectly through these more proximal pathways. The net effect of mediator activation, whatever the septic stimulus, is massive systemic vasodilation, peripheral arteriovenous shunting, and altered cellular oxygen metabolism. The final result is a reduced level of systemic oxygen consumption in the face of a marked increase in oxygen delivery (the product of blood oxygen content and cardiac output). As oxygen consumption falls, oxygen debt develops in specific organs, leading to organ system failure. The pattern of organ failure is fairly predictable, with hepatic and pulmonary failure followed by renal failure and breakdown of the gastrointestinal mucosa. Treatment of septic shock therefore must be directed toward initial replacement of intravascular volume followed by rapid diagnosis and appropriate management of the septic focus. Effort has been directed inappropriately to support failed organ systems in the septic patient. Once progressive multiple organ failure has gained momentum, mortality is inevitable. Aggressive investigation of the nature and location of the septic "motor" of the cascade of organ failure is crucial and it must be followed by immediate intervention. In the case of intraabdominal abscess, for example, surgical drainage is mandatory. Mechanical drainage of mucus plugs and appropriate antibiotic coverage are required in patients with pneumonia.

Hypovolemic shock and septic shock are the most common forms of tissue hypoperfusion in obstetric-gynecologic practice and are frequently found together. The initial hemodynamic insult in sepsis is identical with that in hypovolemic shock because in both cases there is a relative hypovolemia that must be corrected in order to unmask the hyperdynamic state. All forms of shock result in tissue hypoperfusion with resulting oxygen debt. Severe uncorrected oxygen debt leads to immediate organ system failure. Progressive low-grade oxygen debt leads to a complex of failure of multiple organ systems, with mortality proportional to the number of organs involved. All forms of shock require close clinical monitoring of fluid status and insertion of a Foley catheter to measure urinary output. In most cases, especially when response to therapy is not immediate, invasive hemodynamic monitoring is required, with attention to right atrial filling pressures, cardiac output, systemic vascular resistance, and pulmonary capillary wedge pressures. Ultimately, however, attention must be directed to reversal of the process perpetuating the state of shock. Hemorrhage must be controlled, cardiac function must be optimized, a septic focus must be drained, and vital systems must be supported. Emphasis on treatment of the signs and symptoms of shock rather than its cause will delay the specific therapy required to preserve the patient's life.

Hypovolemia must be corrected and central venous pressure monitored to avoid overhydration. Metabolic acidosis must be corrected. Endotoxic shock should be suspected whenever hypotension and oliguria are not promptly reversed by intravenous fluids and blood transfusions. Corticosteroids are often given in the face of an inadequate response to fluids, blood, and antibiotics. The blood pressure must be maintained to assure renal perfusion, although the roles of vasoconstrictors and vasodilators are still somewhat controversial. Pressor amines are often given in the presence of warm, dry skin, and vasodilators in the presence of cold, clammy extremities. Mannitol may be used in an attempt to produce diuresis. The role of heparin in preventing or treating intravascular coagulation in cases of infected septic abortion is still controversial. If necrotic foci in the uterus are not accessible to curettage or if there is evidence of uterine perforation, laparotomy and possible hysterectomy may be required as lifesaving measures. The successful management of endotoxic shock depends upon early consultation with the dialysis team and prompt efforts to prevent permanent renal damage.

TOXIC SHOCK SYNDROME

The toxic shock syndrome (TSS) includes fever of at least 102° F, a diffuse macular erythema, desquamation (particularly of the palms and soles), hypotension, and involvement of three or more of the following organs or systems: gastrointestinal (vomiting or diarrhea), muscular (myalgia or elevated creatine phosphokinase), mucous membranes (vaginal, oropharyngeal, or conjunctival hyperemia), renal (elevated blood urea nitrogen or creatinine, or pyuria in the absence of infection of the urinary tract), hepatic (elevated bilirubin, serum glutamic oxaloacetic transaminase, or serum glutamic pyruvic transaminase), hematologic (decrease in platelets), and central nervous system (disorientation or alterations in consciousness without focal neurologic signs when fever and hypotension are absent). Cultures from blood, throat, and cerebrospinal fluid, if obtained, must be negative, as must serologic tests for Rocky Mountain spotted fever, leptospirosis, and measles.

Toxic shock syndrome has been related to the use of tampons during the menstrual period, particularly brands that are highly absorbent. TSS has also been described in women who did not use tampons, particularly those using the contraceptive sponge, and even in men. The organism most frequently implicated is *Staphylococcus aureus*. An exotoxin is the causative agent and lysogeny, or the presence of temperate bacteriophage, characterizes the virulent strains of the bacterium.

12
CHAPTER

GENETIC DISORDERS AND CONGENITAL ANOMALIES

Examination of the amniotic fluid and cells, chorionic villi, and fetal blood can be used for the following purposes: detection of biochemical disorders (enzymatic defects) such as Tay-Sachs disease; ascertaining fetal blood type; detection of cystic fibrosis; detection of the sex of the fetus (karyotype) in cases of sex-linked disorders such as Duchenne's muscular dystrophy; and detection of chromosomal disorders (karyotype) such as Down's syndrome in fetuses of elderly mothers and others at risk.

GENETIC TERMINOLOGY

In a description of the karyotype, the first item to be recorded is the total number of chromosomes (including sex chromosomes) followed by a comma (,). The sex chromosomal constitution is recorded after the comma:

46,XX — Normal female
46,XY — Normal male
45,X — Turner's syndrome
47,XXY — Klinefelter's syndrome
45,XX,5p− — Cri du chat syndrome

Numeric aberrations of the autosomes are indicated by the individual chromosome number preceded by a plus (+) or minus (−) to indicate an extra or missing chromosome, respectively:

45,XX,−9 — 45 chromosomes, XX sex chromosomes, and a missing chromosome 9

46,XY,+18−21 — 46 chromosomes, XY sex chromosomes, an extra 18 chromosome and a missing 21 chromosome

Chromosomal mosaicism is indicated by two karyotypic designations separated by a diagonal (/):

45,X/46,XY — A chromosomal mosaic with two cell types—one with 45 chromosomes and a single X and the other with 46 chromosomes and XY sex chromosomes

46,XY/47,XY,+21 — A chromosomal mosaic with a normal male cell line and a cell line with an extra chromosome 21

The short arm of a chromosome is designated by the lower-case letter "p" and the long arm by the letter "q." Increase in the length of an arm of a chromosome is indicated by placing a plus (+) sign and decrease in length by placing a minus (−) sign after the designation of the arm:

46,XX,2p+   46 chromosomes with an increase in length of the short arm of chromosome 2

A translocation is indicated by the letter "t" followed by parentheses, which include the chromosomes involved:

46,XY,t(5p−;14q+)   A balanced reciprocal translocation between the short arm of chromosome 5 and the long arm of chromosome 14

or

46,XX,t(5p+;14q−)

A centric fusion (Robertsonian) translocation in which only one translocation chromosome is involved is designated as follows:

45,XX,−14−21+(14;21)   45 chromosomes, XX sex chromosomes, one chromosome 14 and one chromosome 21 missing, the two having united to form a translocation chromosome

Centric fusion results from breaks at or near the centromere in acrocentric chromosomes (13, 14, 15, 21, and 22) with cross fusion of the fragments. One of the most common centric fusions involves chromosomes 14 and 21.

Trisomy 21 (47,XX,+21, or 47,XY,+21) is the most common trisomy compatible with life. It accounts for 95% of all cases of Down's syndrome. Virtually all affected persons are mentally retarded and 30% have congenital cardiac disease (Table 12−1). Less common forms of Down's syndrome involve translocations and mosaicisms.

The risks of having a child with Down's syndrome at various maternal ages are as follows:

Maternal Age	Risk of Down's Syndrome
20	1/1,923
25	1/1,205
30	1/885
35	1/365
40	1/109
45	1/32
49	1/12

The risk of having an aneuploidy of any sort at maternal age 44 or above is of the order of 1 in 10. The empirically calculated risks for several common congenital defects in the general population are as follows: anencephaly and meningomyelocele, 1 — 2/ 1000; cleft lip with or without cleft palate, 1/1000; and cleft palate, 0.4 — 1/1000. The frequencies of the more common chromosomal anomalies found in the newborn are as follows: Trisomy 21, 1/800-1/1000 births; Trisomy 18, 1/8000 births; Trisomy 13, 1/20,000 births; XXY, 1/1000 male births; XYY, 1/1000 male births; XXX, 1/950 female births; and X (XO), 1/10,000 female births. Several of the major syndromes associated with chromosomal anomalies are shown in Table 12−1.

DETECTION OF ANOMALIES

Because congenital malformations account for about 20% of infant deaths in the United States today, the use of amniocentesis, chorionic villus sampling, and percutaneous umbilical blood sampling to detect these defects assumes great importance. The risk of abortion of about 0.5% after amniocentesis precludes its routine use, but certain conditions are clear indications for the procedure including: advanced maternal age, a prior child with a chromosomal anomaly, a parent with a translocation or other chromosomal anomaly, carriers of inborn errors of metabolism (mendelian disorders), and a prior child with a neural tube defect. The rate of pregnancy loss after chorionic villus sampling (CVS) is about 1.2% and after percutaneous umbilical blood sampling (PUBS) it is about 1 to 2%. The information obtained through CVS and amniocentesis is similar except that only amniocentesis can be used to measure α-fetoprotein because fluid is needed for that test.

Alpha-fetoprotein (AFP) is produced by the fetal yolk sac and later the liver and

TABLE 12–1. COMMON CHROMOSOMAL ANOMALY SYNDROMES

Syndrome	Clinical Features	Chromosomal Defect
Trisomy 13	Cleft lip and/or palate, microphthalmia, polydactyly, congenital cardiac disease, death by age 2	80% primary trisomies; 20% mosaic or familial translocation
5p– (cri du chat)	Catlike cry, hypertelorism, micrognathia, microcephaly, wide flat nasal bridge, mental retardation	Most arise de novo; some are parental-balanced translocations
Trisomy 18	Microcephaly, micrognathia, rocker-bottom feet, congenital cardiac defects, death by age 2	Most are primary trisomy 18; a few are mosaic; remainder are double aneuploidies
Trisomy 21	Upward slanting palpebral fissures, bilateral epicanthi, round flat nasal bridge, extra skin at nape of neck, broad short hands, hypotonia, mental retardation, 30% have congenital cardiac disease	Most are primary trisomy; a few are translocations or mosaics
45,X (Turner's)	Short stature, lymphedema of dorsum of fingers and toes, broad chest, prominent ears, webbed neck, low posterior hairline, cubitus valgus of elbow, coarctation of aorta	Usually sporadic
47,XXY (Klinefelter's)	Long limbs, small penis and testes, gynecomastia, sterility, 15% have I.Q. below 80	20% are mosaic
47,XYY	Not well defined; some have increased stature and are more aggressive	Usually sporadic

passes into the amniotic fluid. The α-fetoprotein in the maternal blood rises exponentially early in pregnancy and peaks at 32 weeks (Fig. 12–1). It is not normally found in the adult, but small amounts diffuse into the pregnant woman's blood. At the site of a neural tube defect that is open (not covered by skin), additional AFP escapes, elevating the level of this protein in the amniotic fluid and usually in the maternal plasma as well. The major open neural tube defects that can be detected by an elevated AFP are anencephaly and open spina bifida. Multiple fetuses and fetal death may also elevate the AFP in amniotic fluid and maternal plasma. Additional causes of elevated AFP include omphalocele, congenital nephrosis, and atresias of duodenum and esophagus.

Approximately one to two neural tube defects occur in every 1000 live births in the United States. Ninety to 95% of these disabling and often fatal defects appear in infants with no family history of such disorders. If a couple have had a child with a neural tube defect in a prior pregnancy, there is a 2% chance of having another affected child. The initial screening test, performed at 16 to 18 weeks' gestation, detects elevated values of AFP in maternal blood. The results are expressed as multiples of the median (MOM) so that each laboratory can adjust its values to its own population of patients screened. If the maternal serum α-fetoprotein (MSAFP) is elevated to 2 or more MOM at 16 to 18 weeks of gestation, the test is repeated. Most often the second value is normal. If the second test still shows an elevated value, targeted ultrasound and amniocentesis are recommended. In cases in which ultrasound and amniocentesis yield normal results (unexplained elevation of MSAFP), there may be, according to some investigators, increased risks of premature labor, rupture of the membranes, preeclampsia, intrauterine growth restriction, and congenital defects.

Indications for amniocentesis and measurement of AFP in the fluid include: a prior pregnancy that resulted in an infant with a neural tube defect, a mother or father who has had a neural tube defect, and probably pregnancy in the siblings of the parents of an affected child. Elevation of acetylcholinesterase in the amniotic fluid is an indication that the elevated AFP is a result of a neural tube defect.

Fetal surgery has made possible the correction of certain neural tube defects. Other conditions amenable to this approach include congenital hydronephrosis, congenital diaphragmatic hernia, and obstructive hydrocephalus. The ethical as well as the scientific implications of fetal surgery remain to be elucidated.

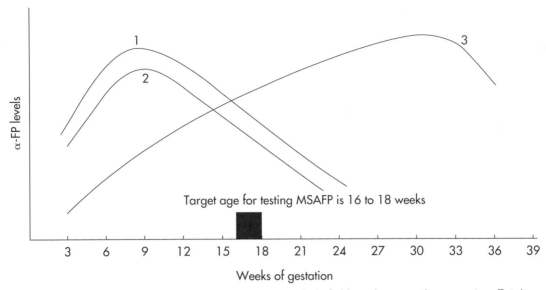

FIG. 12–1. Alpha-fetoprotein (AFP) in fetal blood, amniotic fluid, and maternal serum. 1 = Fetal blood (FB), 2 = Amniotic fluid (AF), 3 = Maternal serum (MS). Note: Graph is not to scale. Ratios at 16 weeks' gestation are:

$$[FB] > [AF] > [MS]$$
$$50,000 : 500 : 1$$

For parents who do not consider abortion an option, prenatal diagnosis offers several potential benefits. The detection of a fetal anomaly may suggest specialized perinatal intervention and may benefit the couple in their psychologic adjustment to the birth of an abnormal infant.

More recently, clinical significance has been attached to the finding of a low value of AFP in maternal plasma. Genetic amniocentesis or CVS sampling in the first trimester in such patients has led to the detection of fetal aneuploidy in women under the age of 30 years. Only 20% of infants with Down's syndrome are born to mothers aged 35 or older. Low values of MSAFP in women under the age of 35, adjusted for maternal age, that indicate a risk of Down's syndrome equal to or greater than 1:270 identify about 30% of the affected fetuses.

To improve the screening for Down's syndrome, a "triple test" has been employed recently. This method of screening includes measurement of human chorionic gonadotropin (hCG), MSAFP, and unconjugated estriol (E_3). In Down's syndrome, the E_3 and MSAFP are low, whereas the hCG tends to be elevated. The triple screening test may detect up to 60% of the affected fetuses.

Use of MSAFP requires several corrections to be of maximal clinical value: maternal weight (dilutional effect in large women), race (higher values in black patients), and diabetic status (lower values in diabetes).

Several classes of inherited biochemical disorders are detectable in the middle trimester through analysis of fluid obtained by amniocentesis. Among the disorders of lipid metabolism are Gaucher's disease, GM_2 gangliosidosis type I (Tay-Sachs disease), and the varieties of Niemann-Pick's disease. The disorders of carbohydrate metabolism include galactosemia, glucose-6-phosphate dehydrogenase deficiency, and the glycogen storage diseases. Disorders resulting from disturbances in mucopolysaccharide metabolism are Hurler's, Hunter's, Sanfilippo's, and Morquio's syndromes. Inborn errors of amino acid and organic acid metabolism include homocystinuria, maple syrup urine disease, methylmalonic acidemia, and phenylketonuria. The Lesch-Nyhan syndrome is listed among the miscellaneous disorders.

Cystic fibrosis is one of the most common autosomal recessive disorders, with a carrier frequency of approximately 1 in 25 in the white population in the U.S. It has been shown recently that about 75% of the mutations in patients with cystic fibrosis correspond to a three-base pair deletion that results in the loss of a phenylalanine residue at amino acid position 508 (ΔF 508) from the coding region of the cystic fibrosis gene on chromosome 7. Carrier testing should be offered to all couples with a familial history of cystic fibrosis. About 75% of the carriers can be detected by analysis of ΔF 508.

Fetoscopy allows direct visualization of the fetus and sampling of fetal tissues, including blood and skin, for the antenatal detection of fetal defects. Diagnosis of α-thalassemia, sickle cell anemia, and some cases of β-thalassemia are possible through analysis of patterns of DNA from cells in the amniotic fluid without fetoscopy. Genetic disorders that require analysis of fetal serum are hemophilia-A (Factor VIII deficiency), Christmas Disease (Factor IX deficiency), and chronic granulomatous disease. Biopsies of fetal skin have led to the prenatal diagnosis of harlequin ichthyosis, epidermolysis bullosa lethalis, and epidermolytic hyperkeratosis. Biopsy of fetal muscle may soon become a reliable method for detection of Duchenne muscular dystrophy.

Prior to fetoscopy, ultrasonographic examination is required to confirm fetal viability, diagnose placental location and plural gestation, verify gestational age, and ascertain fetal position. Diagnosis of disorders of fetal hemoglobin is also possible during the first trimester by means of trophoblastic biopsy in conjunction with restriction endonuclease analysis of fetal DNA.

The role of ultrasound in detection of congenital anomalies is described in Chapter 26. The sensitivity of the technique for this purpose in excellent perinatal centers is in the range of 90 to 95%, depending on the magnitude of the anomaly, the experience of the examiner, and the gestational age at which the test is performed. Sonographic detection of Down's syndrome has utilized measurement of femoral length (FL), ratio of biparietal diameter to femoral length (BPD/FL), and the nuchal skin folds between 15 and 20 weeks of gestation. These tests, however, do not have sufficient sensitivity to replace other methods of detection.

Two important metabolic disorders, phenylketonuria and hypothyroidism, can be detected soon after birth, and both are amenable to treatment. The incidence of phenlyketonuria (PKU) is approximately 1 in 20,000 live births. Phenylketonuria is an autosomal recessive disorder. A high phenylalanine level in the mother induces structural injuries in the fetus. During late gestation, myelination and maturation of the fetal central nervous system are disturbed. The principal abnormalities caused by this disorder include spontaneous abortion, mental retardation in the offspring, microcephaly, congenital cardiac disease, and low birth weight.

Hypothyroidism, which occurs with an incidence of about 1 in 4000 live births, is also associated with mental retardation if the disorder is not detected and treated soon after birth. Hypothyroidism is detected by measurement of TSH in serum. Many states require that tests for phenylketonuria and hypothyroidism be performed routinely.

Maternal hyperthermia, particularly during the period of fetal organogenesis, is associated with increases in spontaneous abortion, stillbirth, prematurity, mental retardation, and neurologic disorders.

13
CHAPTER

MEDICAL, SURGICAL, AND EMOTIONAL COMPLICATIONS IN PREGNANCY

DIABETES MELLITUS

Most medical complications do not alter the course of pregnancy and are themselves not altered by pregnancy. A few major exceptions are discussed on pages 108 through 125. Perhaps the most important is diabetes mellitus. Before the introduction of insulin, diabetic patients rarely carried their pregnancies to term or even became pregnant. At present the incidence of this complication of pregnancy is over 1%. The prevalence of insulin-dependent diabetes in the United States is somewhat under 0.5%, but it varies widely among different ethnic groups. The disorder is often first unmasked during pregnancy. Because of the normal gestational changes in carbohydrate metabolism and renal function, the diagnosis must be made with caution. A 1-hour glucose screen should be performed on all pregnant patients at 24 to 28 weeks of gestation. In patients with a familial history of diabetes mellitus and other risk factors, the screening test should be done at the initial visit and again at 24 to 28 weeks of gestation. If the screening test is abnormal (a value of more than 140 mg/dL), a full 3-hour glucose tolerance test should be performed (Table 13–1). One abnormal value in the glucose tolerance test (GTT) may be sufficient to identify increased perinatal risk. In some institutions, the 2-hour value has proved to

TABLE 13–1. O'SULLIVAN CRITERIA FOR DIAGNOSIS OF GESTATIONAL DIABETES USING TWO OR MORE ABNORMAL VALUES DURING A 100 g, 3-HOUR ORAL GLUCOSE TOLERANCE TEST AFTER AT LEAST AN 8-HOUR OVERNIGHT FAST

Timing of Glucose Measurement	Whole Venous Blood (mg/dL)	Plasma (mg/dL)
Fasting	90	105
1-Hour	165	190
2-Hour	145	165
3-Hour	125	145

correlate best with perinatal risk. A glucose tolerance test (GTT) should be performed on all pregnant patients with a family history of diabetes, a history of large infants (over 4000 g), prior children with congenital anomalies, unexplained stillbirths, habitual abortions, or significant obesity. If the GTT is normal in early pregnancy in these patients, it should be repeated at 24 to 28 weeks' gestation.

Diabetes in pregnancy can be categorized as Type 1, Type 2, and gestational. Type 1 is associated with susceptibility to ketosis. The deficiency in insulin is a result of loss of islet cells. It may occur at any age but is more common in youth. Type 2 diabetes is resistant to ketosis. It too may occur at any age but is more common in adults. Type 2 diabetics invariably require insulin during pregnancy. Gestational diabetes refers to the onset or first recognition of the disease during the present pregnancy. By convention, the definition of gestational diabetes applies whether or not insulin is used for treatment and whether or not the condition persists after pregnancy, but it does not exclude the possibility that the glucose intolerance may have anteceded the pregnancy.

Pregnancy affects the diabetes and diabetes affects the pregnancy. The effects of pregnancy on the diabetes include an alteration in glucose tolerance. There is hyperinsulinemia in normal pregnancy but a decrease in the effectiveness of insulin because of antagonistic factors. The vomiting of pregnancy may lead initially to insulin shock; later, as a result of starvation, ketoacidosis may be produced. The efforts of labor may deplete the glycogen, and the increased likelihood of infection makes the possibility of acidosis greater in pregnancy. Gestational glucosuria may also stem in part from a change in the filtered load of glucose. Insulin is antagonized by human placental lactogen (human chorionic somatomammotropin); the effect of degradation by insulinases is much less significant. Steroid hormones may further decrease glucose tolerance.

The poorly controlled diabetic pregnancy is complicated by an increased incidence of preeclampsia (perhaps fourfold), hydramnios, large babies, fetal death, and congenital anomalies. There is also an increased incidence of maternal urinary tract infection. In most series of poorly controlled diabetics the perinatal mortality rate is increased and there is an increase in respiratory distress syndrome (probably related largely to prematurity) and neonatal hypoglycemia, hypocalcemia, hypothermia, and nonhemolytic hyperbilirubinemia. Less common neonatal complications are polycythemia with thrombosis of the renal vein and the caudal regression syndrome.

The best results in management of the pregnant diabetic are provided by a perinatal team in a tertiary facility. The most important factor is medical control of the disease, ideally beginning before conception. With excellent management, the perinatal mortality may be reduced virtually to that of normal pregnancy and the maternal mortality essentially to zero.

The nonovert (preclinical, Class A) diabetic is managed obstetrically almost the same as a normal pregnant patient. The class A, or chemical, diabetic has an abnormal glucose tolerance test, but is maintained free of symptoms without insulin on dietary management alone.

The diet of the gestational diabetic should provide 36 to 40 calories/kg of ideal weight/day. It should contain 1.3 g of protein/kg/day and 200 to 500 g of carbohydrate/day. The remainder of the calories should be provided by fat. A typical diet of 2350 calories/day should comprise approximately 15% protein, 45% carbohydrate, and 35% fat.

Body mass index (weight/height^2) is a good index of maternal nutritional status. A body mass index (BMI) of less than 19.8 in pregnancy is considered underweight and the total recommended gain in weight is 28 to 40 lbs. A BMI between 19.8 and 26 is considered normal and the recommended gain in weight is 25 to 35 lbs. A BMI between 26 and 29 is considered overweight and the recommended gain in weight is 15 to 25 lbs. A BMI over 29 reflects obesity and the recommended gain in such women is 15 lbs.

Dietary recommendations based on the BMI are as follows. For a BMI between 19.8 and 26, the advice is 28 to 32 kcal/kg during the first trimester and 32 to 38 kcal/kg during the second and third trimesters. For a BMI of 26 to 29, the recommendation is 24 to 30 kcal/kg during the first trimester and adjustments during the second and third trimesters on the basis of the gain in weight. For a BMI above 29, the recommendation is not to exceed 24 kcal/kg throughout pregnancy.

The total caloric intake must be distributed in three regular meals and three snacks. Regular insulin is given 30 minutes before each meal and at bedtime, with some intermediate-acting insulin given with the bedtime snack. For patients beginning insulin therapy, the initial dosage is based on 0.5 to 1.0 units per kg. of body weight, with 40% before breakfast, 30% before lunch, 20% before supper, and 10% at bedtime. Although the recommended goal is to maintain the two-hour postprandial glucose value below 120 mg/dL, experienced investigators have shown that maintaining the 2-hour postprandial value at a higher level but below 150 mg/dL often avoids hypoglycemia and does not jeopardize the perinatal outcome.

Uncomplicated Class A diabetics are generally delivered at term. The overt diabetic is managed by a perinatal team concerned with maintaining strict control of the diabetes and ensuring timely delivery.

The essence of modern management of the pregnant overt diabetic is control of glucose. The best control is accomplished through intensive education of the patient regarding the relation of glucose to insulin and frequent (several times a day) measurements of plasma glucose. These glucose values are then used to determine the amounts of insulin to be given by frequent injections or continuous infusion with a pump. The blood glucose can be measured at home by commercially available techniques. In the best of circumstances, rates of complications in pregnant diabetics who have maintained excellent control of blood glucose before and during pregnancy do not differ significantly from those in nondiabetic pregnant women. Some centers manage the ideally controlled diabetic the same as a normal patient, with respect to timing and route of delivery.

The timing of the delivery depends principally upon degree of metabolic control, fetal maturity, and fetal well-being. Complications to be avoided during pregnancy are infections, acetonuria, and preeclampsia. Dosage of insulin should be regulated according to blood sugars with the aim of maintaining normal glucose levels. It is important to distinguish blood from plasma levels of glucose, for the former are about 87% of the latter. For example, a fasting blood glucose of 90 mg/dL is equivalent to a plasma value of 103 mg/dL. Plasma values are used at most perinatal centers.

The patient should be seen at least once a week throughout pregnancy. Overt diabetics are generally delivered between the thirty-eighth week and term, depending on the severity of the disease and the degree of control of glucose. Earlier delivery may be indicated in the presence of poor control of preeclampsia, repeated ketoacidosis, hydramnios, or advancing retinopathy.

Fetal distress may force early delivery despite prematurity. Nonstress tests, biophysical profiles, and oxytocin challenge tests are helpful in detecting fetal distress.

Despite the often large size of the newborn, its fragile condition requires intensive care in the high-risk or premature nursery. Therapeutic abortion has been performed for progressive renal disease, retinitis with progressive visual loss, and coronary arterial disease.

Class A diabetics have an abnormal glucose tolerance test, but no clinical signs of diabetes. Class B diabetics are those whose disease began after the age of 20 or has been present for as long as 9 years with no vascular disease. Class C diabetics are those whose disease began between the ages of 10 and 19 or has been present for between 10 and 19 years with no vascular disease. Class D diabetics are those whose disease began before the age of 10 or has been present for 20 years or more, with vascular disease, calcification of the vessels of the legs, or background (benign) retinopathy. Class F diabetics have nephropathy, Class H have cardiac disease, and Class R have proliferative retinopathy. The less severe diabetics often have large babies and placentas, whereas the more severe, namely those with vascular disease, often have undergrown babies and small placentas.

The oral glucose tolerance test is more sensitive and physiologic, but because of variations in absorption from the gastrointestinal tract during pregnancy the intravenous test is often easier to interpret. During labor and delivery, because of the changing requirements for insulin, the crystalline (regular) rather than a long-acting variety should be used. Optimal control is achieved through use of an insulin pump and a glucose infusion.

The criteria for diagnosis of diabetes in pregnancy are far from universally accepted and they differ from those used in the nonpregnant state. If the fasting plasma glucose level is less than 100 mg/100 mL in the intravenous test and if the level at 2 hours is not greater than the fasting level, it is unlikely that the patient has diabetes.

In the intravenous glucose tolerance test, the K value, or the rate of disappearance of glucose from the plasma, expressed as percent per minute, is calculated from the formula:

$$K = \frac{0.693}{t_{1/2}} \times 100,$$ where $t_{1/2}$ is the time for the concentration of glucose to decrease 50%.

This value is lower in women with decreased carbohydrate tolerance. Use of the K value allows accurate comparisons of carbohydrate tolerance, with the use of a single number rather than a curve, at various stages of pregnancy.

The patient should be evaluated carefully one week before anticipated delivery in order to regulate her metabolic status and to decide the route of delivery. She is often delivered by cesarean section unless an easy induction can be anticipated. The labor should be monitored and attempts at vaginal delivery abandoned if fetal distress occurs. After delivery, the maternal insulin requirement usually drops.

The problems of the neonate, in addition to those listed on page 109, include birth injuries because of large size and traumatic delivery, and congenital anomalies. The management requires careful regulation of the infant's environmental temperature, oxygen, humidity, and blood glucose. A precipitous fall in neonatal blood glucose may occur if the prior fetal glucose levels, which mirror maternal levels, were elevated as a result of poor control. The fetal prognosis depends on the severity of the maternal diabetes, the medical management and complications of the pregnancy, fetal maturity, and neonatal care. Maternal acidosis may lead to mental retardation in the offspring. The maternal prognosis is influenced by cardiovascular complications, pulmonary emboli, and severe preeclampsia or eclampsia.

During pregnancy, oral hypoglycemic agents should not be used. The lecithin/sphingomyelin ratio is reliable in diabetic pregnancies if a standardized procedure is followed. The dipalmitoyl derivative of lecithin provides an even more reliable index of pulmonary maturity. Phosphatidyl glycerol is the best indicator of pulmonary maturity. If phosphatidyl glycerol is present in the amnionic fluid, delivery can be accomplished without fear of respiratory distress syndrome in the neonate.

Another means of monitoring the diabetic pregnancy is measurement of glycosylated hemoglobin A_{1c}. An increase in this form of hemoglobin suggests poor control of the diabetes in the weeks prior to its measurement and predicts greater difficulties for the fetus. Optimal control of glucose is associated with normal values of hemoglobin A_{1c}.

CARDIAC DISEASE

More than 1% of all pregnant patients have cardiac disease. Of this group, rheumatic heart disease has long been the most common, but congenital heart disease is forming an increasingly large proportion and in some centers is the most commonly found cardiac disease in pregnancy. Diagnosis of cardiac disease in pregnancy is complicated by the normal gestational changes in the cardiovascular system. The maximal rise in cardiac output during pregnancy occurs as early as the end of the first trimester and is not significantly reduced in the last few weeks unless the patient is kept supine. As a result, the patient may decompensate early and at any time up to term. Cardiac failure occurs most commonly at the time of maximal cardiac output.

A systolic murmur may be functional, but diastolic and presystolic murmurs and precordial thrusts must be considered evidence of organic cardiac disease even in pregnancy. Diagnosis of cardiac disease requires at least one of the following: a diastolic, presystolic, or continuous murmur; unequivocal cardiomegaly; a loud harsh systolic murmur especially with a thrill; or an arrhythmia.

Mild cardiac disease may be managed at home with care to correct anemia and prevent or combat infection promptly. The best results are obtained through combined management by a cardiologist and an obstetrician. Treatment varies according to the functional class of the cardiac disease. In general, all patients with cardiac disease should avoid stress and should have increased rest. Preeclampsia, excessive weight gain, and hypertension should be treated vigorously. A cough, rales, or atrial fibrillation should arouse suspicion of impending cardiac failure. Fibrillation should be converted promptly to normal sinus rhythm.

Management of the labor includes well-controlled analgesia and anesthesia to relieve both anxiety and pain. The second stage should be shortened, and antibiotics should be given to prevent subacute bacterial endocarditis. Conduction anesthesia is appropriate for delivery of the patient with cardiac disease. Elevation of the mother's legs from the dorsal lithotomy position may result in an autotransfusion of up to 500 mL of blood and precipitate cardiac failure.

Outlet forceps are indicated to shorten the second stage. Hemorrhage is especially dangerous because the patient with cardiac disease often cannot compensate for sudden hypovolemia. Cesarean section must be reserved for obstetric indications.

The puerperium is also a dangerous period for the patient with cardiac disease. The patient with serious cardiac disease is often kept at bed rest for 7 to 10 days after delivery. Tubal sterilization should be delayed in these patients. For patients with cardiac disease who refuse tubal sterilization or for whom it is not performed for other reasons, effective contraception is mandatory. The patient with severe cardiac disease should be discouraged from becoming pregnant at all.

Abortion is medically indicated for cardiac disease only early in pregnancy, when it can be performed by suction curettage. Later in pregnancy, abortion may be as dangerous as carrying the pregnancy to term on bed rest.

Maternal prognosis depends upon the functional capacity of the heart, other complications that increase cardiac work, the quality of medical care, and psychologic and socioeconomic factors, such as the possibility of hospitalization throughout pregnancy.

The anatomic changes in pregnancy that make the diagnosis of cardiac disease more difficult include elevation of the diaphragm, deviation of the heart to the left, and apparent cardiomegaly on chest film. Pulmonic and apical systolic murmurs are often hemic, presumably caused by lower viscosity of the blood during pregnancy. Dependent edema in pregnancy is not necessarily a sign of cardiac disease, nor are tachycardia and palpitations.

The New York Heart Association classification of cardiac disease is as follows:

Class I—No limitation of physical activity.
Class II—Slight limitation of physical activity. (Ordinary activity produces symptoms.)
Class III—Marked limitation of physical activity. (Less than ordinary exercise produces symptoms.)
Class IV—Complete limitation of activity. (Insufficiency is manifest at rest, that is, cardiac failure.)

Because decreased cardiac output leads to decreased uteroplacental circulation and function, the fetuses of patients with cardiac disease are often undergrown. Patients in Classes I and II may be managed on an ambulatory basis during the early months of pregnancy. Patients in Classes III and IV should remain at bedrest throughout pregnancy. Although pregnant women in Classes I and II rarely go into failure, they must be watched carefully at frequent antepartum visits.

Warning signs include basal rales, dyspnea, tachycardia, and increasing edema. Optimal management includes bed rest for 10 hours a day, rest for half an hour after each meal, household help, avoidance of respiratory infections, and prompt reporting of any so-called cold. Patients must be taught the early symptoms of decompensation and the conditions that may lead to that serious complication. They must also be instructed to report such symptoms immediately to their physicians. If decompensation occurs, morphine, oxygen, digitalis, rotating tourniquets, and diuretics may be lifesaving.

During the puerperium, hemorrhage, infection, and thromboembolism, which are more serious than in normal patients, must be avoided. Class III patients ideally should not become pregnant. If they do, they must remain in bed throughout the pregnancy. Delivery, by any route, of a patient in failure carries a very high mortality.

Any infection in a woman with valvular heart disease must be treated with massive antibiotics after blood cultures are obtained. If the patient requires anticoagulants, heparin is the drug of choice because it does not cross the placenta.

Maternal hypoxia may lead to abortion, intrauterine death, and prematurity. Kyphoscoliotic heart disease may lead to cor pulmonale.

A cesarean section may be indicated in patients with coarctation of the aorta to prevent rupture of the vessel. There is probably no residual cardiac damage or shortening of life expectancy as a result of pregnancy in any patient with cardiac disease.

The cardiovascular surgical risk in pregnancy probably is not greater than it is in the nonpregnant state. The risk to the fetus, however, may be substantial, especially if open-heart procedures with cardiopulmonary bypass are required. Antibiotic prophylaxis is indicated for women with a history of rheumatic fever and for those with rheumatic cardiac disease to prevent streptococcal infections and recurrences of rheumatic fever. Infective endocarditis has been reported in women with prolapse of the mitral valve. No specific treatment is required during pregnancy except prophylactic antibiotics at the time of delivery.

MITRAL VALVE PROLAPSE

This anomaly affects 6 to 8% of women of reproductive age and is thus the cardiac lesion seen most frequently by obstetricians. Prolapse results from degeneration of the leaflets of the mitral valve and disruption of collagen in the chordae tendineae and valvular caps. The chordae tendineae and valvular leaflets thus become more elastic, stretch, and bulge into the left atrium as pressure is generated by the left ventricle during systole. The mitral valve continues to function normally unless the disorder worsens, with resulting mitral regurgitation and rupture of the chordae tendineae.

The primary manifestations of mitral valve prolapse are chest pain and irregularity of cardiac rhythm. The chest pain is retrosternal, of variable intensity, unrelated to physical activity, and unresponsive to nitroglycerin. The most common arrhythmia is supraventricular tachycardia and the most common auscultatory sign is a midsystolic click. As many as 20% of patients with the disorder demonstrate neither a midsystolic click nor a systolic murmur.

During pregnancy, symptoms and auscultatory signs usually decrease, presumably because of the gestational increase in intravascular and left ventricular volumes. Symptomatic patients, especially those with severe or recurrent abnormalities of cardiac rhythm, should be treated. The medication of choice during pregnancy is the β-blocker propranolol. A dosage of 20 to 40 mg, 4 times a day, is usually sufficient.

Antibiotic prophylaxis for mitral valve prolapse remains controversial. In patients with long-standing or severe anatomic changes, the endothelial lining of the atrial surface of the leaflets may rupture and initiate deposition of platelets and fibrin on the valvular surface. Although the benefit of antibiotic prophylaxis is uncertain, the risk is clearly small. It thus seems prudent to administer prophylactic antibiotics at the time of delivery to women with mitral valve prolapse.

RUBELLA

Rubella (German measles) is the most important of the viral diseases known to cause congenital anomalies in the human fetus. In the mother, it is usually a mild disease that causes fever, headache, lymphadenopathy, and a pink, confluent macular rash. The rash appears 1 week after the viremia. The peak of antibody titer follows the rash by 1 or 2 weeks. The fetus is most severely affected when the mother's viremia coincides with the period of organogenesis, or the first 16 weeks. The congenital rubella syndrome, acquired transplacentally, comprises numerous fetal abnormalities, involving the eye (cataracts, microphthalmia, and chorioretinitis), heart, ear, central nervous system, and other organs. The infants may have microcephaly, deafness, major arterial defects, and low birth weight. In addition, there may be osseous and hematologic changes and mental deficiency. Infants born with the congenital rubella syndrome may excrete the live virus.

The diagnosis of maternal rubella is suspected on the basis of clinical signs and symptoms, but confirmed by a rise in antibody titer as demonstrated by hemagglutination inhibition reactions. There is no effective therapy for the disease, but abortion is often performed to prevent birth of a malformed fetus.

The susceptible female population should be identified and vaccinated with a strain of live rubella virus. About 10% of adult women remain susceptible to rubella. Pregnant women, however, must not be immunized with live virus, and pregnancy should be interdicted for at least 3 months after active immunization of the mother.

The earlier in pregnancy the mother contracts rubella, the greater is the likelihood of congenital anomalies in the fetus. Viremia at 4 weeks' gestation is accompanied by a greater than 50% chance of fetal anomalies;

by 12 weeks the likelihood has dropped to 10%. The use of gamma globulin in the mother is controversial, because the clinical signs may be masked without affecting the viremia.

If the titer in the first hemagglutination inhibition test is positive in a 1:10 or greater dilution immediately after clinical signs of the disease, the patient may be considered immune. If it is positive only at dilutions of 1:8 or less immediately after the rash and it rises fourfold or more 10 to 14 days later, the patient very likely has had a viremia, even in the absence of clinical signs and symptoms.

The only rubella vaccine currently available in the United States is prepared from the RA 27/3 strain, a live attenuated virus. Vaccination is indicated in adult women shown to be susceptible with a titer of 1:8 or less on hemagglutination inhibition; the woman must not be pregnant and should be on reliable contraception for at least 3 months if sexually active. Rubella vaccination is not contraindicated in breast feeding mothers or in women in the same household with pregnant family members. The fetal risk in pregnancies complicated by inadvertent vaccination with rubella appears to be very low.

OTHER PERINATAL INFECTIONS

The incidences of the more common perinatal infections per number of live births are as follows: *Herpesvirus hominis,* 1:6000; toxoplasmosis, 1:1000; streptococcal infections, 1:300; cytomegalovirus, 1:75; and *Chlamydia trachomatis,* 1:35.

The TORCH syndrome may result when the fetus is infected in the first trimester. The etiologic agents are the viruses of rubella, cytomegalovirus, and herpes, and a protozoon, toxoplasma. The syndrome comprises microcephaly, chorioretinitis, cerebral calcification, and mental retardation.

Cytomegalovirus is a ubiquitous organism. As the population ages, seropositivity for the virus increases. Diagnosis is made by serologic testing of the mother. Because this is a persistent and latent virus, about 4% of subsequent pregnancies are affected. Of infants who are sick at birth, 5% die early and 85% have neurologic sequelae. Each year in the United States, about 6000 infants are born with cerebral damage and 3000 with deafness caused by cytomegalovirus. There is no effective prevention or treatment.

Herpesvirus hominis is described on page 196. This organism makes a small contribution to the TORCH syndrome, but the major infection with this virus occurs at the time of delivery, when the infant contracts the disease during passage through the birth canal. The syndrome includes gingivitis, stomatitis, keratoconjunctivitis, and encephalitis. Approximately half of the affected infants die and 60% of the survivors have long-term neurologic and ocular sequelae. There is no specific prevention or therapy for perinatal herpetic infection, although cesarean section can prevent transmission to the newborn in many but not all patients whose membranes are intact or only recently ruptured.

Toxoplasmosis is caused by the protozoon *Toxoplasma gondii,* an organism that affects many species of animals. The cat is a primary host, but in addition to cat feces, sources of the organism include raw pork, beef, and lamb. Toxoplasmosis, although deleterious to the fetus, causes only a chronic disease of low virulence in the mother. Investigation of an influenza-like syndrome in a pregnant woman should include serologic TORCH titers during both acute and convalescent phases of the illness.

Fetal infection occurs in 15% of maternal infections in the first trimester and in 25 to 60% in the second and third trimesters. Chorioretinitis, cerebral calcifications, and malformations may be the sequelae of early intrauterine infections. Fetal infection may be confirmed by culture of fetal blood after puncture of the umbilical cord or after amniocentesis in half to two thirds of acutely infected patients.

Human parvovirus-B19 is a DNA virus, which replicates in the nuclei of the late erythroid precursor cells. Its transmission is not well understood, but probable routes of spread include transfusion of blood or blood products, secretions, and vertical transmission from mother to fetus. Outbreaks are most common among school-age children, especially from midwinter through spring, but sporadic cases occur throughout the year. It is known also as fifth disease, or erythema infectiosum. A severe fetal infection may involve the myocardium and erythroid tissues, with subsequent hydrops fetalis and death in 9.2% of infected fetuses. Most fetal parvovirus infections are asymptomatic.

Infection with human immunodeficiency virus (HIV) is diagnosed reliably and indicates an underlying cellular immunodeficiency, usually resulting from a disease that affects the immune system or a drug that alters cellular immunity. The disease (AIDS) presents either as an opportunistic infection or an unusual malignant tumor. Opportunistic infections may include *Pneumocystis carinii* pneumonia, atypical mycobacterial infection, or disseminated toxoplasmosis, cryptococcosis, or other fungal infections. The most common malignant manifestation is Kaposi's sarcoma. Groups at risk for HIV infection include homosexual and bisexual men, prostitutes, users of intravenous drugs, hemophiliacs, sexual partners of high-risk people, and neonates of high-risk mothers. The period of incubation of HIV infection is 6 to 12 weeks, but clinical manifestations of the disease may not appear for 2 to 13 years. Perinatal transmission of HIV occurs in 30% of infected pregnant women. The rate of transmission after a single needle stick from an infected patient is estimated to be about 0.3%. The Western blot assay is used to detect the virus. Therapy includes zidovudine and other newer drugs that are not yet in common use. Further discussion of HIV infection is found on pp. 199–200.

Hepatitis B (HBV) is caused by a DNA virus. Vertical perinatal transmission may occur in patients with acute, chronic, or subclinical infection. Such transmission is not likely during exposure in the first trimester. Certain ethnic groups are at greater risk of chronic HBV carriage, such as Asians, Eskimos, and Haitians. Other women at risk are those who work with patients undergoing renal dialysis or with those who are mentally impaired. Prostitutes and women who use illicit drugs should be tested, as should their sexual partners. Infants born to mothers who are positive for the hepatitis B surface antigen should receive hepatitis B immunoglobulin at birth and at 3 and 6 months of age.

ANEMIA AND THROMBOCYTOPENIA

Anemia is a condition in which circulating red blood cells are deficient in number or in total hemoglobin content. It may be caused by decreased blood formation or increased blood loss or destruction. In the nonpregnant woman, anemia is defined as a hemoglobin concentration of less than 12 g/100 mL. Since there is normally a decline in hemoglobin concentration in pregnancy because of the relatively greater increase in plasma volume than in erythrocyte mass, anemia in pregnancy is defined as a hemoglobin concentration of less than 10 g/100 mL or a hematocrit of less than 30.

The most common cause (95 to 98%) of nondilutional anemia in pregnancy is iron deficiency. Its incidence is much higher in lower socioeconomic groups because of poor diet. Most women enter the reproductive age with low iron reserves because of either dietary deficiencies or blood loss from heavy menstruation. Increased requirements of pregnancy exhaust the reserves of iron and produce anemia. Therefore, supplementary iron is recommended for all prenatal patients.

Maternal complications with severe iron-deficiency anemia include dysphagia, angina pectoris, and congestive heart failure. Perinatal mortality and morbidity are also increased significantly. Diagnosis of iron deficiency depends upon demonstration of a low serum iron content and a high serum iron-binding capacity. Measurement of ferritin provides an even more sensitive index of iron deficiency. In all cases of anemia, a direct blood smear should be examined morphologically. In a mild iron-deficiency anemia, erythrocytes may appear normal. In more severe cases, however, hypochromia and microcytosis are demonstrable. Treatment is aimed at increasing the circulating hemoglobin concentration and total reserves of body iron. To this end, supplementary iron is recommended.

Treatment depends on the severity of the anemia. Ferrous sulfate (300 mg) once a day after breakfast is adequate prevention in normal pregnancy. Ferrous sulfate (300 mg) three times a day after meals may be required for anemia. Parenteral iron in the form of iron-dextran may be given if there is an intolerance to oral iron or poor absorption. A blood transfusion is reserved for only the most serious or refractory cases. Therapy is evaluated by monitoring changes in hematocrit, hemoglobin content, structure of the erythrocytes, and reticulocyte count.

Pregnancy requires about 800 mg of iron (p. 63). Since the maximum absorbed from a usual diet is 1 mg a day, supplementary iron is required. The most common cause of failure to respond to oral iron therapy is negligence in taking the daily supplement. Plural gestations require larger supplements. Occult bleeding is a less common cause. Malabsorption without underlying gastrointestinal disease is rare but may be associated with the use of antacids.

Hereditary anemias (hemoglobinopathies) are associated with increased maternal and fetal morbidity and mortality. The most severe complications are found in patients with sickle cell anemia (SS disease) and SC disease. Five percent of American blacks may have the sickle cell trait (SA), but less than 1% have the true disease (SS). Patients with sickle cell disease have an increased prevalence of infections of the urinary tract and of pneumonitis. As the anemia becomes more intense, pain crises become more common and the frequencies of abortions, stillbirths, and neonatal deaths increase.

Advances in restriction endonuclease technology have made possible the molecular analysis and prenatal diagnosis of several human genetic diseases, notably sickle cell disease and other hemoglobinopathies. Pregnant patients with SC or SS disease should receive supplemental folic acid (5 mg daily). The need for supplemental iron should be individualized.

The treatment of a crisis is oxygen, analgesics, and hydration. Patients may benefit from partial exchange transfusion. Optimally, necessary transfusions should be given before delivery and at least a liter of whole blood should be available during delivery. Since serious complications may occur during pregnancy with these hereditary anemias, family size should be limited by either sterilization or effective contraception.

Megaloblastic anemia caused by a dietary deficiency of folic acid is an uncommon cause of anemia in the United States but is reported to be important elsewhere. Signs and symptoms may include fatigue, anorexia, nausea, vomiting, diarrhea, and glossitis. The diagnosis may be made by demonstration of a low hemoglobin, macrocytosis, hypersegmented polymorphonuclear leukocytes, and a low serum folate level. Specific therapy is oral or parenteral administration of folic acid (1 to 5 mg daily). Most prenatal vitamin tablets contain 1 mg of folic acid. The relation of folic acid deficiency to abruptio placentae has not been demonstrated, nor has the value of folic acid supplementation in prevention of neural tube defects been proved.

If severe immune thrombocytopenic purpura occurs during pregnancy, prednisone (60 to 100 mg/day) should be given; the dose is then tapered to the lowest amount that will produce the desired effect. Splenectomy may be required if severe thrombocytopenia persists despite administration of steroids. Mothers with a diagnosis of autoimmune thrombocytopenic purpura (ATP) antedating pregnancy may produce antibodies in a quantity sufficient to cross the placenta and cause ATP in the fetus. The method of delivery of these fetuses is still debatable, although some authorities advocate cesarean section.

If the platelet count is greater than 100,000/mm^3 and no prior splenectomy has been performed, vaginal delivery is often recommended in the absence of obstetric contraindications. Various methods of assessing fetal platelet counts have been described. If the count is greater than 50,000/mm^3, the patient may be allowed to labor in anticipation of a vaginal delivery. If the platelet count from the fetal scalp is below 50,000/mm^3, cesarean section is often the method of choice for delivery. Percutaneous umbilical blood sampling (PUBS) has been used more recently for assessment of the fetal platelet count.

The neonate with a normal platelet count should be monitored by daily counts for a whole week. The thrombocytopenia is usually self-limited, but prednisone (1-2 mg/kg/day), a transfusion of platelets, or even an exchange transfusion may be required. Splenectomy is contraindicated in the neonatal period.

THYROID DYSFUNCTION

The normal physiologic changes in the maternal thyroid gland during pregnancy are summarized on page 45. Hyperthyroidism in pregnancy is often caused by Graves' disease, which is thought to result from autoimmune phenomena. It is often associated with long-acting thyroid stimulator (LATS), an IgG globulin, which crosses the placenta and may produce hyperthyroidism in the fetus. Signs and symptoms of hyperthyroidism include loss of weight, increased appetite, tremors, increased nervousness, and hyperreflexia. The diagnosis is supported by elevated levels of the free thyroid hormones or the free thyroxine index.

Severe hyperthyroidism during pregnancy must be treated to avoid "thyroid storm" at the time of delivery and possible fetal mortality. Therapy is difficult because antithyroid drugs such as propylthiouracil cross the placenta and may suppress the fetal thyroid. Optimal therapy of hyperthyroidism in pregnancy may be antithyroid medication and iodine to reduce the vascularity of the gland followed by partial thyroidectomy a few weeks later. Radioactive iodine should not be used during pregnancy because it crosses the placenta and is bound in the fetal thyroid.

Hypothyroidism is uncommon in pregnancy and most often results from prior operations on the thyroid or therapy with ^{131}I. Hypothyroid women may have decreased fertility and high rates of abortion and stillbirth. Diagnosis is made by failure of thyroid hormones to rise as usual in pregnancy and by elevated levels of TSH. Patients are treated with full thyroid replacement. Women who become pregnant while on thyroid hormones should receive full replacement for the duration of pregnancy, with normal levels of TSH as the therapeutic goal.

The easiest and least costly screening tests of thyroid function in pregnancy are TSH and total T_4 (TT_4) and T_3 resin uptake. The product of T_3 and T_4 is termed the free thyroxine index (T_7), which is approximately equal to free T_4 and is unchanged during pregnancy. Because of the striking increase in thyroid-binding globulin in pregnancy (an effect of increased estrogen), the concentrations of total T_3 and T_4 (both bound and free) are similarly elevated and somewhat difficult to interpret. Tests utilizing radioactive iodine are contraindicated in pregnancy. Inasmuch as the thyroid gland in pregnancy is not suppressed completely by exogenous thyroid hormone, the usefulness of thyroid suppression tests is limited.

RHEUMATIC DISEASES

The effect of pregnancy on the rheumatic diseases is variable. The group comprises systemic lupus erythematosus, rheumatoid arthritis, scleroderma, polymyositis and dermatomyositis, Sjögren's syndrome, amyloidosis, necrotizing arthritis, rheumatic fever, relapsing polychondritis, and ankylosing spondylitis. The most important rheumatic diseases that coexist with pregnancy are systemic lupus erythematosus (SLE) and rheumatoid arthritis (RA).

Most patients with SLE have normal fertility, but there are increased prevalences of abortion, stillbirth, prematurity, and small-for-dates babies, especially in patients with renal disease.

Treatment of SLE must be individualized, but generally consists of aspirin or corticosteroids. Patients with RA may have clinical remissions during pregnancy with postpartum exacerbations. RA generally has little effect on the pregnancy. Aspirin and corticosteroids are the mainstays of therapy.

Clinical estimates of the prevalence of renal involvement in SLE range from 45 to 75%. The prognosis for pregnancy in patients with lupus nephropathy is best judged by the presence or absence of signs of activity in the 6 months before conception. In the absence of such signs the fetal prognosis is good and two thirds of the mothers will remain in remission. If the SLE has been clinically active within the 6 months before conception, the perinatal loss is about 25%, signs are aggravated in about 50% of the mothers, and few undergo remissions during the pregnancy. Contrary to earlier teaching, when exacerbations occur, they do so predominantly during pregnancy rather than after abortion or delivery. Lupus anticoagulant in the plasma of a pregnant woman and anticardiolipin antibodies identify her as a patient at high risk for fetal wastage and thrombosis. There is no good evidence that therapeutic doses of prednisone or azathioprine, an immunosuppressant, are teratogenic in human pregnancy. A patient with a prolonged PTT and a history of recurrent fetal wastage should be screened for anticardiolipin antibodies and lupus anticoagulant.

THROMBOPHLEBITIS

Thrombophlebitis complicates only about 1 in 300 to 400 pregnancies, but is more common in the puerperium (p. 147). The patient may present with palpable, indurated tender cords in the lower extremities or vulva. Deep calf tenderness, tachycardia, and fever may also be found. Treatment of superficial thrombophlebitis includes bed rest, elevation of the legs, heat, and anti-inflammatory agents. If the thrombophlebitis fails to improve or worsens with the aforementioned treatment, anticoagulant therapy is indicated, usually in the form of heparin for 10 days. Coumarin derivatives, which cross the placenta, are contraindicated during most of pregnancy. In the first trimester, they may be teratogenic. In the later stages of pregnancy, particularly during labor and delivery, they may cause fetal hemorrhage, most seriously in the brain. Deep thrombophlebitis of the legs or pelvis requires heparinization. Pulmonary emboli may necessitate ligation or plication of the vena cava and ligation of the ovarian veins.

BRONCHIAL ASTHMA

Asthma is the most common obstructive pulmonary disease that coexists with pregnancy, complicating about 1% of all gestations. The effect of pregnancy on the course of asthma is difficult to predict. Approximately one third of patients with asthma react differently in subsequent pregnancies, irrespective of the sex of the fetus. The risks of perinatal morbidity and mortality are increased only minimally in the asthmatic patient, especially if adequate medical care is received. Beta-mimetic drugs are the mainstay of therapy for the pregnant asthmatic, and evidence is lacking that these drugs are teratogenic. Terbutaline, the most commonly prescribed beta-mimetic agent, is administered in the usual dosage of 2.5 to 5 mg four times a day. Aerosolized β-mimetic agents such as metaproterenol are important therapeutic additions because of their local action and lack of systemic side effects.

Corticosteroids play an important role in the management of asthma in pregnancy. They should be administered without hesitation to patients who are not controlled adequately with β-mimetic agents. Theophyllines also may be considered in the treatment. Status asthmaticus requires immediate therapy to avoid potentially life-endangering complications.

APPENDICITIS

Appendicitis is the most common acute surgical condition that complicates pregnancy. Its incidence is 1 in 2000 births. It is encountered with equal frequency in all three trimesters of pregnancy. The diagnosis is often more difficult and more likely to be delayed because the clinical presentation is altered by the symptoms and physical changes of pregnancy. Factors confusing the diagnosis are the nausea, vomiting, and abdominal discomfort of early pregnancy, the upward displacement of the appendix by the enlarging uterus, the laxity of the abdominal wall, the physiologic leukocytosis, and the elevated sedimentation rate. The signs and symptoms of appendicitis in pregnancy, however, are similar to those in nonpregnant patients. If the appendix ruptures, either peritonitis or a localized abscess may follow. For these reasons, early diagnosis and operation in all suspect cases is urgent. The differential diagnosis includes pyelonephritis, renal colic, abruptio placentae, torsion of an ovarian cyst, degenerating myoma, pancreatitis, and cholecystitis.

ACUTE CHOLECYSTITIS

Cholecystitis is more common in pregnancy, presumably because of uterine pressure, which interferes with the circulation and drainage of the gallbladder. The clinical picture is not different from that in the nonpregnant woman. The attack usually begins with biliary colic, nausea, vomiting, and tenderness in the right upper quadrant. In most cases, medical therapy suffices. Appropriate antibiotics such as cephalosporins, along with intravenous fluids, nasogastric suction, antispasmodics, and analgesics, usually lead to resolution of the acute attack within 48 hours. If obstruction of the common duct complicates the clinical picture, cholecystectomy or cholecystotomy should be performed without delay.

TRAUMA

Uterine injury as a result of trauma is highly unlikely in early pregnancy, but later in pregnancy the uterus becomes an abdominal organ, which is injured more easily. The fetus is usually well protected by its cushion of amniotic fluid, but placental separation may occur as a result of a direct blow or hypovolemic shock. Traumatic injuries should be managed as necessary for the mother, with care to minimize damage to the fetus.

ANXIETY AND DEPRESSION

The psychologic reactions of women during childbirth include the common, relatively mild, and transient "maternity blues" (50 to 70% incidence); the more prolonged affective disorders that are regarded as postpartum depressions (10 to 15% incidence); and true puerperal psychosis (0.14 to 0.26% incidence). Although etiologic factors in this spectrum of psychologic complications are known but poorly, they cannot be said to form continuum of progressively severe manifestations of a single underlying disorder. The most common psychologic manifestations during pregnancy include a transient state of fearfulness, anxiety, irritation, and restlessness, described collectively as maternity blues or postpartum blues. This common response of the parturient very likely can be considered normal. It occurs mainly within the first week after delivery and usually disappears by the tenth postpartum day. Because the syndrome is transient and of short duration, no treatment is indicated. Anticipatory explanation and a sympathetic attitude on the part of the family members and the obstetrical team are important in averting or ameliorating these troublesome but common complaints.

Postpartum depression may occur in 3 to 34% of parturients, for as long as 1 year after delivery. No association has been found with later depression, social class, marital status, or parity. There is a high risk of recurrence in subsequent pregnancies. Furthermore, 20 to 30% of postpartum depression occurs in women who had a previous depressive reaction unassociated with pregnancy. The signs and symptoms of postpartum depression are not different from those in the nonpregnant patient. Tricyclic antidepressants are useful in treatment of this disorder.

A psychosis specific to postpartum women has been described. Its signs and symptoms in general do not differ from those of acute nonpuerperal psychosis, but the frequency of symptoms differs substantially. Most patients with puerperal psychosis are manic-depressive, with confusion and disorientation figuring prominently in the clinical presentation. Postpartum psychosis is said to carry a prognosis more favorable than that occurring in the nonpuerperal state, and it frequently lasts only 2 to 3 months. All patients with puerperal psychosis require hospitalization at least for the initial evaluation and initiation of therapy, which should be supervised by an experienced psychiatrist.

The effects of drugs and alcohol on pregnancy are discussed on pages 63–67.

14
CHAPTER

HYPERTENSIVE AND RENAL DISORDERS

A figure for the combined incidences of the various hypertensive disorders in pregnancy is unavailable, but it is estimated frequently to be between 5% and 15%. It varies among different populations and chiefly with the observation and recording of blood pressures, urine analyses, careful physical examinations, and the diagnostic criteria. The hypertensive disorders are major causes of maternal and fetal morbidity and mortality. They are often associated with spontaneous or iatrogenic premature delivery, which leads to an increased rate of neonatal death.

CHRONIC HYPERTENSION

Presumably, pregnant women may have any of the forms of hypertension that are found in nonpregnant women. Essential hypertension accounts for about 85% of the cases. Characteristically, pregnant women have decreases in diastolic blood pressure that average about 10 mm Hg in early and midpregnancy. The decrease is often exaggerated in hypertensive women, and many, even those with severe hypertension, may be normotensive when first seen. Typically, the pressure rises in the third trimester and gives the false impression of an acute onset of hypertension.

Most women with uncomplicated chronic hypertension do well in pregnancy, al-

though there is an increased risk of intrauterine death of mature fetuses. The real hazard is the risk of superimposed preeclampsia, to which such women are predisposed. The diagnosis of superimposed preeclampsia is made by the specific increases in blood pressure together with proteinuria.

PREECLAMPSIA-ECLAMPSIA

Preeclampsia-eclampsia, characterized by hypertension, edema, and proteinuria, characteristically develops after the twentieth week of gestation and appears with increasing frequency as pregnancy progresses. Hypertension and at least one of the other signs are required for the diagnosis. Eclampsia is preeclampsia with convulsions, which may occur ante partum, intra partum, or post partum. The cause of preeclampsia is still unknown, although numerous hypotheses have been advanced. It is predominantly a disorder of primigravidas, or more accurately, nulliparas. The diagnosis in multiparas is likely to be erroneous, and when it does occur, there usually is some predisposing factor. Preeclampsia is often confused with essential hypertension or renal disease, either latent and revealed by pregnancy, or frank but unobserved because the patient was not seen until late in gestation. A blood pressure of 140/90 or higher before the twentieth week suggests chronic hypertension antedating pregnancy. Preeclampsia may be superimposed on chronic hypertension. Gestational (pregnancy-induced) hypertension without either proteinuria or edema and with disappearance after delivery is called transient.

Gestational (transient) hypertension is highly likely to recur in some or all later pregnancies and has been the usual basis for the erroneous diagnosis of preeclampsia in multiparas. Gestational hypertension, especially in primigravidas, may occasionally be incipient preeclampsia, but more often it is a sign of latent essential hypertension unmasked by pregnancy.

Pregnancy is a screening test for future hypertension. Gestational hypertension indicates a great likelihood of future chronic hypertension, probably of early onset. Normotensive pregnancies are predictive of a greatly reduced likelihood of hypertension; furthermore, if hypertension develops subsequently, it will be less severe because the age of onset will be greater than the average for all women. Preeclamptic and eclamptic hypertension have no remote prognostic significance because women destined to become chronically hypertensive are neither more nor less likely to develop preeclampsia than are women in general. Except for the intercurrent preeclampsia, the woman may have had either normotension or transient hypertension.

A major aim of prenatal care is to detect incipient preeclampsia early in its course, for its progression to eclampsia usually can be prevented. Although the only specific treatment is termination of pregnancy, early signs are treated by bed rest. Restriction of sodium, which has been part of the management of preeclampsia for many years, is often recommended although there is no proof that it is beneficial, particularly in the mild forms of the syndrome. The objectives are to prevent convulsions and to salvage the infant with minimal trauma to the mother. With bed rest, the blood pressure, weight, and proteinuria should decrease. If they do not and the patient is within 4 weeks of term, delivery is desirable. If the patient is several weeks from term and the preeclampsia is mild, temporization may be justified. The diagnosis of "mild" pre-

eclampsia must never lead to complacency. Nearly 25% of women who develop eclampsia have apparently mild preeclampsia until the onset of convulsions, and some of them die. The risks of allowing the pregnancy to continue include aggravation of the preeclampsia, convulsions, fetal death, and abruptio placentae. Signs and symptoms of aggravation call for delivery despite prematurity.

Antihypertensive drugs are used only if the hypertension is so severe as to be dangerous in itself, as with a diastolic pressure sustained at 100 to 110 mm Hg. Reduction of maternal blood pressure, however, will probably decrease uterine blood flow, which is at most half of normal in hypertensive pregnancies. The fetus will thus be deprived of its supply of nutrition. Therefore, the diastolic pressure should not be reduced below 85 to 90 mm Hg. Hydralazine is the drug of choice in preeclamptic hypertension. An anticonvulsant agent, preferably parenteral magnesium sulfate, is used in the treatment of severe preeclampsia and eclampsia. It is used also in patients with moderately severe preeclampsia at the onset of spontaneous or induced labor. In eclampsia, oxygen should be administered and digitalis given at the onset of pulmonary edema. It is traditional practice that, as soon as the patient is conscious and oriented, labor be induced or cesarean section performed. Similarly, in patients with severe preeclampsia, pregnancy should be terminated as soon as the clinical condition is stable. Some recent studies have shown, however, that in the presence of fetal immaturity and the absence of maternal hepatic dysfunction, coagulopathy, and renal compromise, expectant management can be attempted. Other senior investigators believe, however, that temporization to gain fetal maturity in the face of severe preeclampsia is always risky. Furthermore, the patient is most likely to be a young nullipara whose later pregnancies are likely to be far less complicated. Usually the uterus is sensitive to oxytocin and labor can be induced even with an "unfavorable" cervix, but cesarean section may be preferable if vaginal delivery does not appear easy and imminent. Anticonvulsant therapy should be continued for at least 24 hours after delivery. Convulsions are associated with a significant increase in maternal mortality and perinatal loss; a major factor in perinatal loss is prematurity.

Patients with severe preeclampsia are at risk for water intoxication if oxytocin is given in 5% dextrose or a similar salt-free solution. The antidiuretic effect of oxytocin is evident even in doses too low to affect uterine contractions. Patients tend to lie supine, furthermore, a position that greatly reduces urinary output.

Hypertension is a sustained rise, over the usual levels, of 30 mm Hg in the systolic or 15 in the diastolic readings, or a sustained pressure of 140/90 or higher. "Sustained" means on at least two occasions 6 or more hours apart. Generalized edema, rather than pedal edema, is a diagnostic sign, although it occurs in many normal pregnant women. Proteinuria means one plus or more.

In superimposed preeclampsia, diagnosed by the specified increases in blood pressure together with proteinuria, the perinatal loss is four times as great as in either preeclampsia or chronic hypertension alone, and there is a severalfold increase in abruptio placentae. Low socioeconomic status and geographic and racial differences are alleged to be factors in the development of preeclampsia, although proof is lacking. There is strong evidence that a single recessive gene may determine the development of the disorder. The frequency of the putative gene appears to be about 25%. If the sister of a nulliparous patient had preeclampsia-eclampsia, the patient has a 37% chance of developing the syndrome; if her mother was affected, she has a 25% chance; and if her grandmother was affected, she has a 16% chance, assuming an incidence of preeclampsia of about 6% in the population in general.

In differential diagnosis, chronic hypertension rather than preeclampsia is suggested by (1) previous hypertensive pregnancy, (2) multiparity, (3) retinal angiosclerosis, or hemorrhages and exudates, (4) cardiomegaly, (5) exorbitant hypertension, and (6) little or no proteinuria.

Factors predisposing to preeclampsia are (1) nulliparity, (2) familial history of preeclampsia-eclampsia, (3) plural gestation, (4) diabetes, (5) chronic hypertension, (6) hydatidiform mole, with which preeclampsia may occur as early as the fourteenth week, (7) fetal hydrops, (8) extremes of age, and (9) collagen vascular diseases.

Inconstant signs of incipient preeclampsia are gains of three or more pounds per week, increasing edema of the hands and face, and a trend to rise in blood pressure. Occasionally the onset of preeclampsia is explosive. The presence of one or more of the following marks preeclampsia as severe: (1) sustained blood pressure of 160/100 or higher, (2) proteinuria of more than 5 g/liter, (3) urinary output of less than 400 ml/24 hours, (4) cerebral or visual disturbances, and (5) cyanosis or pulmonary edema. Others are hemoconcentration, epigastric pain, coagulopathy, and increases of certain hepatic enzymes in the plasma (e.g., SGOT, SGPT, and lactic dehydrogenase). Whether hyperreflexia also indicates severe preeclampsia is not certain.

Magnesium sulfate is given intravenously as an initial dose of 3 or 4 g in 10% solution, followed by either (a) continuous infusion of 1 to 2 g or more/hour or (b) 10 g in 50% solution by deep intramuscular injection, with later injections of 5 g doses at intervals of 4 hours. The initial dose is safe, but subsequent doses, or the continuous infusion, may not be unless (1) the knee jerk is active, (2) the urinary output is at least 100 mL/4 hours, and (3) the respiratory rate is 12 or more/minute. Dosage of magnesium sulfate should be adjusted to maintain a plasma level of magnesium between 4 and 6 mg/dL. Calcium gluconate, 10 mL of 10% solution, is an antidote to magnesium toxicity and should always be available. If the urinary output falls below 20 mL/hour, mannitol is infused but not repeated unless the urinary volume rises to about 100 mL/hour. Furosemide may be given intravenously (but it is usually contraindicated, as are all diuretics) for pulmonary edema.

Thiazides are best avoided in pregnancy. Adverse effects of these drugs, particularly in preeclampsia, include further depletion of an already diminished plasma volume, hypokalemia and hyponatremia, hemorrhagic pancreatitis, depression of placental function, and in the newborn, thrombocytopenia.

Complications of preeclampsia and eclampsia include restriction of fetal growth, abruptio placentae, acute renal failure, thrombocytopenia, cerebrovascular accidents, hemolysis, jaundice; and rarely, disseminated intravascular coagulation (DIC), retinal detachment, hepatic rupture, and trauma incurred during convulsions. The major causes of maternal death in eclampsia and superimposed preeclampsia are cerebral hemorrhage and cardiac failure. The combination of hemolysis, elevated liver enzymes, and low platelets has been designated the HELLP syndrome, which carries a grave prognosis.

Anatomic lesions in fatal cases of eclampsia are widespread arteriolitis, thrombosis of small vessels, hemorrhage, and necrosis. A characteristic but not wholly specific renal lesion is found in biopsies from preeclamptic women; the glomerular capillary endothelial cells are swollen, there is an increase in size and possibly number of mesangial cells, and fibrin derivatives are deposited, accounting partially for the reduction in renal blood flow and the still greater decrease in glomerular filtration.

Another characteristic but not entirely pathognomonic lesion is found in the uterine arteries in the placental bed. In preeclampsia, as opposed to normal pregnancy, the "physiologic" dilation of the uterine arteries is restricted to the decidual segments and there is an atherotic change in the vessels. Similar lesions have recently been described, however, in nonpreeclamptic pregnancies complicated by restriction of intrauterine growth and in cases of chronic hypertension.

The fundamental derangements are an abnormally large retention of sodium and arteriolar spasm. There is no good evidence that diuretics and limitations of weight gain and sodium intake prevent preeclampsia; once severe preeclampsia has developed, however, restriction of sodium seems to be beneficial. The arterioles are sensitized to pressor substances, but no such agent has been identified as causing preeclamptic hypertension. Despite the generalized vasoconstriction, the total blood flows to most regions of the body are often normal or nearly so. In normal pregnancy, the placenta produces equivalent amounts of thromboxane and prostacyclin, but in preeclamptic pregnancy, the placental production of thromboxane is 7 times that of prostacyclin. The result is vasoconstriction, with reduction in placental blood flow. Low-dose aspirin has been used to increase the ratio of prostacyclin to thromboxane. Recent data suggest that endothelial damage is responsible for the manifestations of preeclampsia.

Almost the only helpful laboratory tests are serial measurements of proteinuria, which increases with severity, and of the hematocrit as an index to the hemoconcentration occurring in severe preeclampsia and eclampsia. Progressive or irreversible hemoconcentration, low platelet counts, and elevated hepatic enzymes denote a bad prognosis. Hyperuricemia supports the diagnosis of preeclampsia. Significant increases in blood or plasma creatinine point to renal disease.

Ambulatory treatment of severe preeclampsia is unsatisfactory. A patient with minimal signs may be treated at home, but must be seen 2 or 3 times each week. Once the diagnosis seems definite, she should be in the hospital. A convulsion in a pregnant woman must be regarded as eclampsia until proved otherwise. Among conditions to be differentiated are epilepsy, lesions in the central nervous system, and water intoxication. The edema and usually the proteinuria clear within a few days after delivery. In half the cases, the blood pressure returns to normal within 10 days but may be unstable for as long as 6 months. In the other half, the pressure subsides more slowly, but unless the patient has underlying hypertension, it will return to normal within a few weeks.

About one third of primigravidas with preeclampsia-eclampsia have a recurrence of hypertension in later pregnancies, usually without more than mild increases; such women are likely to develop essential hypertension later. The recurrence is usually merely transient hypertension, but roughly 10 to 15% may have recurrent preeclampsia or eclampsia. It is improbable that preeclampsia-eclampsia causes so-called residual hypertension. The earlier the onset of preeclampsia, the more likely there is to be some underlying predisposing factor, such as renal disease, and the greater the likelihood of recurrent preeclampsia in later pregnancies.

PYELONEPHRITIS

Acute pyelonephritis is the most common renal disease in pregnancy. It is usually bilateral, although the right side is said to be affected more often than the left. The onset, which is frequently abrupt, is heralded by fever, chills, and flank pain. Because it is an ascending infection, it may be preceded by signs and symptoms of lower urinary tract infection, such as dysuria, frequency, and urgency. Diagnosis is made on the basis of leukocytes and bacteria in the urine in the presence of suggestive clinical findings. Antibiotic therapy, directed against the common pathogens, is usually begun empirically. Cultures and sensitivity tests are performed to confirm the correct choice or to indicate the necessary change of antibiotic. The organisms implicated most commonly are *Escherichia coli,* Klebsiella, Proteus, Pseudomonas, and other gram-negative bacilli.

Antibiotic therapy should be intensive and continuous for at least 10 days because persistent or recurrent pyelonephritis may lead to permanent renal damage. Therapy should not be discontinued until two successive sterile urine cultures are obtained. Suppressive therapy after a single bout of pyelonephritis may be indicated throughout the duration of pregnancy. Ampicillin (0.5 g q.i.d.) was formerly the most frequently employed first drug, but resistance to that antibiotic appears to be increasing. Ampicillin with sulbactam, a cephalosporin, or a combination of ampicillin and gentamicin provides popular alternative initial antibiotic coverage. The antimicrobial drugs cross the placenta, and most of them may affect the fetus. If there is no response to antibiotics, a urologic investigation, including cystoscopy, is indicated. An intravenous pyelogram may be indicated post partum to rule out obstructive uropathy or a urologic anomaly.

Dilation of the ureters and renal pelves and decrease in peristalsis, primarily as a result of the hormonal changes of pregnancy, predispose to urinary stasis. Increased renal excretion of glucose and amino acids, furthermore, provides a medium for favorable growth of bacteria. Introduction of bacteria into the bladder (bacilluria) leads to cystitis, which may progress as an ascending infection to involve the ureters and kidneys. Routine catheterization of the bladder in pregnant women is therefore to be avoided.

Bacteriuria is defined as 10^5 or more colony counts per mL of urine in a clean midstream specimen. About 6 to 7% of pregnant patients have asymptomatic bacteriuria; of these women about one quarter, or 1 to 2% of all gravidas, subsequently develop pyelonephritis. It is believed that pyelonephritis, but not necessarily asymptomatic bacteriuria, leads to an increase in the rate of prematurity. Despite the cost of screening for asymptomatic bacteriuria, it is recommended so that appropriate antibacterial therapy may be instituted to minimize the risk of pyelonephritis.

Sulfonamides, such as sulfisoxazole, and ampicillin have been used widely on an outpatient basis for mild urinary tract infections. Sulfonamides, by competing with bilirubin for albumin binding and conjugation by glucuronyl transferase, may cause jaundice and kernicterus in the newborn, particularly the premature. They are not recommended during the first and third trimesters. The first-generation cephalosporins have become popular because of emerging resistance of *E. coli* and Klebsiella to ampicillin.

Aminoglycosides such as gentamicin and kanamycin may be ototoxic and nephrotoxic to the mother. Tetracyclines administered to the mother in the third trimester may lead to discoloration of the infant's deciduous teeth, and, rarely, may cause jaundice in the mother. Administered in the first trimester, tetracyclines may cause micromelia and other skeletal deformities. Chloramphenicol may produce the "gray baby syndrome" and, rarely, bone marrow depression in the mother. Nitrofurantoin should be used only for mild infections or for maintenance after the primary infection has been eradicated by an antibiotic. Such maintenance should be continued on a daily basis throughout pregnancy. In patients with a glucose-6-phosphate dehydrogenase deficiency, nitrofurantoin may cause hemolysis. Methenamine mandelate is inadequate therapy for frank pyelonephritis. The newer quinolones are contraindicated in pregnancy because of their possible adverse effect on developing cartilage.

CHRONIC RENAL DISEASES

The most common chronic renal disease in pregnancy is "glomerulonephritis," a broad term applied to several entities. Others include nephrosclerosis, interstitial nephritis, pyelonephritis, and a scattering of less common disorders. In general, if the plasma concentration of creatinine is less than 1.5 mg/dL, pregnancies are likely to be successful, with no lasting adverse effect on the course of the disease. Higher levels of creatinine indicate advanced renal impairment, which is associated with increased fetal loss and often a significant aggravation and progression of the maternal disease. The degree of hypertension is a significant determinant of perinatal mortality. The normotensive nephrotic syndrome entails almost no increased loss.

15
CHAPTER
RH-ISOIMMUNIZATION

Pregnancy may initiate immunologic sensitization of a mother to tissues of her fetus. The usual cause of isoimmunization is the Rh factor. In this situation, an Rh-negative mother is sensitized by transfer of fetal erythrocytes to the maternal circulation, usually at the time of delivery but occasionally earlier in pregnancy. The Rh-positive fetal cells enter the maternal circulation through breaks in the placenta. Sensitization may also be produced by transfusion of Rh-positive cells into an Rh-negative mother. In both cases, the maternal anti-Rh antibodies are transferred back to the fetus and cause hemolysis. An Rh-negative mother should have serial titers during pregnancy. The antibody titers are not good indications of the severity of erythroblastosis but provide a good screening test. Once the indirect Coombs' test is positive in a titer of higher than 1:16, an amniotic fluid analysis (amniocentesis) must be done to detect the bilirubin levels.

OBSTETRIC MANAGEMENT

In a sensitized mother, obstetric management is directed toward improvement of fetal survival. The management and prognosis of the fetus are related to the amniotic fluid analysis and to the histories of prior pregnancies. The unsensitized Rh-negative mother should receive 300 μg of anti-D (Rho) gamma globulin (RhoGAM) intramuscularly within 72 hours of premature or term delivery if her infant is Rh-positive or if its blood type is unknown. Rh-immune globulin likewise should be administered after abortion, ectopic pregnancy, or amniocentesis. After a large transplacental hemorrhage or a mismatched transfusion of blood, more than 300 μg may be required. A dose of 300 μg protects against a hemorrhage of 15 mL of D-positive erythrocytes or 30 mL of fetal blood. Whether Rh-immune globulin is needed after delivery of a hydatidiform mole is still debatable. All Rh-negative mothers must have fetal cord blood tested after abortion or delivery to assess the fetal Rh-status and the presence of sensitivity. Administration of Rh-immunoglobulin to Rh-negative women in the third trimester at 28 weeks' gestation further reduces the likelihood of isoimmunization of the fetus in subsequent pregnancies.

In each pregnancy, the mother should have blood group and Rh-type tested and an irregular antibody screen performed as early as practicable. The woman who is Rho(D)-negative but not Rho(D)-isoimmunized should have anti-D antibody tests repeated at 28, 32, and 36 weeks' gestation. If the tests show no anti-D antibody, she should receive Rh-immunoglobulin after delivery; if the tests are positive, she should be managed as an Rho(D)-sensitized mother. The most common cause of Rho(D)-isoimmunization is the delivery of an Rho(D)- or (D^u)-positive infant by an Rho(D)-negative mother. Rho(D^u)-antigen is a weakly reacting Rh-antigen. When an Rho(D)-negative woman, whether D^u-positive or D^u-negative, delivers an Rho(D)- or D^u-positive infant, she should receive Rh-immunoglobulin after delivery.

The first pregnancy in an Rh-negative woman who has not received a transfusion of incompatible blood usually produces an unaffected child. With each successive pregnancy with an Rh-positive fetus, the prognosis becomes worse. A history of prior Rh-disease or a positive maternal antibody titer requires amniocentesis at 26 weeks to detect levels of bilirubin derivatives. An optical density graph of the amniotic fluid is prepared and the peak at 450 nm is read (Fig. 15–1).

If the graph indicates isoimmunization with hemolysis before 34 weeks, an intrauterine transfusion may be required. Later in gestation, early delivery and exchange transfusion are preferable. Because of gross prematurity, intrauterine transfusion is appropriate therapy only after the twenty-fifth week. After the thirty-second week, premature delivery is safer and more appropriate. Intrauterine transfusion thus finds its great-

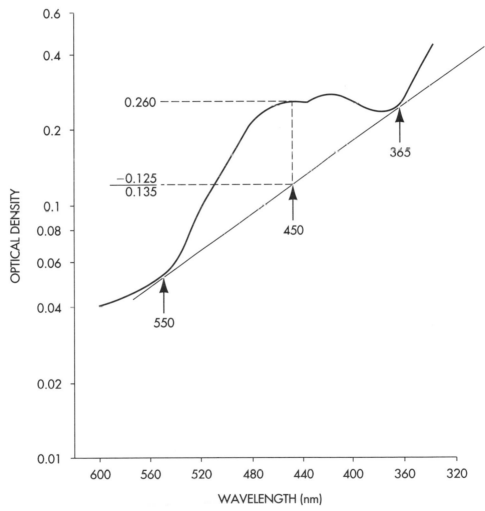

FIG. 15–1. Graph showing optical density of amniotic fluid plotted against wavelength. Note the peak at 450 nm.

est place between the twenty-fifth and thirty-second weeks of pregnancy.

The terms Rh-positive (DD or Dd) and Rh-negative (dd) refer essentially to the presence or absence, respectively, of the antigen D, although other isoantigens such as C and c or E and e may be involved.

FETAL COMPLICATIONS

Not all Rh-incompatibility results in hemolytic disease of the newborn (erythroblastosis or isoimmunization). ABO-incompatibility may protect against Rh-disease. Hemolytic disease on the basis of major blood group incompatibilities is uncommon because of the wide distribution of fetal A and B antigens, as a result of which antibodies are bound elsewhere than the erythrocytes. Type O women have anti-A and anti-B antibodies, which hemolyze A and B erythrocytes before maternal sensitization to the Rh-antigens takes place.

Intrauterine death with isoimmunization may occur with cardiac failure, edema (hydrops), and ascites. The neonate may have anemia, hyperbilirubinemia, and kernic-

terus. The placenta in hydropic forms of erythroblastosis is large. The Langhans layer is prominent, and nucleated erythrocytes are found in fetal vessels (Fig. 15–2). The fetus is not jaundiced because the placenta clears its plasma of bilirubin.

In hemolytic disease of the newborn, prompt clamping of the umbilical cord is recommended and the end is left long for possible exchange transfusions. A positive direct Coombs' test on the cord blood means an affected fetus. A hemoglobin level less than 10 g or an unconjugated bilirubin value greater than 5 mg suggests the possible need for exchange transfusion. The bilirubin level should be kept below 20 mg%. Phototherapy is useful to decrease the bilirubin.

Nonimmune fetal hydrops may be caused by cardiovascular disorders (arrhythmias and structural defects), congenital infections, chromosomal anomalies, and the twin-to-twin transfusion syndrome. It may result also from pulmonary and renal disorders of the fetus, placental thrombosis and angiomas, and maternal diabetes mellitus or pregnancy-induced hypertension. A significant proportion of nonimmune fetal hy-

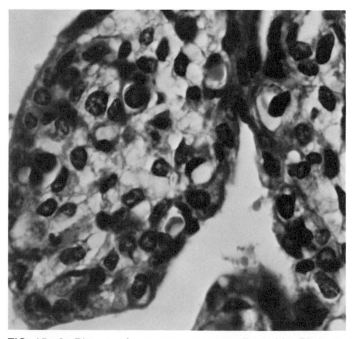

FIG. 15–2. Placenta from pregnancy complicated by Rh-isoimmunization (erythroblastosis fetalis), showing nucleated erythrocytes in fetal vessels.

drops is idiopathic. Ultrasound is the key to prenatal diagnosis.

Under ultrasonic guidance, the umbilical cord can be punctured and its blood sampled. With percutaneous umbilical blood sampling (PUBS), the umbilical vein is punctured near the insertion of the cord onto the placenta. Fetal blood thus obtained can be analyzed for hemoglobin and hematocrit, mean corpuscular volume, ABO and Rh status, and direct Coombs reaction. If the hematocrit is below 25, intravascular transfusion can be performed through the same catheter. Before resorting to PUBS, it is appropriate to test the father's zygosity (Rh-negative or homozygous or heterozygous Rh-positive) and the presence or absence of atypical blood groups. If the father is Rh-negative, further evaluation is unnecessary. If the father is heterozygous Rh-positive, there is a 50% chance that the fetus may carry the antigen and thus may be at risk for hemolytic disease. If the father is homozygous for the Rh-antigen, the fetus may be assumed to be isoimmunized and serial amniocenteses are performed to detect derivatives of bilirubin (see Fig. 15–1). As prophylaxis with Rh-immune globulin has reduced the prevalence of isoimmunization to that antigen, the atypical blood groups have become relatively more important. The antigens most frequently encountered are Kell, Lewis, and Duffy.

16
CHAPTER
PLURAL GESTATIONS

Plural gestations (twins and higher multiples) occur in more than 1% of all pregnancies. The fetuses may lie in any combination of presentations. Initial diagnosis or confirmation of clinical findings may be made by sonography (Fig. 16–1). The prevalences of hydramnios, preeclampsia, maternal anemia, and prematurity are increased with plural gestation. The second twin should be delivered within 15 to 30 minutes of the first twin. After delivery of the first infant, the uterine end of its cord should be clamped. Oxytocin and blood should be available in such situations to prevent or combat postpartum hemorrhage, which may complicate any pregnancy with an overdistended uterus.

TYPES OF TWINNING

The rate of monovular twinning is constant in all maternal age groups and races. Dizygotic (binovular, fraternal) twins are more common in the black population. With twins, the uterus is usually larger, and more than the usual number of fetal small parts may be palpated. Two fetal heartbeats differing by more than 10 beats per minute suggest twins. The infants in plural gestation usually deliver before term. Death of one or both twins during labor or delivery may result from operative interference, prolapse of the cord, or premature separation of the placenta.

When the morula splits during the first 4 days of gestation, dichorionic diamnionic twins develop. The placentas may fuse or remain separate. When the blastocyst splits at a later stage before implantation, during the first week of gestation, the twins develop a common chorion but two separate amnions. The single placenta resulting therefrom is monochorionic diamnionic. When the blastocyst splits after implantation, during the second week of gestation, the amnion will have already differentiated and monochorionic monoamnionic twins develop.

Monochorial twinning may lead to the transfusion syndrome, with the donor twin malnourished and the recipient twin plethoric. Monoamnionic twins may have knotted cords, which may lead to death of one or both fetuses. Twins have a greater prevalence of vasa previa and velamentous insertions of the cord, which may result in injuries to the umbilical vessels and fetal hemorrhage. In vasa previa, the umbilical vessels traverse the lower uterine segment in advance of the presenting part. Rupture of the membranes in cases of vasa previa may result in laceration of the fetal vessels with fetal hemorrhage or death. In cases of

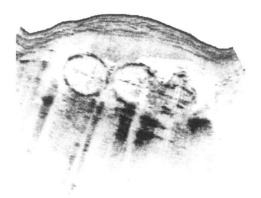 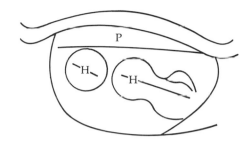

FIG. 16–1. Longitudinal sonogram showing twin intrauterine gestation. The two fetal heads (H) are identified. The torso of one fetus and the placenta (P) are also visible.

velamentous insertion of the cord into the fetal membranes, the umbilical vessels course between amnion and chorion unprotected by Wharton's jelly.

MANAGEMENT OF PLURAL GESTATION

If the outcome of plural gestation is to improve, the problems of recognition and management of fetal growth restriction and premature delivery must be solved. Early detection of twins or higher multiples results in improved perinatal outcome. Prior to the widespread use of obstetric ultrasound, fewer than 50% of plural gestations were recognized before the end of pregnancy. Today, with ultrasonic detection and referral to a specialized tertiary obstetric service, the results with plural gestation are improved. Patients with twins or higher multiples should be advised to obtain additional rest. Examinations by ultrasound should be performed every 3 weeks beginning at the twenty-sixth week of gestation to monitor the growth of the fetuses. If restriction of growth is detected, antenatal monitoring such as the nonstress test is indicated beginning at the thirty-fourth week of gestation. The method and timing of the delivery are based on the presentations of the twins, the gestational age, the superimposition of maternal or fetal complications (such as preeclampsia), the experience of the obstetrician, and the availability of expert anesthesiologic and neonatal care. With viable triplets and higher multiples, the method of choice for delivery is usually cesarean section.

17

CHAPTER

DYSTOCIA

Dystocia (difficult labor or failure to progress in parturition) is caused by one of three main factors or combinations of them: abnormalities of uterine contractions (uterine dysfunction); abnormalities of size, presentation, or development of the fetus; and abnormalities of pelvic size or architecture. Relative pelvic contraction is often associated with uterine dysfunction. Together they are the most common cause of dystocia.

Management of all forms of dystocia includes clinical assessment of pelvic dimensions and architecture, electronic monitoring of the strength of uterine contractions, careful clinical observation and recording of the progress of labor (effacement and dilatation of the cervix and station of the presenting part), and electronic monitoring of fetal well-being by continuous recording of the fetal heart rate. If the diagnosis of cephalopelvic disproportion is made, stimulation by oxytocin is contraindicated and a cesarean section is performed.

UTERINE DYSFUNCTION

Uterine dysfunction may result from subnormal or abnormal contractions. Subnormal (weak or infrequent) contractions are the most frequent indication for stimulation by oxytocin. In abnormal contractions, there is a lack of fundal dominance (gradient from top to bottom of the uterus) or asynchrony of uterine contractions. Uterine dysfunction is most commonly confused with false labor, which requires no treatment. Primary uterine dysfunction is present from the onset of labor. It is essentially a prolongation of the latent phase of the first stage of labor. Prolongation of either the first or the second stage increases perinatal mortality. Secondary dysfunction usually occurs after labor has begun normally. It results from an overdistended uterus, disproportion, premature administration of anesthesia and analgesia, and maternal exhaustion. Secondary dysfunction is usually associated with contractions that are subnormal in amplitude or frequency. It is often designated hypotonic, although the term is physiologically inaccurate. Hypertonic dysfunction is often primary and the contractions are abnormal, with a reversal of gradient or asynchrony of impulses from the cornua. There may possibly be emotional factors in the causation of uterine dysfunction. Graphs of normal and abnormal patterns of labor are shown in Figure 17–1.

True labor should not be diagnosed until the cervix has reached at least 3 cm dilatation. During an effective uterine contraction, the uterus cannot be indented. Pain is

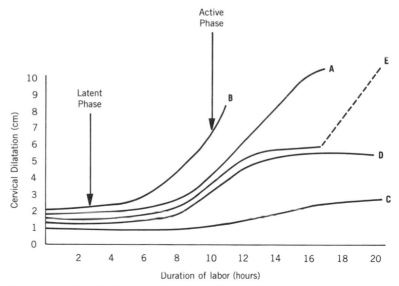

FIG. 17–1. A. Normal labor in primigravida; B. Normal labor in multipara; C. Prolonged latent phase (primary dysfunction); D. Prolonged active phase (secondary dysfunction); E. Effect of oxytocin on secondary dysfunction (dotted line).

not a good indication of the effectiveness of labor. In the latent phase, effacement may occur without much cervical dilatation.

Subnormal uterine contractions complicate about 4% of all labors. The strength of a uterine contraction is best measured by means of an intrauterine catheter. Fetal distress occurs late; oxytocin is specific therapy; and rest is of no value.

Hypertonic uterine dysfunction complicates about 1% of all labors. It involves mostly the latent phase and may appear to be painful out of proportion to the stage of labor. Fetal distress occurs early. Oxytocin is probably of no value, but rest and sedation for a short period of time may be tried before resorting to cesarean section.

In the management of subnormal uterine contractions, it is important to prepare a timetable of action, which includes precise objectives to be achieved by specific points in time. A cesarean section is indicated when these objectives are not met or when disproportion is discovered. The pelvic measurements, cervical dilatation, and fetal station and position must be known precisely. When using oxytocin the physician should remain with the patient, electronically monitoring the fetal cardiac rate and uterine contractions and recording the maternal

vital signs. An intravenous infusion of crystalloid and water must be started and the solution of oxytocin (10 units/liter) run into the tubing of the first infusion. The infusion should be started slowly and increased to a maximum of 20 to 30 milliunits per minute, preferably with control by an accurate pump. Higher concentrations are unnecessary and potentially dangerous. When used for proper indications, oxytocin is effective at low concentrations and after only a short period of infusion. The intravenous route is the only accurate, safe, and easily controlled method of administering oxytocin. Prostaglandins also have been used successfully for stimulation of labor in other countries, but ergot alkaloids and other drugs should not be used for this purpose.

A long latent period may be defined as 20 hours in the primigravida and 14 hours in the multigravida. During the active phase the cervix normally dilates at the rate of about 1.2 cm per hour in the primigravida and 1.5 cm in the multipara. A minimal pressure of 15 mm Hg is required for an effective contraction. The pressure exerted during an average uterine contraction is about 50 mm Hg.

Contraindications to oxytocin are absolute and relative. Absolute contraindications include fetopelvic disproportion and transverse lie. Relative contraindications include advanced age (over 35 years), high parity (greater than 5), and overdistension of the uterus (as with twins and hydramnios). If doubt about the propriety of using oxytocin in a particular situation remains, it is safer to avoid using the drug.

ABNORMAL PRESENTATIONS

Fetal causes of dystocia include excessive size or malpresentations of a normal-sized infant (for example, transverse lie at term in a normal pelvis). This group also includes fetal anomalies such as hydrocephalus, double monsters, and fetal tumors. Fetal causes of dystocia are managed by cesarean section as soon as the diagnosis is made.

Breech presentation, in which the sacrum or one or both feet may be the presenting part, occurs in 3 to 4% of all pregnancies at term. A breech presentation should be suspected on the basis of physical examination (abdominal and pelvic). The suspicion is usually confirmed sonographically. Since the largest part of the fetus (the head) passes through the pelvis last, the route of delivery (abdominal or vaginal) must be decided early, for there can be no trial of labor. Complications of breech presentation include increased incidence of prolapse of the cord and increased perinatal mortality and morbidity. Cesarean section is indicated in all cases of breech presentation with pelvic contraction or oversized fetus (estimated weight greater than 3500 g). Fetal weight is estimated sonographically by measuring the biparietal diameter of the fetal head and the abdominal circumference or by measuring fetal femoral length and abdominal circumference. Since the breech often does not fit the pelvis well, the likelihood of premature rupture of the membranes is increased. A vaginal examination should be performed immediately after this event to rule out prolapse of the cord. Premature rupture of the membranes should be managed aggressively (p. 143) to minimize intrauterine infection and perinatal morbidity and mortality. Because breech presentation is associated with a twofold to threefold increase in congenital anomalies, compared with cephalic presentation, it is important that each fetus presenting by the breech be subjected to thorough sonographic examination. If fetal anomalies incompatible with life are found, cesarean section should be performed only for maternal indications.

The most common type of breech is the frank breech (knees extended and thighs flexed on the abdomen). With full, or complete, breech, both knees and hips are flexed. In frank and full breeches, the presenting part is the sacrum. In footlings, one or both hips and knees are extended. The fetal head does not have time to mold and may be trapped by the cervix if delivery begins before full dilatation. Since the cord is inevitably compressed against the inlet by the fetal head by the time the fetal umbilicus reaches the introitus, delivery must be completed within several minutes of this time to avoid fetal hypoxia.

Although prolapse of the cord commonly occurs with breech presentation, the accident may be associated with any factor that interferes with adaptation of the presenting part to the inlet, such as transverse lie, face presentation, plural gestation, small fetus, or contracted pelvis. Treatment of prolapse of the cord depends upon the dilation of the cervix. With full dilation, a forceps delivery of a vertex or a breech extraction may be performed if there are no obstetric contraindications. When the cervix is incompletely dilated and the fetus is alive, cesarean section should be performed.

The use of cesarean section for delivery of breeches has increased markedly in recent years. Some obstetricians recommend abdominal delivery of virtually all primigravidas with breech presentations because their pelves are untried. Other indications for cesarean section include footling breeches (to prevent prolapse of the cord), premature breeches (to prevent entrapment of the head by an incompletely dilated cervix), and a hyperextended fetal head (to prevent mechanical difficulties during delivery). Vaginal delivery of a term breech remains an acceptable option for the experienced obstetrician when the fetus weighs less than 3500 g, the pelvis is of normal size and shape, the breech is frank, and the head is not hyperextended. The upper and lower limits for which cesarean section is indicated in breech presentation are still controversial. Many large centers in this country choose cesarean section as the method of delivery for the fetus that weighs between 750 and 1500 g.

Breech presentation may be associated with hydramnios, hydrocephalus, placenta previa, uterine septa, prematurity, and twinning. Since about 40% of fetuses present by the breech at the twenty-eighth week, whereas only 3 to 4% present by the breech at term, it is evident that 90% turn spontaneously during that third trimester. The perinatal mortality associated with breech presentation at term is three times that of vertex presentation.

External version (p. 162) may be attempted in the last 6 weeks of pregnancy, with tocolysis. The preferred method of delivery is partial breech extraction, or assisted breech delivery. In this procedure the breech delivers spontaneously to the umbilicus. In spontaneous breech delivery, the entire fetus is born without assistance, as commonly happens with prematures. Total breech extraction is performed only for difficulties such as fetal distress or a prolonged second stage. The procedure requires deep uterine relaxation and is replaced safely by cesarean section in most cases.

Oxytocin must be used with caution in any breech presentation. Complete breech extraction requires appropriate anesthesia. Fetal injuries associated with breech delivery include fractures of the clavicle, femur, humerus, and spine; injuries to the brachial plexus; hemorrhage in the adrenal, kidney, liver, and spleen; intracranial bleeding; and hypoxia leading to brain damage. The perinatal mortality and morbidity are increased by these factors as well as by prematurity, congenital anomalies, and associated maternal conditions such as placenta previa.

In transverse lie, the long axis of the fetus is perpendicular to that of the mother, and the shoulder is the presenting part. This presentation occurs once in about 300 labors. Vaginal delivery of a term-sized fetus in this presentation is usually impossible, and cesarean section is therefore required. Transverse lie is associated with a relaxed abdominal wall (high multiparity), pelvic contraction, placenta previa, prematurity, plural gestation, and uterine myomas.

The mother's prognosis in transverse lie is worsened because of spontaneous and traumatic (version) uterine rupture and associated conditions such as placenta previa and advanced age. The fetal prognosis is poor because of traumatic delivery, hypoxia, infection associated with premature rupture of the membranes, and prolapse of the cord. A neglected transverse lie may lead to serious intrauterine infection, which may require cesarean hysterectomy (p. 159).

With face presentations, the head is completely extended and the chin is the presenting part. This presentation occurs once in about 400 labors. It should be recognized early and cephalopelvic disproportion, which is frequently associated with face presentation, excluded. A cephalic prominence on the same side as the fetal back suggests face presentation. If the chin is anterior and there is no disproportion, vaginal delivery may be expected. If the chin remains posterior during labor, cesarean section is required for delivery.

Brow presentation is usually transitional from a fully extended (face) to a fully flexed (occiput) presentation. It persists in only 1 in 1000 to 1 in 1500 deliveries. A persistent brow with a term fetus or any cephalopelvic disproportion requires delivery by cesarean section. The perinatal mortality of brow presentation is several times that of vertex presentation.

Occiput posterior is essentially a normal positional variant often associated with anthropoid and android pelves. This position may be associated with a prolonged second stage and incomplete flexion of the head. Most occiput posteriors turn spontaneously to occiput anterior positions. Persistent occiput posteriors may be delivered by rotation (manual or forceps) to an anterior position or as occiput posteriors (face to pubis). Cesarean section should replace difficult midforceps delivery of occiput posteriors.

PELVIC CONTRACTION

Absolute contraction of the pelvic inlet of midpelvis prevents vaginal delivery of a normal-sized infant. An unusual pelvic configuration, even without absolute contraction, may necessitate cesarean section. When the major diameters of the pelvis are at or below critical values, oxytocin must be used with great caution in the presence of a normal-sized fetus. Minor degrees of pelvic contraction are often associated with uterine dysfunction.

The critical diameters, in centimeters, of the pelvis are as follows:

	Anteroposterior	Transverse
Inlet	10.0	12.0
Midplane	11.5	9.5

A contracted pelvis may result from malnutrition, injury, or congenital anomalies. Maternal complications include prolonged labor, premature rupture of the membranes, uterine rupture, and fistulas. Fetal complications include infection, prolapse of the umbilical cord, and intracranial hemorrhage.

The ideal obstetric pelvis has a roundish inlet with a broad and deep posterior segment. The lateral walls slope gently toward the symphysis to form a broad and deep forepelvis. The sacrosciatic notch is wide; the pubic arch is wide; and the bones are light. A flat, or platypelloid, pelvis favors a transverse position of the head and a long, or anthropoid, pelvis favors a posterior mechanism of labor.

18
CHAPTER

THIRD-TRIMESTER BLEEDING

PLACENTA PREVIA

Placenta previa and abruptio placentae are the two most common causes of serious third-trimester bleeding. Placenta previa is characterized by painless vaginal bleeding in the third trimester. It is an important example of the principle that the incompletely separated placenta leads to maternal hemorrhage. If the fetus is judged to be under 2500 g and neither subsequent bleeding nor labor ensues, expectant management may be attempted; that is, no attempt at delivery is made until an estimated weight of 2500 g is attained. If severe or continuous bleeding occurs, if the patient goes into labor, or if the fetus is already mature, expectant management is inapplicable and the patient must be delivered promptly, usually by cesarean section.

In the most extensive variety of placenta previa (total), the entire internal os is covered by placenta. In the partial variety, only a portion of the internal os is covered. In the least extensive varieties (marginal placenta previa and low-lying placenta), the placenta barely encroaches upon the internal os.

Although the initial presumptive diagnosis is made most often by ultrasound (Fig. 18–1), definitive diagnosis is made only by digital palpation of the placenta. Transvaginal sonography has been valuable in the diagnosis of extent of placenta previa. In experienced hands, this technique has not been associated with excessive bleeding. Nevertheless, the definitive diagnosis of placenta previa still requires digital palpation of the placenta. This examination must not be performed, however, except in the operating room, where immediate cesarean section may be accomplished if placenta previa is found. This is the double setup for examination and possible cesarean section. No vaginal or rectal examinations are permitted in a patient with suspected placenta previa except in the operating room.

Placenta previa occurs once in about 200 pregnancies. Its incidence increases with increasing maternal age and parity. It is associated with defective vascularization of the decidua and occasionally with partial placenta accreta. Abnormal presentations (transverse lie and breech) and twins are found more commonly with placenta previa. There is a tendency to repetition in subsequent pregnancies. Bleeding from placenta previa must be distinguished from heavy "show." In case of doubt, the patient should be hospitalized for diagnosis.

With placenta previa, the uterus is of normal consistency and is nontender, unlike that of typical abruptio placentae. Placenta previa rarely occurs before the seventh month, and the first hemorrhage is rarely, if ever, fatal. On initial examination, a speculum should be inserted gently into the

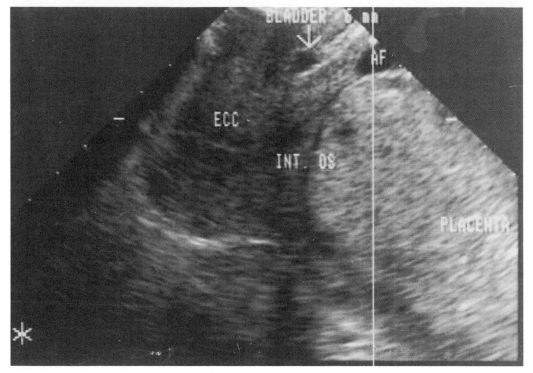

FIG. 18–1. Complete placenta previa, as detected by transvaginal sonography in a mid-sagittal view.

vagina to rule out nonobstetric causes of vaginal bleeding such as carcinoma of the cervix or lacerations. For all bleeding patients, blood should be typed and cross-matched and an intravenous infusion should be started through a large-bore needle. If the patient is anemic, blood should be transfused.

Most patients with placenta previa, including all primigravidas and all patients with total and partial varieties, are delivered by cesarean section. Vaginal delivery by simple rupture of the membranes may occasionally be indicated in a case of low-lying placenta in a multipara with minimal bleeding. Cesarean section reduces both antepartum bleeding and traumatic bleeding at delivery and post partum from injury to the friable lower segment. Less than half of all cases of placenta previa may be managed expectantly. The maternal mortality of well-managed cases should approach zero, but the perinatal mortality remains high because of prematurity and fetal hypoxia.

ABRUPTIO PLACENTAE

Abruptio placentae, the premature separation of the normally situated placenta after the twentieth week of gestation, is the other major cause of third-trimester bleeding. Abruption is classified as either severe or mild, depending upon the degree of separation of the placenta from the uterine wall. The bleeding may be confined to the uterus, as in a retroplacental hematoma with no external bleeding (concealed hemorrhage), usually the more serious form of the disorder. If blood escapes into the vagina, external hemorrhage results.

Signs and symptoms depend on the degree and the duration of the separation. Maternal signs and symptoms may include vaginal bleeding, shock (if the bleeding is severe), and uterine tenderness and rigidity. With severe or rapid bleeding, fetal distress or fetal death may occur. Electronic monitoring of the fetal heart rate for signs of fetal distress is thus critical to management. If only slight external bleeding occurs in the absence of uterine pain or rigidity or fetal distress, bed rest and careful observation may suffice temporarily. A hard uterus, usually indicating retroplacental bleeding, and fetal distress suggest severe abruption and the need for rapid delivery.

The route of delivery is determined by obstetric factors and the speed with which vaginal delivery may be anticipated. If there is no contraindication to oxytocin, it should be used together with rupture of the membranes when delivery through the vagina can reasonably be expected within 6 to 8 hours. In all other circumstances, cesarean section is required. Severe abruption may be complicated by grave fetal distress or death and by maternal hypofibrinogenemia and acute renal failure.

The primary reason for rapid delivery is to forestall these serious complications, which may increase as the interval between abruption and delivery is prolonged. Aggressive management of abruption, based on the presumptive danger of time-related maternal complications, is not, however, universally practiced. Excellent results have been obtained in many institutions that do not require delivery within 8 hours, as long as the maternal blood pressure and renal perfusion remain normal.

Abruptio placentae occurs in about 1% of all pregnancies. The exact frequency depends on the criteria for diagnosis. The precise cause is unknown, although a vascular lesion of the decidua frequently appears to be an underlying factor. Hypertension is associated with abruptio placentae in about one third to one half of cases, chronic hypertension more often than preeclampsia. Maternal mortality should not exceed 1% in well-managed cases, but fetal mortality depends primarily on the extent and acuteness of the separation and the degree of fetal maturity.

Management includes monitoring of maternal blood loss, pulse rate, and blood pressure; typing and crossmatching of blood; monitoring of urinary output and infusion of crystalloids in solution to maintain a urinary flow of 100 ml/hr; monitoring of central venous pressure to avoid overhydration (over 12 cm of water); administration of blood when indicated by prior maternal hemorrhage or a fall in the level of fibrinogen to 100 mg%; and most important, emptying the uterus within 6 to 8 hours by amniotomy and oxytocin or by cesarean section. The use of heparin in treating the consumptive coagulopathy that may occur in the severe forms of this disorder is controversial and potentially dangerous. Effusion of blood within the uterus in cases of severe abruption may produce a bluish discoloration (Couvelaire uterus). It is not necessary to remove the uterus except in the rare event that it fails to contract in response to oxytocin.

Trauma, short cord, and folic acid deficiency are not important etiologic factors. The earlier in pregnancy an abruption occurs, the more it resembles a late incomplete abortion. During the past several years, the use of cocaine by pregnant women has resulted in a greatly increased incidence of abruption. The vasoconstriction and hypertension related to cocaine may lead to premature separation of the placenta. Between 5 and 20% of all women with abruption at the University of New Mexico have toxicologic screens that are positive for cocaine. Maternal smoking of cigarettes is associated with vascular necrosis, and pregnant women who smoke more than ten cigarettes a day have a decided increase in the incidence of abruption. The risk of recurrence of abruption in subsequent pregnancies may be as high as 15%, or about 20 times the rate in the general population.

The most trivial degrees of separation may include rupture of the marginal sinus. There is about a 10% likelihood of recurrence of abruption in subsequent pregnancies.

Other obstetric conditions in which hypofibrinogenemia occurs include amniotic fluid embolism, fetal death, and severe postpartum hemorrhage. Epsilon-aminocaproic acid is generally contraindicated unless unequivocal excessive activator activity or hyperplasminemia can be demonstrated. Successful management of the renal failure depends on close cooperation with the "dialysis team."

19
CHAPTER
PRETERM LABOR

Prematurity is the leading cause of perinatal mortality and morbidity.

DEFINITIONS OF PREMATURITY

A fetus is considered mature by weight at 2500 g. A fetus that weighs between 1000 and 2499 g is considered premature, and one between 500 and 999 g is immature. A fetus that is born weighing less than 500 g (the lower limit of viability) is an abortus.

Preterm birth, however, refers not to weight but to completed weeks of gestation. A preterm birth is one that occurs before 37 weeks from the first day of the last normal menstrual period. Labor or delivery before 20 weeks is considered abortion rather than preterm labor and accordingly is managed differently (see Chapter 11).

Home monitoring of uterine activity by means of a portable tocodynamometer has been recommended as a way to detect premature contractions. The patient wears the sensor and the record of uterine activity is transmitted by telephone. Uterine activity should be recorded for an hour twice a day. Preliminary reports suggest that this method of detecting preterm labor may aid in reduction of preterm births, particularly in groups of patients at high risk for this complication. A definitive cost benefit analysis, however, remains to be completed.

ETIOLOGY AND TREATMENT

The basic cause of premature labor is unknown, although it is often associated with premature rupture of the membranes. Less commonly, premature labor may be ascribed to maternal systemic disorders including infections, second and third trimester uterine bleeding, and uterine anomalies.

Treatment of premature labor includes bed rest, hydration, mild sedation, and tocolysis. The tocolytic agent used most frequently in the United States is terbutaline, although the FDA originally approved only ritodrine hydrochloride for this purpose. Both drugs are β-sympathomimetic agents that act primarily on the β_2 receptors of the uterus. A second β-sympathomimetic agent, hexoprenaline, received FDA approval in 1991. It is likely that terbutaline and other β_2-mimetics will receive FDA approval for use as tocolytic agents in the near future.

Patients who qualify for tocolytic treatment are those with uterine contractions leading to progressive effacement or dilatation of the cervix and whose fetuses are of 20 to 37 weeks' gestation. Patients who do not qualify include those with amnionitis, vaginal bleeding, eclampsia or severe preeclampsia, a dead fetus or a major fetal malformation, maternal cardiac disease or hyperthyroidism, and any obstetric or medical complication that contraindicates prolongation of pregnancy. The chances of successful tocolytic therapy are limited by an incompetent cervix, ruptured membranes, advanced labor, and untreated infections.

When ritodrine is used intravenously, the maternal and fetal cardiac rates as well as maternal blood pressure and uterine activity must be monitored. The most common side effect is tachycardia. Additional effects include decrease in diastolic blood pressure, transient elevation of blood glucose and insulin, occasional elevations of free fatty acids and cAMP, and reduction of potassium. The initial dose is 0.1 mg/minute. The dose is then increased by 0.05 mg/minute every 10 minutes until contractions stop or unacceptable side effects occur. The dose should be reduced if side effects are poorly tolerated. The maximal dose is 0.35 mg/minute. Ritodrine should be discontinued if labor persists with the maximal dose, but if labor is successfully arrested, the infusion should be continued for at least 12 hours.

When ritodrine is given orally, the initial dose should be 10 mg administered 30 minutes before the infusion is stopped. The drug is then given in doses of 10 mg every 2 hours for 24 hours. If contractions do not decrease, 10 to 20 mg are given every 4 to 6 hours until tocolysis is no longer indicated. The maximal oral dose should be 120 mg/day. If labor recurs during oral administration of ritodrine, an infusion may be repeated if it is clinically appropriate.

Magnesium sulfate is another tocolytic agent that has been used extensively in recent years. The method of action of magnesium is presumed to be as an antagonist to calcium, thus decreasing free intracellular calcium, which is required for contraction of uterine smooth muscle. Other tocolytic agents that have been receiving attention recently are the prostaglandin synthetase inhibitors. Success with these agents has been reported to be as high as 80% in many clinical trials. Postpartum hemorrhage and maternal gastrointestinal side effects have been reported, however. There is also the possibility that the prostaglandin synthetase inhibitors such as indomethacin may cause constriction of the fetal ductus arteriosus and perhaps lead to pulmonary hypertension in the neonate. Calcium channel blockers and diazoxide have also been used in the management of preterm labor.

Although attempts to stop premature labor are not always successful, they should always be made unless there are specific contraindications or the fetus is sufficiently mature. Narcotics that cross the placenta and depress the fetus should be avoided whenever possible. Delivery should be conducted under regional or local anesthesia, usually with episiotomy; it should be accomplished spontaneously or with elective outlet forceps. Fetal hypoxia and trauma must be avoided. The fetal prognosis depends on maturity and obstetric management. Expert neonatal care is a major factor in successful outcome. Preterm labor in a prior pregnancy is associated with repetition of the complication in subsequent pregnancy.

About 5 to 10% of all labors are premature. Prematurity is the cause of about two thirds of all cases of perinatal mortality and morbidity. In addition, it is a major etiologic factor in cerebral palsy and mental retardation. In only a minority of cases can a cause for prematurity be found. Conditions known to be associated with prematurity include prior preterm delivery, chronic vascular disease of the mother, preeclampsia-eclampsia, abruptio placentae, placenta previa, hydramnios, plural gestation, uterine malformations and tumors, and certain fetal anomalies.

Maternal genital infections are an important cause of potentially preventable prematurity. Increased rates of prematurity have been associated with maternal infection by Group B streptococci, *Neisseria gonorrhoeae, Chlamydia trachomatis,* and the virus of herpes simplex. Decreased birth weight, chorioamnionitis, and stillbirth have been associated with *Ureaplasma urealyticum;* febrile spontaneous abortion with *Mycoplasma hominis;* and prematurity and stillbirth with *Treponema pallidum.* Certain microorganisms, including *M. hominis, Gardnerella vaginalis,* and *Bacteroides* species, produce phospholipase A_2, an enzyme capable of cleaving arachidonic acid from the phospholipids of fetal membranes. The arachidonic acid thus released may result in the production of prostaglandins, which stimulate uterine contractions and premature labor.

Infants of mothers who smoke weigh less than those of mothers who do not, although the infants of smokers may not be premature by dates. Low socioeconomic status, poor nutrition, and stress appear to be conducive to prematurity.

20
CHAPTER

PREMATURE RUPTURE OF THE MEMBRANES

Premature rupture of the membranes is defined as rupture that occurs more than an hour before the onset of labor. Preterm rupture of the membranes is defined as rupture before term, associated or unassociated with labor. Premature and preterm rupture may coexist. Although premature rupture of the membranes may occur at any stage of pregnancy, its incidence increases as term is approached. The basic cause is unknown, but the condition is associated with premature delivery, maternal sepsis, and increased perinatal morbidity and mortality. Near term, it is followed by the onset of labor within 24 hours in about 80% of cases, but the earlier in pregnancy premature rupture of the membranes occurs, the longer is the latent period (time between rupture and onset of labor). The reported incidence of premature rupture of the membranes varies from 3 to 18% of all deliveries.

ETIOLOGY

Factors contributing to premature rupture include incompetent cervix, cervicitis, placenta previa, genetic abnormalities, amnionitis, hydramnios, fetal malpresentation, trauma, plural gestation, and other conditions associated with an overdistended uterus.

DIAGNOSIS

Premature rupture of the membranes usually presents as loss of fluid through the vagina. Diagnosis, however, can be difficult. Direct visualization of fluid escaping from the cervix, on speculum examination, is the most reliable method of diagnosis. It is not necessary for the examiner to insert a finger into the cervix. When the amniotic fluid, which is normally alkaline, escapes into the vagina, there is a change in vaginal pH, which can be detected by a change in the color of Nitrazine (phenaphthazine) paper from yellow to blue. This change in color usually occurs in the range of pH between 4.5 and 7.5. If the vaginal secretions are contaminated with blood, urine, or antiseptic solutions with an alkaline pH, a false-positive test can result. When allowed to dry on a clean slide, the amniotic fluid forms a "fern" (arborization). Other indications of ruptured membranes are fetal epithelial cells, hair, or globules of fat in the vagina.

Once the diagnosis of ruptured membranes has been made, the gestational age of the fetus must be assessed. Ultrasonography is quite useful in this regard. External fetal monitoring is performed at this time to detect distress, which may occur as result of compression or prolapse of the umbilical cord.

When premature rupture of the membranes occurs in the presence of a preterm fetus, the risks associated with preterm delivery must be balanced against those of infection. Early in gestation, the mother is at risk for failed induction because of the status of the cervix. Fetal complications of preterm premature rupture of the membranes before 26 gestational weeks include pulmonary hypoplasia and positional anomalies of the skeleton.

TREATMENT

When premature rupture of the membranes occurs after 36 weeks and the cervix is favorable, labor should be induced. If the cervix is unfavorable, expectant management for 24 hours may be justified to minimize the risks of failed induction and maternal morbidity. When the decision is made to attempt expectant management in the patient with preterm premature rupture of the membranes, attention must be directed to fetal pulmonary maturity and possible chorioamnionitis. Amniotic fluid can be obtained by amniocentesis or collection from the pool in the posterior vagina for detection of phosphatidyl glycerol or analysis of the lecithin/sphingomyelin ratio. The presence of the former and a ratio of 2 or higher in the latter indicate the likelihood of pulmonary maturity. Additional laboratory tests of value in the management of these patients include cervical cultures for Group B streptococci, Chlamydia, and *Neisseria gonorrhoeae*. Chorioamnionitis may present with high maternal fever and an irritable, tender uterus. Subclinical intraamniotic infection often presents with subtler findings, such as fetal tachycardia. The presence of pathogenic bacteria in a Gram stain of the amniotic fluid correlates with maternal infection in half the cases. Prophylactic antibiotics remain debatable in management of premature rupture of the membranes. Also controversial is the use of tocolysis and corticosteroids to induce fetal pulmonary maturation in preterm premature rupture of the membranes.

21

CHAPTER

POSTPARTUM HEMORRHAGE AND OBSTETRIC INJURIES

Postpartum hemorrhage is defined as a loss of more than 500 mL of blood during the first 24 hours after delivery. It is the most common variety of severe hemorrhage in obstetrics and a major factor in maternal mortality. Effective hemostasis after separation of the placenta depends on myometrial contraction and compression of uterine vessels. The three principal causes of postpartum hemorrhage are uterine atony, trauma to the genital tract, and retained secundines (placenta and membranes). Uterine atony, the most common cause, may result from any condition that leads to overdistension of the uterus. Injuries result primarily from traumatic deliveries and inadequately repaired episiotomies. Retained secundines usually result in a somewhat more delayed hemorrhage.

DIAGNOSIS AND TREATMENT

Diagnosis and treatment must be performed with minimal delay. As soon as excessive bleeding is recognized, a large-bore needle is inserted into a vein for administration of fluids, and blood is crossmatched and made available. In a healthy young woman, the blood pressure and pulse rate may remain almost normal until a great deal of blood has been lost, at which point shock may develop suddenly.

Transfusion should always be instituted before the patient has lost 1000 mL of blood. The first step in management is uterine massage. An oxytocic agent is administered if the uterus is hypotonic. If bleeding continues from a firmly contracted uterus, injuries to the genital tract are a more likely cause. After any difficult delivery, the vulva, vagina (including episiotomy site), and cervix should be inspected and any lacerations repaired. The uterus should be explored manually, especially if the cervix is deeply lacerated, to rule out injury and to remove any placental fragments. Anesthesia provides for a more thorough examination. The delivered placenta should be examined carefully to rule out incomplete removal. In the unusual event of placenta accreta the placenta, or more commonly a part thereof, cannot be separated from the uterus (Fig. 21–1). Hysterectomy may then be required to control hemorrhage. The blood should be observed to see whether it clots and to rule out hypofibrinogenemia, which is generally treated by administration of cryoprecipitate. If the uterus is still bleeding after lacerations have been repaired and after oxytocic agents have been administered, the uterus should be compressed bimanually and the patient prepared for laparotomy. The Anti-G or MAST (military antishock trousers) suit is also a frequently effective means of combating uterine hemorrhage caused by atony.

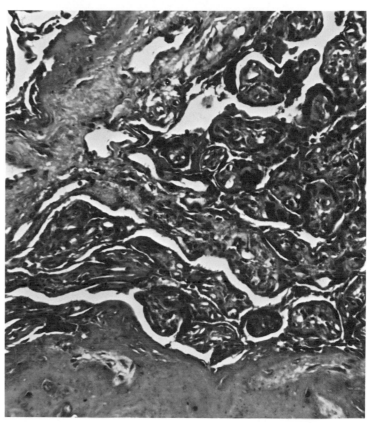

FIG. 21–1. Placenta accreta, showing villi in direct contact with myometrium without an intervening decidual cushion.

Packing the uterus hides rather than stems the hemorrhage.

ETIOLOGY AND MANAGEMENT

Uterine atony accounts for about 90% of all cases of immediate postpartum hemorrhage. It should be anticipated in prolonged labor, high multiparity, and general anesthesia with agents that relax the uterus. It is more common with plural gestation, hydramnios (2000 mL or more of amniotic fluid), excessively large infants, myomas, and amnionitis. The likelihood of uterine atony is greatly reduced by the proper use of oxytocic agents. Ten to twenty units of oxytocin in physiologic saline solution may be administered by intravenous drip after delivery of the infant, but not directly into the vein in a single rapid injection. Methylergonovine maleate (0.2 mg) may be given intravenously or intramuscularly after delivery of the placenta. Maternal hypertension is a relative contraindication to this drug. Another drug used successfully to treat uterine atony postpartum is prostaglandin $F_{2\alpha}$. A synthetic 15-methylated derivative of this prostaglandin is also effective. The drug is given is doses of 0.25 mg injected into the deltoid muscle every hour or 2. Up to five doses may be given without adverse effect.

Trauma to the genital tract results from tumultuous labor, difficult forceps delivery and internal podalic version, injudicious use of oxytocin before delivery, and mismanagement of the third stage (forceful attempts to remove the placenta prematurely). After any difficult labor or delivery, the genital tract should be inspected systematically. If a uterine rupture is encountered or suspected, the patient should be transported without delay to the operating room. Ligation or embolization of the internal iliac arteries or hysterectomy may be required for hemostasis.

The delivered placenta should be inspected carefully to rule out retention of a cotyledon, as indicated by a defect in the maternal surface. A torn vessel at the edge of the placenta suggests retention of a succenturiate lobe. Retained secundines and sub-involution of the placental site usually lead to postpartum hemorrhage that is delayed (from the second day to a month after delivery). Placental fragments may then be removed by polyp forceps and the subinvoluted site curetted.

Hypofibrinogenemia is a much less common cause of postpartum hemorrhage. It is often associated with severe abruption of the placenta, retention of a dead fetus for more than a month, and amniotic fluid embolism.

Uterine rupture may occur through a scar (usually cesarean section) before and during labor or through an intact organ after difficult labor or delivery. Rupture should be suspected when the uterine contractions cease and the fetal heart tones are lost in the presence of severe abdominal pain. A classical cesarean section scar may rupture early (before the onset of labor), whereas a low-segment scar more often ruptures during labor.

22
CHAPTER

DISORDERS OF THE PUERPERIUM

Puerperal morbidity is defined as any fever of 100.4° F (38° C) or higher on any 2 of the first 10 days post partum, excluding the first 24 hours, as detected with an oral thermometer using a standard technique at least 4 times daily. Unless another cause is found, puerperal infection, often manifested by chills, fever, and tachycardia, is assumed to be endomyoparametritis (often abbreviated to metritis). The other common causes of fever in the puerperium are urinary tract infection, mastitis, thrombophlebitis, and infection of an episiotomy site. Low-grade fever is common post partum and often resolves spontaneously. Frank postpartum infection complicates 1 to 8% of all deliveries.

METRITIS

Introduction of bacteria into the genital tract by attendants is one of the main causes of metritis. Another common cause is rupture of the membranes with contamination and colonization of the amniotic cavity by organisms that are indigenous to the vagina and cervix. Frequent vaginal examinations, internal fetal monitoring, and trauma to the cervix and vagina predispose to infection. Cesarean section, especially after prolonged rupture of the membranes, is another major factor predisposing to postpartum infection. The most common pathogens are Group B streptococci, *Escherichia coli,* Group D enterococci, Bacteroides, and Peptostreptococcus. Confirmation of the diagnosis of metritis is made by cultures of the uterine cavity and blood before administration of antibiotics. The diagnosis is suspected on the basis of fever, malaise, abdominal pain, and purulent discharge.

Treatment of metritis includes cefoxitin or a similar cephalosporin or broad-spectrum penicillins. For more serious cases of metritis, a combination of clindamycin and gentamicin may be used. In addition to blood counts, blood cultures, and uterine cultures, Gram stains of material from the genital tract may be useful when hemolytic streptococci, Clostridia, and other anaerobes are suspected.

PELVIC THROMBOPHLEBITIS

Metritis may lead to pelvic abscess or femoral thrombophlebitis. Pelvic abscesses are suggested by manual examination and confirmed by ultrasound. Drainage may frequently be accomplished by transcutaneous aspiration or culdocentesis under sonographic guidance. After pelvic abscess is ruled out, pelvic thrombophlebitis should be suspected in any puerperal patient who does not respond to treatment of presumptive metritis. Thrombophlebitis may first appear

147

7 to 10 days after delivery. Pain and swelling of the leg suggest femoral thrombophlebitis. Pelvic thrombophlebitis is suspected on the basis of pain and tenderness on pelvic examination. Pulmonary emboli are occasionally the first signs of deep phlebitis. The treatment usually requires intravenous heparin for 10 days and occasionally ligation of the inferior vena cava. Puerperal infection and its sequelae may be minimized by elimination of infections before labor, correction of anemia, appropriately timed delivery after rupture of the membranes, aseptic technique, restriction of the number of vaginal examinations, and avoidance of trauma and loss of blood during delivery.

URINARY TRACT INFECTION

Infection of the urinary tract may follow trauma and catheterization superimposed on urinary stasis and bacteriuria. Treatment is discussed on page 123.

MASTITIS

Mastitis occurs infrequently after delivery. *Staphylococcus aureus* is the most important offending organism. Group A and Group B streptococci also may be involved. The initial antibiotic of choice is either a penicillinase-resistant semisynthetic penicillin such as dicloxacillin or a cephalosporin. Support of the breast and ice packs or heat, depending on the duration of the swelling, in addition to analgesics, are required frequently. The mother may continue to nurse unless an abscess forms.

SUBINVOLUTION OF THE UTERUS

Subinvolution of the uterus may be caused by retained secundines, metritis, or myomas. It produces prolonged lochia and occasionally delayed postpartum hemorrhage. Ergot derivatives are useful. If infection supervenes, antibiotics are administered. A curettage is usually required to remove retained tissues or a subinvoluted placental site, but it must be performed gently to avoid removal of excessive endometrium with resulting Asherman's syndrome.

23
CHAPTER

MATERNAL AND PERINATAL MORTALITY

The principles and practice of regionalization of perinatal care have decreased maternal, fetal, and neonatal mortality and morbidity. The concept of regionalization includes levels of obstetric and pediatric services, perinatal centers, and maternal transfers of high-risk patients.

The maternal mortality rate is the number of maternal deaths per 100,000 live births as a direct result of the reproductive process. According to some definitions, the term includes all deaths of pregnant women from any causes, including those unrelated to pregnancy. The rate for nonwhites is several times that for whites. Although both rates are continuing to fall, the differential is increasing, primarily as a result of social and economic factors. The last full year for which figures are available in the United States reflected a remarkably low maternal mortality rate of 7.8 per 100,000 live births.

MATERNAL MORTALITY

The most common causes of maternal deaths are hemorrhage, infection, hypertensive disorders, embolism, anesthesia, and cardiac disease. Deaths associated with abortion continue to account for significant maternal mortality in jurisdictions where the procedure is governed by restrictive laws. Ectopic pregnancy continues to ac-

count for an increasing number and proportion of maternal deaths.

Deaths may be related directly to pregnancy or to coincident diseases that are affected by pregnancy or may be caused by factors unrelated to pregnancy. Deaths from hemorrhage, preeclampsia-eclampsia, infections, vascular accidents, and anesthesia may be considered directly related to pregnancy. Deaths from hemorrhage have been reduced by blood transfusion and hospital delivery. Those from infection have been reduced by asepsis, hospital delivery, and antibiotics; and those from preeclampsia-eclampsia have been reduced by prenatal care and early delivery in the hospital. Embolism involving amniotic fluid, air, and thrombi may be considered direct results of the reproductive process. Coincident conditions that may be exacerbated by pregnancy include cardiac disease, diabetes, and anemia. Important causes unrelated to pregnancy include infections and malignant diseases, suicide, and accidents.

PERINATAL MORTALITY

Perinatal mortality is the sum of stillbirths (fetal deaths) and neonatal deaths (deaths of liveborn infants in the first 28 days of life). A stillbirth is defined as an infant with no heartbeat who neither breathes nor cries nor

149

shows any other signs of movement. The fetal death rate is the number of fetal deaths (deaths of fetuses weighing 500 g or more) per 1000 births (live births plus stillbirths). (A weight of 500 grams corresponds roughly to 20 weeks' gestation.) The neonatal death rate and the infant mortality rate (deaths under 1 year of age) are calculated per 1000 live births.

Perinatal deaths are divided almost equally between stillbirths and neonatal deaths. Many stillbirths are caused by maternal diseases such as diabetes, but in a larger percentage of cases there is no obvious cause. The most common cause of neonatal death is prematurity. Other causes of perinatal mortality include congenital malformations, obstetric trauma, intrauterine hypoxia, infection, hematologic disorders (including Rh-isoimmunization), pulmonary dysfunction (atelectasis and respiratory distress syndrome), and other iatrogenic causes. In many cases there is no sufficient pathologic diagnosis. Disseminated intravascular coagulation has been reported (rarely) in mothers with prolonged retention of a dead fetus.

GRIEVING

A perinatal death requires special attention to the grieving mother and her family. Grief may follow the actual death of a fetus or infant or the loss of an idealized child, as in the case of malformations or birth injuries. Some centers have specialized teams of physicians, nurses, social workers, and counselors to manage the difficult problem of grief resulting from perinatal loss. The father's grieving may take a form different from that of the mother in cases of loss of an infant or fetus. Emotional support must be provided for the mother and her family as she moves from antepartum setting to labor and delivery to postpartum setting and finally returns to her home.

ETIOLOGY

Between 1950 and 1986, the total perinatal mortality rate in the United States fell from 40 per 1000 to less than 12 per 1000. The most recent year for which figures are available (1987) reflects a neonatal mortality rate of 6.5. University hospitals and referral centers may have higher mortality rates because of the greater numbers of high-risk patients. Many northern European countries have lower incidences of prematurity and lower perinatal death rates, which may reflect their more stable populations, lower prevalences of poverty, and important possible differences in reporting.

One factor in perinatal mortality, congenital malformations, may be genetically or environmentally induced. Intrauterine hypoxia may result from preeclampsia-eclampsia; abruptio placentae; placenta previa; prolapse, knots, or entanglement of the cord; maternal hypotension; anesthesia and analgesia; shoulder dystocia; delayed delivery of the aftercoming head; and prolonged labor.

Infections may be intrauterine or extrauterine and are usually of viral or bacterial origin. Most neonatal viral infections are acquired when the infant passes through the birth canal. Important iatrogenic causes of perinatal mortality include premature and traumatic deliveries. Maternal diseases associated with increased perinatal loss include hypertensive disorders, glomerulonephritis, urinary tract infection, diabetes mellitus, and symptomatic cardiac disease.

24
CHAPTER

POSTTERM PREGNANCY

Pregnancy is considered postterm when its duration exceeds 294 days, or 42 weeks, from the first day of the last menstrual period. This complication is associated with a significant increase in perinatal mortality and morbidity. A postterm infant is considered postmature, a form of dysmature (p. 153), when he shows clear evidence of intrauterine nutritional deprivation.

When pregnancy progresses beyond term, the placenta may fail to supply the nutrition and oxygenation necessary for continued fetal survival. Furthermore, oligohydramnios, which may complicate postterm pregnancy, contributes to fetal morbidity through increased likelihood of compression of the umbilical cord. The frequency of postterm pregnancy is between 7 and 12%, but most of the postterm fetuses are not dysmature.

The logical management of postterm pregnancy requires accurate dating of the pregnancy. Pregnancies that are postterm are classified as those with certain and those with uncertain dates. The two groups require different clinical management. Good dating may be achieved by: a positive β-hCG within 6 weeks of the last menstrual period, a bimanual examination in the first 10 weeks of pregnancy, fetal heart tones detected by Doppler at 12 weeks of gestation, quickening between 16 and 18 weeks of gestation, and gestational age confirmed by ultrasound before 28 weeks. A pregnancy is considered to be of uncertain gestational length when the dates cannot be substantiated by these criteria.

In uncomplicated postterm pregnancy, both aggressive and expectant forms of management play a role. Expectant management requires careful fetal surveillance. When a high-risk pregnancy, such as one with preeclampsia or diabetes, is allowed to continue past term, the fetus is jeopardized, even when fetal surveillance is reassuring. Thus, high-risk pregnancies should not extend beyond term. Even when the pregnancy is not complicated, if the cervix is favorable, labor should be induced at or before 42 weeks. If the cervix is not favorable and the pregnancy is not high-risk, close fetal surveillance should begin by 41 weeks. When the dates are uncertain, fetal surveillance must be initiated at the best estimate of term. Fetal compromise or the superimposition of a maternal complication demands termination of the pregnancy. If the pregnancy remains uncomplicated, it is terminated by 43 weeks in any case. Accepted methods of fetal surveillance include the fetal kick count, the contraction stress test, and the nonstress test (p. 154). The optimal perinatal outcome seems to result when nonstress tests are performed twice weekly along with simultaneous measurements of amniotic fluid. Alternatively, serial biophysical profiles may be employed. Delivery is indicated by decrease in volume of amniotic fluid and evidence of more acute fetal distress. The intrapartum period is hazardous in postterm pregnancy even when antepartum complications are absent. Intrapartum management requires attention to prevention of aspiration of meconium and traumatic delivery. Continuous electronic monitoring during labor and delivery is the standard of care in postterm pregnancy. To prevent traumatic vaginal delivery of a macrosomic infant, ultrasonic estimation of fetal weight is indicated. If macrosomia is detected in a postterm fetus, serious attention should be given to cesarean section as the safest method of delivery. A summary of one suggested method of management of the postterm pregnancy is found in Table 24–1.

TABLE 24–1. MANAGEMENT OF POST-TERM PREGNANCY OF KNOWN DATES

A. Establish dates
B. Perform fetal surveillance
   1. Weekly contraction stress test or twice-weekly nonstress test
   2. Estimation of amniotic fluid volume or biophysical profile weekly
   3. Estimation of fetal weight
C. Decide route and timing of delivery
   1. Decreased amniotic fluid: deliver
   2. Fetal distress: deliver
   3. Superimposed maternal complications: Deliver
   4. Ripe cervix: Deliver
   5. Macrosomia: Consider abdominal delivery
   6. Normal with unripe cervix: Expectant management

25
CHAPTER

ABNORMALITIES OF FETAL GROWTH

Dysmaturity is a discrepancy between birth weight and gestational age. It is associated with increased perinatal mortality and morbidity. The obstetrician must identify predisposing factors and affected fetuses. Dysmaturity may be of the small-for-gestational-age (SGA) or the large-for-gestational-age (LGA) varieties. In SGA, which complicates 3 to 7% of all pregnancies, the fetal weight is at or below the tenth percentile of the weight appropriate for that gestational age. In LGA, the fetal weight is greater than the 90th percentile. The former is often called intrauterine growth restriction (retardation) and the latter, fetal macrosomia. Both are disorders of the third trimester. Serial measurements of fundal height in centimeters above the symphysis (obtained by tape measure at each antepartum visit) provide clinical assessment of fetal growth. If these clinical measurements suggest an abnormality (a difference of more than ± 3 cm), ultrasonic assessment of the fetal biparietal diameter, abdominal circumference, and femoral length, as well as estimation of fetal weight, provide accurate information. The sonographic examination should be performed at least every 3 weeks. All diagnoses of abnormalities of fetal growth depend on accurate knowledge of the gestational age (p. 59).

INTRAUTERINE GROWTH RESTRICTION

Fetuses with intrauterine growth restriction (IUGR) are at increased risk for the adverse effects of hypoxia. As neonates, they have deficient subcutaneous fat and are at increased risk for hypoglycemia, hyponatremia, hypocalcemia, aspiration of meconium, hypothermia, and polycythemia.

One third of all cases of IUGR are of the symmetric type and two thirds are of the asymmetric type. Symmetric IUGR is caused by a fetal insult early in gestation, such as infection, a chromosomal anomaly, or radiation. Approximately 25% of fetuses with symmetric IUGR have chromosomal anomalies. The ratio of circumference of the head to that of the abdomen is below the 95th percentile, and both number of cells and content of DNA in the brain are reduced. Such a fetus has a guarded prognosis. Asymmetric IUGR is caused by an insult later in gestation, such as preeclampsia, chronic hypertension, or diabetes. The ratio of circumference of the head to that of the abdomen is above the 95th percentile, and the number of cells is decreased but the DNA content of the brain is normal. "Catch-up" growth is possible in these infants and, although intrapartum distress may occur, the prognosis is usually good.

Many maternal, placental, and fetal factors are associated with IUGR. The more important include: hypoperfusion of the placenta; maternal undernutrition and hypoxia; low maternal socioeconomic status; small placenta; maternal smoking, strenuous exercise, and consumption of alcohol and drugs during pregnancy; high altitude; maternal disorders, including cardiac disease, anemia, pulmonary insufficiency, essential hypertension, preeclampsia-eclampsia, chronic renal and vascular disease, and some hemoglobinopathies; transplacental viral infection, for example rubella or cytomegalovirus; infection with mycoplasmas or *Chlamydia trachomatis;* chromosomal abnormalities in the fetus, including trisomies and deletion syndromes; fetal congenital anomalies; plural gestation; and pregnancies prolonged beyond 42 weeks. Women who have had a baby with IUGR in a prior pregnancy are at risk for repetition of that complication.

The nonstress test should be initiated twice weekly as soon as the diagnosis of growth restriction is suspected. Antepartum evaluation of fetuses with IUGR requires close surveillance, including, in addition to nonstress testing, the contraction stress test, biophysical profile, measurements of the volume of amniotic fluid, and tests for pulmonary maturity. More recently, umbilical arterial velocimetry by Doppler has been employed for evaluation of ''downstream'' resistance. An elevated systolic:diastolic ratio and absent or reverse diastolic flow are correlated positively with intrauterine growth restriction (Figs. 25–1 and 25–2). Optimal management entails close surveillance of fetal well-being and delivery as soon as the fetus approaches maturity.

LARGE-FOR-GESTATIONAL-AGE FETUSES

Large-for-gestational-age, or macrosomic, infants are those with a birth weight over 4000 g. Another definition of macrosomia uses the figure of 4500 g. This complication affects male fetuses more frequently. The two most common obstetric complications are postpartum hemorrhage and shoulder dystocia. Detection of macrosomia before delivery would avert these complications, but such efforts have not been highly successful to date. Estimation of fetal weight in this group of large fetuses is fraught with an error of ± 10%, largely because the fetal head is too deeply engaged in the pelvis to allow an accurate measurement of its circumference.

Infants may be large for gestational age for the following reasons: constitutionally large by heredity, transposition of the great vessels, recipient twin in the transfusion syndrome, and overproduction of insulin. Infants who produce an excess of insulin include those born to diabetic mothers and those with certain cases of erythroblastosis fetalis. Fetal macrosomia secondary to maternal diabetes can be diminished greatly, but not eliminated, by strict control of the diabetes during the antepartum period.

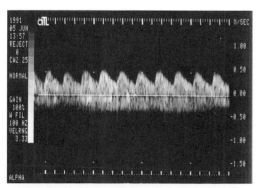

FIG. 25–1. Normal fetal arterial umbilical flow, as detected by Doppler velocimetry.

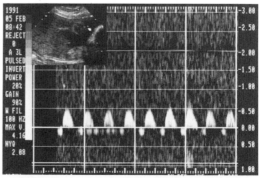

FIG. 25–2. Reverse diastolic flow in a case of intrauterine growth restriction, as detected by Doppler velocimetry.

OBSTETRIC PROCEDURES

26
CHAPTER

ULTRASOUND

The application of sonography (diagnostic ultrasound) to obstetrics and gynecology is probably the most important technologic advance in the specialty during the second half of the twentieth century. Although it is not routinely indicated in all pregnancies, there is no documented harm to either mother or fetus when it is used according to accepted guidelines. The most important applications of diagnostic ultrasound are listed in Table 26-1.

Real-time ultrasound creates images within a fraction of a second. When the image of the fetus is compounded at a rate faster than that of the eye, the fetus appears to be moving in real time. As the frequency of the sound waves becomes higher, the resolution becomes better but the depth of penetration becomes shallower. Obstetricians most often use linear array and sector scanning transducers. Routine sonographic evaluation includes location of the placenta, assessment of the volume of amniotic fluid, documentation of the number and viability of fetuses, evaluation of gross anatomic features of the fetus, measurement of the crown-rump length or biparietal diameter and femoral length, documentation of fetal presentation, and detection of fetal anomalies. Initial ultrasonic examination should include, in addition, measurement of fetal abdominal circumference, assessment of the ventricular system in the fetal brain, estima-

tion of fetal weight, and identification of malformations.

Assessment of gestational age during the first 18 weeks is highly accurate. Measurement of fetal crown-rump (CR) length between 6 and 10 weeks of pregnancy pinpoints gestational age to within 3 to 5 days (see Fig. 5-14). After 12 weeks of pregnancy, the curvature of the fetal body destroys the accuracy of the crown-rump measurement for ascertaining gestational age. Between 12 and 18 weeks of pregnancy the biparietal diameter (BPD) achieves its greatest usefulness in assessing gestational age. The transverse BPD is obtained ideally at the level of the thalamus and the cavum septi pellucidi. (see Fig. 5-13). Measurements of fetal abdominal circumference and femoral length have been used to monitor fetal growth as well as to assess gestational age. Use of multiple criteria after 18 weeks of pregnancy identifies fetal age better than does any single measurement. In most centers, sensitivity of ultrasound for detection of major fetal malformations is 95%. Those identified easily include hydrocephaly, anencephaly, cardiac anomalies, defects of the abdominal wall, and skeletal dysplasias.

Transvaginal, or endovaginal, sonography permits closer evaluation of the pelvic contents than does the transabdominal technique because less tissue need be pene-

TABLE 26–1. INDICATIONS FOR DIAGNOSTIC ULTRASOUND

1. Estimation of gestational age
2. Evaluation of fetal growth
3. Vaginal bleeding of uncertain cause
4. Diagnosis of fetal presentation
5. Suspected plural gestation
6. Adjunct to amniocentesis and chorionic villus sampling
7. Discrepancy between uterine size and clinical dates
8. Pelvic mass
9. Suspected hydatidiform mole
10. Adjunct to repair of incompetent cervix
11. Suspected ectopic pregnancy
12. Adjunct to special procedures
13. Suspected fetal death
14. Suspected uterine anomaly
15. Localization of intrauterine device
16. Surveillance of ovarian follicular development
17. Biophysical evaluation for fetal well-being
18. Observation of intrapartum events
19. Suspected polyhydramnios or oligohydramnios
20. Suspected abruptio placentae
21. Adjunct to external cephalic version
22. Estimation of fetal weight or presentation in premature rupture of membranes or preterm labor
23. Abnormal value of serum α-fetoprotein
24. Follow-up of identified fetal anomaly
25. Follow-up of placental location in identified placenta previa
26. Follow-up of prior congenital anomaly
27. Serial evaluation of fetal growth in plural gestation
28. Evaluation of fetal maturity in patients who register late for prenatal care

trated. Most major fetal anatomic features can be visualized transvaginally between 9 and 15 weeks of gestation. Transvaginal sonography is advantageous for the early detection of intrauterine pregnancy, the diagnosis of ectopic pregnancy (p. 93), and the assessment of follicular development in an evaluation of infertility (p. 345). It is of additional value in the diagnosis of cervical incompetence (p. 98) and placenta previa (p. 137).

Doppler ultrasound has been used for many years to assess blood flow and cardiac motion. The development of real-time frequency spectrum analyzers now permits a detailed visual display of the Doppler frequency shift as a function of time. The two methods of display are continuous wave Doppler (CW) and pulsed-wave Doppler (PW). Analysis of the systolic:diastolic ratio, the pulsatility index, and the resistance index has permitted evaluation of downstream impedance, or resistance, in the fetal

circulation. Fetuses with increased downstream resistance as a result of placental insufficiency may show absent or reverse diastolic flow in the umbilical artery, a predictor of poor perinatal outcome. (Compare Figs. 25–1 and 25–2.)

Estimation of gestational age in patients with uncertain dates or those who are scheduled to undergo elective repetition of a cesarean section, induction of labor, or other elective termination of pregnancy permits proper timing of delivery and avoids the hazard of premature delivery. Monitoring of fetal growth permits assessment of the effect of a complication of pregnancy on the fetus and guides management of the pregnancy. Such monitoring is indicated when there is an identified cause of uteroplacental insufficiency, such as severe preeclampsia, chronic hypertension, chronic renal disease, and severe diabetes mellitus, and in other medical complications of pregnancy in which restriction of intrauterine growth or macrosomia is suspected. In cases of vaginal bleeding, ultrasound often permits assessment of the source of the bleeding and the condition of the fetus. When the identity of the presenting part is not certain, ultrasound permits accurate diagnosis and guides management of the delivery. When plural gestation is suspected by detection of more than one fetal heartbeat, a fundal height greater than expected for dates, or knowledge or prior use of drugs to stimulate ovulation, ultrasound may identify the number of fetuses and guide management.

In the course of amniocentesis, ultrasound permits guidance of the needle to avoid the fetus and placenta, to increase the likelihood of obtaining amniotic fluid, and to decrease the chance of fetal loss. When there is a discrepancy between the size of the uterus and the clinical dates, ultrasound permits dating of the pregnancy and detection of complications, such as oligohydramnios, polyhydramnios, plural gestation, restriction of intrauterine growth, and fetal anomalies. Sonographic examination of a pelvic mass aids in diagnosis of its location, size, and consistency. Ultrasound permits accurate diagnosis of a hydatidiform mole and differentiation of this growth from fetal death. The diagnosis is often suspected on the basis of hypertension, proteinuria, ovarian cysts, or failure to detect a fetal heartbeat with Doppler after 12 weeks. Ultra-

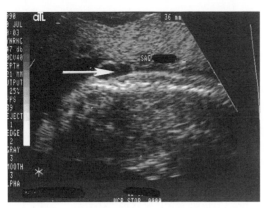

FIG. 26–1. Sagittal ultrasonic view of the fetal spine, showing a cystic structure (arrow) in the lumbar area, compatible with an open neural tube defect.

sound aids in timing and proper placement of the stitch or tape in the repair of an incompetent cervix. When ectopic pregnancy is suspected or when pregnancy occurs after surgical procedures on the fallopian tube or prior ectopic pregnancy, ultrasound is valuable for ruling out this complication. Ultrasound facilitates guidance of the appropriate instruments and increases the safety of special diagnostic procedures such as chorionic villus sampling, fetoscopy, intrauterine transfusion, placement of shunts, and in-vitro fertilization and embryo transfer. In cases of suspected fetal death, use of ultrasound provides rapid diagnosis and facilitates optimal management. Sonographic serial surveillance of fetal growth and condition improves fetal outcome in cases of suspected

uterine abnormality, such as clinically significant leiomyomata or congenital structural anomalies.

Ultrasound facilitates the removal of an intrauterine device, thus reducing complications that might result from a misplaced contraceptive device. Surveillance of ovarian follicular development by sonography is valuable in the treatment of infertility. Assessment of the volume of amniotic fluid and tone, movements, and breathing of the fetus after 28 weeks of gestation (biophysical evaluation of fetal well-being) assists greatly in the management of high-risk pregnancies. Intrapartum procedures such as version and extraction of a second twin and manual removal of the placenta may be done more safely with ultrasonic visualization. Confirmation of suspected polyhydramnios, as well as identification of the cause of the condition in certain pregnancies, can be accomplished with ultrasound. Confirmation of the diagnosis and extent of suspected abruptio placentae likewise may be accomplished. Visualization provided by ultrasound facilitates external version from breech to cephalic presentation. Information provided by ultrasound facilitates estimation of fetal weight and presentation in premature rupture of membranes and preterm labor and aids management regarding timing and method of delivery.

In evaluation of the significance of abnormal α-fetoprotein values in the serum, ultrasound provides an accurate assessment of gestational age for comparison with standards and identifies several conditions such as twins, anencephaly, and open neural

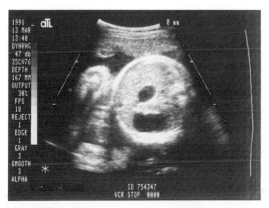

FIG. 26–2. Transverse ultrasonic view of the fetal abdomen, showing the "double bubble" sign, consistent with duodenal atresia.

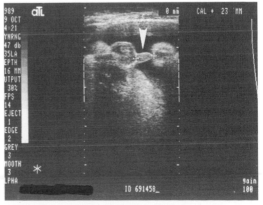

FIG. 26–3. Male genitalia, as detected by ultrasound. Arrowhead indicates fetal penis.

tube defect (Fig. 26–1) that may cause elevation of the level of AFP. Ultrasound may be used to follow the change in location of the placenta with respect to the internal os in cases of placenta previa identified earlier in pregnancy. Ultrasound may be employed to assess a fetal anomaly (Fig. 26–2) and to detect recurrence (or lack thereof) of congenital anomalies in a patient who had an affected fetus in a prior pregnancy.

The psychologic benefits of knowledge that the fetus is normal are obvious. Ultrasound permits recognition of the sex of the fetus in X-linked chromosomal disorders (Fig. 26–3) and of discordant fetal growth in plural gestation, thus aiding management and timing of delivery. Finally, in the case of a patient who registers late in pregnancy for her prenatal care, ultrasound provides information concerning fetal maturity.

Currently about half of all pregnant women have at least one sonogram. The equipment is available in virtually all hospitals and many obstetricians' offices in the United States. As experience with the technique and knowledge of its safety increase, it seems likely that ultrasound will play an even greater role in obstetrics in the future.

Continuous wave Doppler ultrasound has been used in assessment of uterine blood flow. Analysis of waveforms and velocities may predict or detect the growth-restricted fetus at a relatively early stage and thus lead to appropriate clinical management.

27
CHAPTER

OTHER COMMONLY PERFORMED PROCEDURES

CESAREAN SECTION

Delivery of a fetus through incisions in the abdomen and uterus is called cesarean section. The essence of the operation is the hysterotomy. As a result of improvement in surgical technique, antisepsis, blood replacement, and anesthesia, cesarean section has become a safe operation, which has replaced difficult vaginal deliveries. The two main types of cesarean sections are the classical, which involves incision of the upper contractile portion of the uterus, and the low-segment operation, which involves incision of the lower uterine segment after dissection of the vesicouterine peritoneum. The low-segment incision is usually transverse, although it may be vertical. Cesarean section may be combined with hysterectomy when it is desirable to remove the uterus for disease.

In the United States today, about half of all cesarean sections are primary and half are operations that are repeated because of a uterine scar. Indications for primary cesarean section may be fetal or maternal. A major factor in the perinatal mortality associated with cesarean section is prematurity. Ascertaining fetal maturity (p. 59) before elective or repeated cesarean section will minimize this threat.

Most cesarean operations in the United States are low transverse procedures. The indications for classical section are restricted mainly to certain cases of anterior placenta previa and transverse lies. With premature breeches, because the lower uterine segment is poorly developed, it may be less traumatic to the infant to deliver him through a vertical incision, which may be extended upward if necessary to provide more room. Disadvantages of a classical section include greater likelihood of rupture, especially before the onset of labor, in subsequent pregnancies, and a greater incidence of infection, bleeding, and adhesions. Cesarean section-hysterectomy may be indicated for neglected transverse lie with an infected uterus, myomas, carcinoma in situ of the cervix, and postpartum hemorrhage with atony.

Many primary cesarean sections are performed for dystocia related to pelvic contraction or a large fetus. Other important maternal indications include abnormal presentations, uterine dysfunction, placenta previa, abruptio placentae, preeclampsia-eclampsia, hypertension, isoimmunization, diabetes, prior vaginal plastic surgical procedures, and possibly the elderly primigravida (over the age of 35). Fetal indications include prolapsed cord and fetal distress. Fetal monitoring has provided a more logical basis for selection of cesarean section for fetal indications, such as post-term pregnancy (p. 151).

159

The frequency of cesarean section in the United States in the last 20 years has quadrupled, from a rate of a little over 5% in 1970 to about 21 to 25% in 1989, or even higher, depending on the proportion of complications in the obstetric population and the local medical attitudes toward repeating all cesarean sections. Complications of the procedure include hemorrhage (the average blood loss during cesarean section is between 800 and 1000 mL), infection, anesthetic accidents, and separation of the uterine and abdominal wounds. Maternal mortality has been reduced to 0.1%, or even less in some series. It is related largely to the indication for the operation, the presence of infection, the duration of labor, and anesthesia. Abdominal delivery per se, nevertheless, involves a distinctly greater risk of maternal mortality and morbidity than does vaginal delivery. Each decision to perform a cesarean section, particularly a primary section, must therefore be made with this increased risk in mind. Perinatal mortality is related to the indication for the operation and in the case of repeated cesarean sections, to the prevalence of prematurity.

The rate of maternal morbidity after cesarean section is approximately 25 to 30%. The prophylactic use of antibiotics in that operation thus seems justified. The drug of choice should be both safe for mother and fetus and effective against the offending organisms. The cephalosporins are often appropriate for this purpose. For metritis after cesarean section, clindamycin and an aminoglycoside may be the combination of choice. Other therapeutic regimens include a cephalosporin of the second or third generation or ampicillin together with an aminoglycoside.

In response to concern about the rapidly rising rate of cesarean section in the United States, much attention has been directed to the indications for the procedure and the means of reducing the number of abdominal deliveries. There seems little doubt that the medicolegal climate in the United States has contributed substantially to the high rate of cesarean section. Current emphasis is placed on a careful analysis of dystocia, uterine scars, breech presentation, and fetal distress as the major factors contributing to the rise in the rate of abdominal delivery.

The causes of dystocia are fetopelvic disproportion and dysfunctional labor (p. 132). Disproportion, which should be recognized easily, has not contributed greatly to the rise in cesarean section, but the diagnosis of abnormalities of uterine contraction is the basis for a significant proportion of abdominal deliveries. Before resorting to cesarean section for uterine dysfunction, the obstetrician should consider other methods of treatment such as rest and oxytocin, for abnormal and subnormal contractions, respectively.

The precept of routine repetition of all cesarean sections has been abandoned. A trial of labor is an option for patients who have: nonrepetitive indication, uterine incision known to be low-segment transverse, singleton pregnancy, vertex presentation, estimated fetal weight less than 4500 g, and absence of all other contraindications to vaginal delivery. Many centers have liberalized the indications for a trial of labor after cesarean section even further. Capability for continuous monitoring of the fetal cardiac rate and uterine activity are prerequisite to attempted vaginal delivery of patients with a uterine scar. The patient must understand that cesarean section may become necessary during the course of labor. Availability of an operating room for immediate cesarean section and appropriate anesthetic and pediatric personnel are required when a trial of labor after cesarean section is attempted. Some centers are now delivering vaginally 60 to 70% of patients who had prior cesarean section, but the patient should be apprised of the risks and through informed consent be allowed to participate in the decision regarding route of delivery.

Abdominal delivery may remain the safest course when the patient has had more than one prior cesarean section and, of course, is required when the cephalopelvic disproportion is absolute. In each of the last few years, about 3.5 million babies have been born in the United States. With a cesarean section rate of about 20%, or 700,000 abdominal deliveries, and a prior uterine incision the indication for about 25% of those operations, almost 200,000 cesarean sections are done each year on that basis alone. If a significant proportion of these 200,000 women can be delivered vaginally with safety, a great medical and economic advantage would result. Nevertheless, the seriousness of uterine rupture for both mother and fetus requires careful selection of patients for vaginal delivery after cesarean section.

Breech presentation also has contributed to the large increase in the rate of cesarean section. Vaginal delivery of the term breech should remain an option when the following conditions are satisfied: fetal weight less than 3500 g, normal pelvic size and shape, frank breech presentation without hyperextended head, and delivery under the supervision of an obstetrician experienced in the technique. The use of external version with tocolysis has reduced the numbers of breech presentations at term and, consequently, of cesarean sections.

The diagnosis of fetal distress should be documented more carefully. Ideally employed, fetal monitoring should not in itself increase the rate of cesarean section, for it may not only identify jeopardized fetuses that require prompt abdominal delivery but may also prevent operations that might otherwise have been performed unnecessarily. With proper surveillance, the rate of cesarean section should be kept to 15% or below, with minimal maternal and perinatal mortality and morbidity.

FORCEPS

The obstetric forceps is an instrument used primarily for traction and rotation of the fetal head. Each pair of forceps consists of two branches. Each branch comprises a handle, a shank, a lock, and a blade. The blade, which may be solid or fenestrated, has two curves. The cephalic curve corresponds to the fetal head, and the pelvic curve corresponds to the pelvic axis. All forceps applications must be cephalic, that is, according to the position of the fetal head.

The forceps may be applied for fetal or maternal indications or electively. The classification of forceps deliveries according to station and position of the fetal head was changed by the American College of Obstetricians and Gynecologists in 1988. The current classification replaces the one in use since 1965 and is probably more consistent with obstetric practice.

An outlet forceps delivery is performed when the fetal scalp is or has been visible at the introitus without separating the mother's labia. The fetal skull has reached the pelvic floor and the sagittal suture is either (a) in the anteroposterior diameter of the outlet or (b) requires rotation of 45° or less.

A low forceps delivery is performed when the fetal head has not yet reached the pelvic floor but is at station +2 cm or below. Low forceps operations include those that require (a) rotation of 45° or less and those that require (b) rotation of more than 45°.

A midforceps delivery involves a procedure performed when the head is engaged but above station +2 cm. Difficult midforceps operations have been replaced in modern obstetrics by cesarean section. A high forceps operation is performed on an unengaged head. It has no place in modern obstetrics because of its potential dangers to mother and fetus and is not included in the current classification of forceps deliveries. For several reasons, not the least of which is medicolegal, forceps procedures are employed less commonly today than in prior decades.

About 20% of deliveries in this country entail the use of forceps. The prerequisites to the application of forceps include the following: fully dilated cervix, engaged head, exact knowledge of the position and station, absence of disproportion, ruptured membranes, proper positioning of the patient on the table, appropriate anesthesia, and preferably, empty bladder and rectum. The procedure should be performed only by an experienced operator who is committed to abandoning the attempt at forceps delivery if difficulty is encountered. Application of forceps is usually accompanied by an episiotomy.

Maternal indications include a prolonged second stage, cardiac disease (to shorten the second stage), acute emergencies such as pulmonary edema and abruptio placentae, and anesthesia that prevents voluntary expulsive efforts in the second stage. Fetal indications include prematurity (to prevent trauma to the fetal head on the perineum) and fetal distress (a heart rate lower than 100 or higher than 160 per minute between contractions, irregularity of the fetal heart, or passage of meconium). The use of forceps for fetal distress is justified only when delivery thereby can be accomplished as safely as and more expeditiously than with cesarean section.

The recent suggestions of the American College of Obstetricians and Gynecologists (ACOG) regarding the shortening of the second stage have not generated unanimity among experienced obstetricians but are included as follows. Outlet forceps may be used to shorten the second stage for maternal or fetal reasons, provided that all the criteria for outlet forceps are met. When the second stage is prolonged, the risks and benefits of allowing labor to continue should be assessed and documented on the chart. The ACOG's suggestions of the definition of prolongation include, for a nullipara, more than 3 hours with a regional anesthetic or more than 2 hours without anesthesia, and for a multipara, more than 2 hours with a regional anesthetic and more than 1 hour without anesthesia.

EPISIOTOMY

Episiotomy may be median (from fourchette directly posteriorly through the midline of perineum), or mediolateral, which involves an incision from the fourchette into the perineum at about 45 degrees from the midline. A midline (median) episiotomy is technically a perineotomy. The operation is performed frequently in first deliveries and in subsequent deliveries after repair of a prior episiotomy. The operation is intended to prevent lacerations of maternal tissues and injury to the fetal head. It is generally used with forceps deliveries. Immediate complications of inadequate repair include hematomas, urinary retention, and shock. Rectovaginal fistula may be a delayed complication of unrecognized or improperly repaired extension of the episiotomy into the rectum.

First-degree obstetric lacerations involve only the vaginal mucosa or perineal skin. Second-degree lacerations involve the underlying muscle and connective tissue but not the sphincter ani. A third-degree laceration involves the anal sphincter in addition. When the rectal mucosa is torn as well,

a fourth-degree, or complete, laceration results.

Median episiotomy entails less blood loss, is easier to repair, and is more comfortable for the patient. It may be used in most spontaneous or low forceps deliveries in any patient with an adequate perineum. The main advantage of a mediolateral episiotomy is the decreased likelihood of its extension into the sphincter ani or rectum, a complication that is usually managed easily by an experienced obstetrician. If an extension of the episiotomy occurs, the injury should be repaired immediately by a skilled obstetrician.

VACUUM EXTRACTION

The vacuum extractor, or ventouse, is more popular in Europe than in the United States. The instrument consists of a disk-shaped cup through which a vacuum of up to 0.8 kg/cm^2 is applied to the fetal scalp. The suction produces a caput succedaneum, to which traction is applied during uterine contractions. Both metal and silastic cups are available, and both manually and electrically induced vacuums are employed. The vacuum should be maintained for a maximum of 30 minutes to avoid injuries to the scalp, a major drawback of the procedure. Vacuum extraction can be used only when the fetus presents by the vertex and should not be used for delivery of premature infants. Successful use of the vacuum extractor depends largely on the obstetrician's experience with the instrument.

VERSION

Version is manual turning of the fetus by the obstetrician from one presentation to another. Cephalic version is turning of the breech or transverse to a head, or cephalic, presentation. This procedure is done externally under tocolysis and ultrasonic guidance without anesthesia before the onset of labor. The fetus may revert to its original presentation after the maneuver. Podalic version is turning of the cephalic or transverse presentation to breech. It is performed internally during the second stage of labor under deep general anesthesia. Its current indications seem restricted to delivery of a second twin or rare cases of transverse lie in the multipara with a fully dilated cervix and intact membranes. Internal version may cause traumatic rupture of the uterus and has been supplanted largely in the United States by cesarean section. Version is contraindicated in the presence of marked oligohydramnios, placenta previa, premature rupture of the membranes, and possibly a uterine scar.

AMNIOCENTESIS

Amniocentesis, or tapping the amniotic sac and withdrawing fluid for analysis through a needle or catheter, is used early in pregnancy (between 15 and 17 weeks' gestation) for prenatal diagnosis by means of examination of the fluid and cells. Late in pregnancy, it is used for ascertaining fetal maturity. A sonographic examination, preferably with dynamic imaging, is used concurrently in fetal diagnosis to measure the biparietal diameter, ascertain the position of the placenta and the location and amount of amniotic fluid, detect fetal cardiac motion, and ascertain the number of fetuses. A 22-gauge needle is inserted through the maternal abdomen into the amniotic cavity and 20 to 30 mL of fluid are removed. The fluid is sent for cytogenetic evaluation of the cultured cells and the supernatant for analysis of α-fetoprotein (p. 104). Recent advances have permitted detection of cystic fibrosis and certain forms of muscular dystrophy through evaluation of the amniotic fluid. Several centers have been performing amniocentesis as early as 10 to 15 weeks of gestation. The dangers of the procedure to mother and fetus are small. The risk of abortion after midtrimester amniocentesis is estimated to be 1 in 200 or less. Evaluation of fetal pulmonary maturity is made on the basis of the lecithin/sphingomyelin ratio, the "shake" (foam stability) test, and the amniotic fluid turbidity.

CHORIONIC VILLUS SAMPLING

Sampling of chorionic villi (CVS) involves transcervical insertion of a catheter of 1.5 mm diameter under ultrasonic guidance. The procedure can be performed earlier in pregnancy than can amniocentesis and therefore can provide an earlier and safer decision about termination of the pregnancy. In experienced hands, the procedure-related rate of abortion is about 0.8%, or slightly higher than that of amniocentesis. CVS does not provide fluid for biochemical analysis, for example, of α-fetoprotein. Sampling can be performed transabdominally as well. The rates of procedure-related abortion with transcervical and transabdominal sampling or chorionic villi are equal.

INDUCTION OF LABOR

Labor may be induced medically (by oxytocin or prostaglandin) or surgically (amniotomy, or rupture of the membranes). Medical induction is accomplished by means of an infusion containing 10 units of oxytocin/1000 mL of 5% dextrose in Ringer's lactate or isotonic or half-isotonic saline, administered at the same rate and with the same precautions as used for stimulation of labor (p. 132). The hazards of induction with oxytocin include rupture of the uterus, premature separation of the placenta, and fetal hypoxia. Additional complications include prematurity, uterine infection, and prolapse of the umbilical cord. Several European clinics have found parenteral prostaglandins to be suitable alternatives to oxytocin for medical induction of labor. Vaginally administered prostaglandin has been used successfully to evacuate the uterus in cases of fetal demise toward the end of the second trimester.

Prostaglandin gels, administered intravaginally or intracervically, have been used in many centers as adjuvants in the induction of labor. Their use, however, has not been accompanied by a reduction in the rate of cesarean section for failed induction. "Ripening" the cervix with natural Laminaria or tents made of a synthetic hygroscopic polymer has been shown to increase the rate of success of medicinal induction of labor.

A few of the important indications for induction of labor are erythroblastosis fetalis, diabetes mellitus, preeclampsia-eclampsia, and premature rupture of the membranes. Induction of labor in a multipara who lives some distance from the hospital and has a history of rapid labors may be considered obstetrically indicated. When induction of labor is medically indicated, delivery should usually be accomplished within 48 hours after initiation of attempts at induction and within 24 hours after rupture of the membranes.

Strictly elective inductions may appear convenient for the patient and the obstetrician, but their advisability as a routine procedure is at best questionable. Induction is most likely to succeed if rupture of the membranes is accompanied by simultaneous initiation of an infusion of oxytocin. Success of induction is further increased when the cervix is effaced, at least 2 cm dilated, and anterior, and the fetus is mature. An unengaged head is not an absolute contraindication to amniotomy, but before the procedure is performed, the fetal head must be brought as deeply as possible into the pelvis by fundal and suprapubic pressure and facilities for immediate cesarean section should be available to cope with the possibility of prolapse of the umbilical cord.

NEONATAL CIRCUMCISION

Circumcision of the newborn male infant in the United States is performed most commonly with the Gomco clamp or a similar instrument. The procedure is relatively safe and bloodless. Other instruments are popular, each with its advantages and inconveniences. Whether to use local anesthesia routinely is still debatable and there is no national standard of care with respect to this issue. The procedure is discussed further in Chapter 8.

III

GYNECOLOGY

CONTROL OF REPRODUCTION

28
CHAPTER

CONTRACEPTION

The exponential increase in the populations of the nation and the world has placed family planning and population control in the forefront of medical and social problems. The justification for detailed discussion of this subject is thus obvious.

Contraception may be either temporary or permanent. Permanent contraception is often referred to as sterilization. The effectiveness of a contraceptive technique is determined by the pregnancy rate (PR), which is defined as follows:

$$PR = \frac{\text{Number of pregnancies} \times 1200}{\text{Patients observed} \times \text{months of exposure}}.$$

The pregnancy rate in a population that does not use contraception is about 80 to 90. The birth rate is the number of births per 1000 population. The fertility rate is the number of live births per 1000 female population between the ages of 15 and 44 years. The marriage rate is the number of marriages per 1000 population.

By 1991, the world's population had reached well over 5 billion. This is considerably more than twice the number of people on earth at the end of World War II (1945). By the year 1850, the population of the world had reached one billion; the second billion were added in less than a century. With an annual birth rate of 29 and a death rate of 11, the current rate of growth is 1.8%.

The time required for doubling the world's population at its present rate of growth is about 35 years. Although the rate is smaller in highly developed countries, the life expectancy at birth is greater there. In the United States, life expectancy is 75 years.

The crude birth rate, death rate, and natural increase (annual percentage) for the United States are 16, 9, and 0.7, respectively. These figures correspond to a doubling time of the population of 95 years. Thus, the projected population of the United States for the year 2000 is over 270 million.

The effectiveness of a contraceptive is defined by its theoretical effectiveness and its use-effectiveness. Theoretical effectiveness is the antifertility action of any contraceptive method under ideal conditions with no omissions or errors in use. Use-effectiveness, or actual effectiveness, is the protection achieved under realistic conditions of life. It depends on motivation, cultural characteristics, and socioeconomic status of the population.

No ideal contraceptive is currently available. The characteristics of a perfect contraceptive include effectiveness, safety, low cost, esthetic qualities, ease of use, lack of relation to coitus, and absence of the requirement for repeated motivation.

Because patients are often receptive to discussions of contraception during pregnancy, it is wise to initiate these discussions at that time, immediately post partum, and again at the 4-week postpartum examination.

Contraception may be divided into folk (primitive), conventional (traditional), modern, and experimental methods.

FOLK METHODS

The important primitive techniques include coitus interruptus (withdrawal), extravaginal intercourse, abstinence, prolonged lactation, and postcoital douches.

Coitus interruptus, or withdrawal, is still a common practice throughout the world. Its pregnancy rate is 15. The contraceptive effectiveness depends on prevention of ejaculation into the vagina. It requires, however, male control over ejaculation and the prevention of the preejaculatory dribble of spermatozoa-laden fluid. The technique is often inapplicable or unsatisfying to one or both partners.

The postcoital douche as a sole means of contraception is to be discouraged because it has a failure rate almost equal to that of unprotected intercourse. The lack of effectiveness results from the rapid entrance of the sperm into the cervical canal.

The failure rate of prolonged lactation as a contraceptive technique is unknown. The delay of ovulation post partum is highly variable and has been known to occur early during breastfeeding. The advantages of this technique are its lack of cost and ready availability.

Extravaginal intercourse is widely practiced, sometimes for purposes of contraception. Intertriginous, oral, and anal intercourse are effective only when not accompanied by vaginal intromission. Receptive anal intercourse, furthermore, carries the risk of AIDS when the active partner is infected with the virus.

Abstinence is time-honored and effective but obviously inapplicable to most couples.

TRADITIONAL METHODS

The traditional contraceptive techniques include rhythm; intravaginal spermicides such as jellies, creams, tablets, sponges, and foams; and mechanical (barrier) methods including the condom, diaphragm, and cervical cap.

RHYTHM

Aside from abstinence, the rhythm method is the only means of contraception in compliance with all religious doctrines. It depends on the avoidance of coitus during the fertile period, which requires prediction of ovulation. Because of uncertainties in the duration of viability of the sperm and the egg, intercourse must be avoided for a week before and 3 days after ovulation. A clinically useful method of predicting ovulation that is independent of the length of the cycle is based on measurements of viscosity of cervical mucus. The pregnancy rate with this method is about 20.

Rhythm, or calendar, methods of predicting ovulation are dependent upon length of the prior cycle. Thus, historic data are needed to predict satisfactorily a future ovulation. The success of the method depends upon the regularity of the menses and requires strong motivation. For maximal safety, long periods of abstinence are required. Although menstruation occurs fairly regularly at 14 days after ovulation, the length of the preovulatory phase is quite variable. A rise in basal body temperature of about 0.5° C during the luteal phase of the cycle can be used to detect ovulation, but it is necessarily a retrospective finding.

The symptothermal method of contraception combines features of the techniques that depend on detection of the rise in temperature and prediction of ovulation. The signs and symptoms of impending ovulation include thinning and flow of the cervical mucus, tenderness of the breasts, abdominal cramps, vaginal spotting, and changes in position and consistency of the cervix. This method requires abstention from intercourse from the time that vaginal wetness is first detected until the third day after the rise in temperature or the fourth day after the time of maximal production of mucus.

SPERMICIDES

The use of spermicidal jellies, creams, tablets, and foams as the sole contraceptive technique is accompanied by a pregnancy rate of about 20, which is much higher than that of the most effective forms of contraception but only one quarter of the rate associated with the use of no contraception. These agents may be used to advantage in the woman who has infrequent intercourse, but are unesthetic, must be used just before coitus, and may taste objectionable to those who perform cunnilingus. Allergic reactions to certain components of the products may occur in one or both partners. The Encare Oval tablet provides a foaming viscous barrier and contains the most commonly employed spermicide, nonoxynol-9. Rates of pregnancy with this preparation are similar to those with the older vaginal spermicides. Spermicidal agents are used most effectively in conjunction with the diaphragm. All of these products are available in the United States without prescription (over the counter).

BARRIER METHODS

The vaginal diaphragm is an occlusive device with a diameter of 65 to 90 mm. The theoretical pregnancy rate with the diaphragm alone is about 7, but it can be reduced by use in conjunction with a spermicidal agent. The realistic failure rate of this method, however, is about 18. This form of contraception is inexpensive and it may render intercourse during menstrual periods more esthetic. The disadvantages of the diaphragm are the need for recurrent motivation, the association with coitus, and the requirement for fitting by a physician. For maximal effectiveness, it is necessary to refit the diaphragm annually and post partum. Many women find the required vaginal manipulation unesthetic, but the sexual partner may be taught to insert the diaphragm. It may be inserted many hours before intercourse, but for maximal safety it should remain in place at least 8 hours after the last intercourse. This technique is not suitable with severe degrees of pelvic relaxation. Emphasis in the lay press during the 1980s on adverse effects of the oral and intrauterine contraceptives has resulted in increased utilization of the diaphragm in the last decade in certain populations.

An occlusive technique that may be used in cases of vaginal relaxation is the cervical cap, which adheres by suction. The pregnancy rate with the cervical cap is about 7. Its principal disadvantage is the need for frequent removal, but it requires no manipulations during the cycle. Current experimental designs utilize one-way valves, which permit escape of menstrual efflux while excluding the entrance of spermatozoa into the cervix.

The condom, with a pregnancy rate of about 7, is still the most important traditional method of contraception throughout the world. Its realistic failure rate is about 12. It is also a mechanical device with an additional advantage of providing protection against sexually transmitted diseases. The latex varieties in particular decrease greatly the risk of transmission of HIV. Its principal disadvantages are the relatively high cost, the need for interruption of the sexual act, and the requirement for high motivation. Failures with the condom are related to poor timing of its application, breaks or leaks, and spillage of semen during removal. Some condoms decrease penile sensitivity, an effect that is generally but not always considered a disadvantage. A female condom, though not widely used, is available. It lines the vaginal cavity and provides an additional option for the woman to take responsibility for contraception and prevention of disease.

MODERN METHODS

Intrauterine devices and hormonal contraception are the two modern methods, which have the lowest pregnancy rates.

INTRAUTERINE DEVICES

The intrauterine devices (IUDs) regained popularity as contraceptives during the 1960s and early 1970s. The newer varieties are made of inert plastics. The pregnancy rate is about 6. The theoretical effectiveness is about 99% and the use-effectiveness about 94%. The mechanism of action is incompletely known, although the most popular current hypothesis involves an antizygotic or antinidational effect produced by a subclinical endometritis. Advantages include the low cost and the lack of relation to coitus. For further safety the patient should feel for the string, which projects through the cervix into the vagina. Additional protection is provided by the use of a spermicidal agent at midcycle.

Recently the manufacturers of all but one of the popular IUDs ceased distribution of their products within the United States. The decision was made for medicolegal rather than medical reasons. The inert loop (Lippes loop) was removed from the market in the autumn of 1985 and the major copper-containing devices (Copper-7 and Copper-T) were removed early in 1986.

Intrauterine contraception is a reversible technique that involves only a single decision on the patient's part. It requires a physician or another trained health professional to perform a pelvic examination to ascertain size and position of the uterus. The insertion is facilitated by application of a tenaculum to the anterior lip of the cervix. The larger devices have a lower rate of expulsion but generally cause more bleeding and cramps. The likelihood of uterine perforation is about 1 in 2000. Open (loop or coil) rather than closed (bow or ring) devices are the only forms currently used in the United States because perforation by the closed types is more likely to cause intestinal obstruction. An important advance in the field of intrauterine contraception was the addition of metallic copper to the plastic device. The ionization of the copper produces a spermicidal or antizygotic effect, which is in proportion to the amount of metal wrapped around the device. The formerly available Copper-7 and Copper-T required replacement every 3 years.

Another intrauterine contraceptive technique involves the impregnation of the device with a slowly released steroid. The Progestasert device releases progesterone and combines the action of an inert IUD with local effects of the steroid on the endometrium. It requires annual removal and replacement by a new device. The Progestasert has been associated with a higher rate of ectopic pregnancies than have some other IUDs, but for a short while it was the only intrauterine device distributed in the United States. Devices containing epsilon-aminocaproic acid are available in other countries; through inhibition of fibrinolysis they are designed to decrease the amount of blood lost.

In the 1990s, a new copper-containing intrauterine device (ParaGard) was introduced in the United States. It has the advantage of effectiveness for as long as 8 consecutive years. Current investigations of the device suggest that it is toxic to sperm and is therefore by definition contraceptive rather than abortifacient. This distinction is of major significance in relation to the acceptability of this technique to large groups of women.

Contraindications to the use of any IUD include pregnancy or suspicion of pregnancy; abnormalities of the uterus that cause distortion of the uterine cavity; acute pelvic inflammatory disease or a history of repeated bouts of pelvic inflammatory disease; postpartum endometritis or infected abortion in the preceding three months; known or suspected endometrial or cervical cancer and abnormal Papanicolaou smears without histologic confirmation; genital bleeding of unknown cause; and untreated acute cervicitis. In addition, copper-containing devices are contraindicated in patients with Wilson's disease or a known allergy to copper.

Insertion of an IUD should be performed, if possible, during or shortly after a menstrual period to avoid placement within a pregnant uterus. To reduce the risk of perforation or expulsion, insertion after delivery or abortion should be delayed until the uterus has returned to its normal size. The patient with an IUD in place should receive an annual pelvic examination and Papanicolaou smear, although it is not necessary to remove the inert device periodically. For maximal protection, it may be desirable to use another form of contraception for the first few months that the device is in place.

Disadvantages of the IUD include difficulty of insertion and undesirability in the nullipara, and the possibility of uterine perforation, bleeding, and cramps, especially in the first few cycles. In addition, there is a rate of initial expulsion of about 10%. A major complication of the IUD is an increased relative risk of pelvic inflammatory disease and consequently of ectopic pregnancy. The relative risk of infection in parous women in monogamous relationships is low, however. The risk of tubal infection is greatest during the first month after insertion or reinsertion of the device, although patients with IUDs are at higher risk for salpingitis up to 12 months after the device has been removed. Among users of

IUDs, about 1 pregnancy in 20 results in an ectopic implantation, in part because of the greater effectiveness of IUDs in preventing uterine as compared with ectopic pregnancies.

Unilateral nongonococcal adnexal abscesses, some of actinomycotic origin, have been described (Fig. 28–1). Because of the risks of infection and ectopic pregnancy, it is generally inadvisable to prescribe the IUD for a nullipara to whom other contraceptive techniques are available, or for a patient who has already had one ectopic pregnancy.

When a woman becomes pregnant with an IUD in place and wishes to keep the pregnancy, the device should be removed if the strings are visible. If the strings are not visible and the device cannot be readily removed, the patient is asked whether she wishes to continue with the pregnancy. If she does, she is informed of the increased risks of spontaneous abortion, infection, and ectopic pregnancy. If she does not want to continue with the pregnancy, the IUD is removed and the pregnancy is terminated. Intrauterine infection demands termination of the pregnancy in any case.

If a closed or a medicated IUD perforates the uterus, it should be removed by laparotomy or laparoscopy. An inert open device is generally innocuous, although it too should be removed to preclude perforation of an adjacent viscus.

HORMONAL CONTRACEPTION

Hormonal contraception (pill, injection, and implant) is the most effective form of birth control presently available. For the most part, these drugs are used orally (oral contraceptives), but they are also effective parenterally. Before any of these drugs is used, a complete history and physical examination must be performed and pregnancy excluded. Particular attention must be paid to the breasts, the thyroid, and the blood pressure. A Papanicolaou smear should be obtained and the urine tested for protein

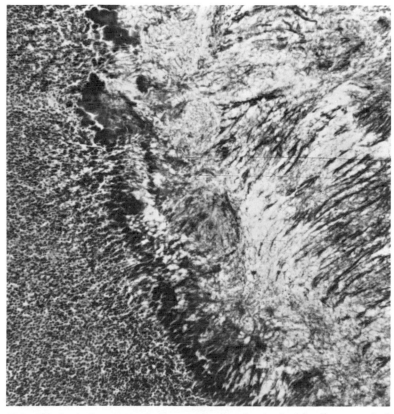

FIG. 28–1. Actinomyces in the ovary, showing typical "sulfur granule."

and sugar. Young women should be examined at least annually and older women at even more frequent intervals.

The most popular oral contraceptive pills currently available are monophasic and triphasic combination products, which contain various formulations of both a synthetic estrogen and a synthetic progestin. Most of the pills contain ethinyl estradiol (EE) in doses of 20 to 50 μg. A few still contain mestranol, the methylated derivative of EE, which is demethylated before becoming physiologically active. During the last three decades, the doses of estrogen in the pill have been reduced gradually and substantially so that both the mild and serious side effects reported with the higher-dose preparations occur much less frequently today. There are currently about eight progestins used worldwide in oral contraceptives. Although the compounds may be synthesized from three parent molecules (pregnanes, estranes, and gonanes), only progestins from the latter two groups are available at present in oral contraceptives. The five progestins in use in the United States today are norethindrone, norethindrone acetate, levonorgestrel, norethynodrel, and ethynodiol acetate. The remaining progestins, which are available in Europe and elsewhere but are not yet approved for distribution in the United States, are gestodene, desogestrel, and norgestimate. The decreased androgenicity of desogestrel and norgestimate and the more favorable effects on blood lipids, compared with other progestins, make them attractive alternatives for contraception. As with the synthetic estrogens, the doses of the constituent progestins have decreased progressively with no loss of effectiveness but with considerable reduction in side effects.

The effects of the specific combined preparations depend on the doses and ratios of the estrogen and the progestin. All conventional combined oral contraceptives inhibit ovulation. They may also effect a change in cervical mucus, which results in decreased penetrability by spermatozoa. Furthermore, these drugs may affect the endometrium or tubal and uterine fluids. In the combined form of oral contraception, a pill containing estrogen and progestin is taken every day for 20 or 21 days starting on Day 5 of the cycle. Bleeding normally occurs 3 or 4 days after the last pill is taken. In the 21-day regimen no pill is taken for 7 days. In the 28-day regimen a placebo is taken for 7 days after the last active pill.

With the traditional combined pills, the amounts of estrogen and progestin in each pill remain unchanged during the cycle. With the newer triphasic methods, only the amount of estrogen remains fairly constant and the amount of progestin is increased on about Day 12 and again on about Day 17. The lower steroid content of the triphasic oral contraceptive, as compared with the fixed-dose combination pill, ideally lessens systemic side effects and interference with normal hypothalamic-pituitary function without decreasing contraceptive efficacy.

In one of the popular triphasic preparations, the dose of ethinyl estradiol is kept constant at 35 μg but that of norethindrone is raised from 0.5 mg in the first week, to 0.75 mg in the second week, to 1 mg in the third week. In another triphasic regimen, the dose of estrogen varies from 30 to 40 μg and the progestin (levonorgestrel) is increased from 0.05 mg to 0.075 mg to 0.125 mg. Biphasic and triphasic pills are available in 21-day and 28-day regimens.

A new hormonal agent described as an antiprogesterone and named RU-486 was introduced in France in 1982. This drug is capable of expelling from the uterus any ovum fertilized during that month. The conventional oral contraceptives must be taken for 3 weeks each month, whereas RU-486 is effective when taken only once a month in the form of a pill or an injection. The drug competes with and displaces progesterone from its endometrial receptors, renders the uterus deficient in progesterone, and causes progesterone-withdrawal bleeding. The dual potential action of RU-486 as both contraceptive and abortifacient has led to the designation of the drug as a "contragestive." In 1991, New Hampshire became the first state to allow testing of this drug. RU-486 is particularly effective when used together with prostaglandins to expel the uterine contents.

The advantages of all forms of oral contraception are their lack of relation to coitus and their extreme effectiveness. The disadvantages are their relatively high cost, the need for constant motivation, the mild common side effects, and the rare but serious hazard of thromboembolism and other cardiovascular complications.

Mild and inconstant complications of the pill include nausea and occasional vomiting, bloating, enlargement and tenderness of the breasts, melasma (irregular brownish discoloration of the skin of the face), weight gain, hypomenorrhea, benign cervical hyperplasia, and altered metabolic functions, among which may be increase in binding globulins, increase in triglycerides and total phospholipids, decrease in glucose tolerance, and possibly jaundice. The estrogen in the combined pill may lead to increase in high-density lipoprotein (HDL) cholesterol, whereas some progestins may cause the reverse. There is a small increase in coronary occlusion, a disease that is ordinarily rare in women of reproductive age.

Additional possible complications include a reversible hypertension (perhaps of the renin-dependent variety), uncommon neurologic or ophthalmologic problems, a change in libido (increase or decrease), and occasional increase in vaginal discharge.

Less common complications include an increase in gallbladder disease and urinary tract infections, presumably as a result of hormonal effects similar to those of pregnancy. Unusual complications, associated particularly with mestranol-containing compounds, are focal nodular hyperplasia of the liver and hepatic adenomas. Although most of the hepatic adenomas related to the pill are benign, they may rupture and produce serious hemorrhage. The association of hepatic carcinoma with use of the pill has not been confirmed.

The most serious complication that has been documented is thromboembolism. The causes of the increased risk of deep venous thrombosis and thromboembolism are not well understood. Vascular intimal and medial lesions with occlusive thrombi have been described. In addition, use of combined estrogen-progestin pills may lead to acceleration of platelet aggregation and reduction in activity of both plasma antithrombin III and endothelial plasminogen activator. The incidence of thromboembolism associated with use of oral contraceptives is directly related to the dose of estrogen. Pills containing less than 50 μg of synthetic estrogen are associated with a low risk of thromboembolism and, in some

studies, no increased risk at all in women not otherwise predisposed to these complications.

The FDA requires detailed information in the package labeling of oral contraceptives. All mortality and morbidity rates, however, must be compared with those associated with pregnancy itself. Furthermore, the seriousness of the cardiovascular complications is proportional to the prevalence of those diseases in the geographic area under consideration. The risks are therefore greater in western Europe and the United States than they are in parts of Africa, for example, where the rate of thromboembolism is low.

Anterospective studies report that the cardiovascular effects of oral contraceptives are synergistic, rather than simply additive, with those of hyperlipidemia, diabetes mellitus, hypertension, obesity, and cigarette smoking. The date from these studies, furthermore, indicate that the increased risk of death from cardiovascular disease in women is greater than that suggested in prior retrospective studies and that it occurs at an age somewhat lower than previously reported. Women who have taken the pill for more than 5 years and who smoke are at particular risk. Again, diabetes, hypertension, and obesity add to the danger. These studies show that even if the pill is stopped, there is an increased likelihood of later death from cardiovascular disease. For women under 35, there occurs only one death per year per 20,000 women on the pill. The risk rises sharply over this age. Between the ages of 35 and 44, the rate is one per 3000 women, and for women over 45, the rate is one in 700. The overall annual rate is one death per 5000 women on the pill.

In addition to pulmonary embolism, myocardial infarction, and stroke, several other cardiovascular complications have been associated with the pill: subarachnoid hemorrhage, malignant hypertension, cardiomyopathy, mesenteric arterial thrombosis, and exacerbation of congenital and rheumatic cardiac diseases. Logical recommendations based on this new information are as follows. For women under the age of 30 there is no need to stop oral contraception, although cessation of smoking is advantageous. Between the ages of 30 and 35, the risk gradually increases. Some women in this group, for example those who have used oral contraceptives continuously for 5 years and smoke cigarettes, should reconsider the use of the pill. Nonsmokers could probably continue the pill. Women over the age of 35, particularly those who have used the pill continuously for 5 years or more or who smoke, would do well to consider other forms of contraception. Inasmuch as the pill takes several years to affect the cardiovascular system, there is no reason to stop it suddenly. The pill should not be stopped without an alternate temporary contraceptive method or sterilization.

In 1990, the FDA made a significant change in its recommendations for use of oral contraceptives. It is now considered safe for a woman at age 40 or beyond to continue the use of oral contraceptives if she has no other risk factors. In fact, it may be in the best interests of some women to continue oral contraceptives until their fertile years are over, at which time they may switch to estrogen replacement therapy. It has become clear in the last few years that many of the alleged hazards of oral contraceptives were, in fact, results of the concomitant effects of smoking cigarettes. It is probably fair to suggest that cigarettes are a far greater hazard to health than oral contraceptives ever were.

Two factors associated with the use of oral contraceptives appear to increase the likelihood of venous thrombosis and thromboembolism: decreased activity of antithrombin III and lower levels of epithelial plasminogen activator. Among users of the pill, furthermore, those with blood types A, B, or AB have three times the likelihood of thromboembolic and other cardiovascular disease than do those with blood type O. This finding suggests a genetic predisposition to thromboembolism.

Except for history of thromboembolic disorder or actual thrombophlebitis, most contraindications to the pill are relative. There are no data to support the relation of combined oral contraceptives to the development of carcinoma of the cervix. A prospective study, however, of women with dysplasia of the cervix showed an increase in severity of dysplasia and of conversion to carcinoma in situ in users of the contraceptive pill compared with users of other non-barrier contraceptive methods, although factors such as smoking, age at first intercourse, and number of sexual partners were more significant. The incidences of endometrial and ovarian carcinoma are actually decreased by use of the pill.

Whether a woman's past use of oral contraceptives increases her risk of mammary cancer remains controversial. Multiple epidemiologic studies as well as a meta-analysis of pooled data fail to yield a consensus regarding increased relative risk for mammary cancer in women who have ever used oral contraceptives. The confounding variables of age at first use, duration of use, variety of oral contraceptive formulations ingested, fertility status, and independent familial risks have made the analysis difficult. Several large case-controlled studies of mammary cancer and use of oral contraceptives tend to suggest that prior use of oral contraceptives does not increase a woman's relative risk of developing mammary cancer. Studies that have examined the data carefully within several subgroups of users of oral contraceptives, however, have concluded tentatively that patients with a prior history of benign mammary disease, patients with first-degree relatives with mammary cancer, and patients presenting with confirmed mammary cancer before age 45 may have unidentified cofactors that, in conjunction with use of oral contraceptives, have increased slightly their relative risk of developing cancer of the breast.

The oral contraceptives should not be used in a patient with undiagnosed uterine bleeding. Relative contraindications include hypertension, obesity, cardiovascular and venous diseases, hepatic disorders, a strong familial history of thromboembolism, diabetes mellitus, and possibly migraine headaches. Pills with a large dose of estrogen may cause myomas to increase in size. Use of steroidal contraception during lactation may, rarely, cause jaundice in the newborn.

The main cause of failure of oral contraception is irregular or incorrect use of the pills. With this form of birth control, the use-effectiveness is considerably lower than the theoretical effectiveness. The pregnancy rate based on theoretical effectiveness of the standard combined pills is 0.1, which is equivalent to virtually complete effectiveness. The pregnancy rate based on use-effectiveness, however, is close to 3.0.

The patient should not depend on the oral contraceptives for complete protection for the first 7 to 10 days of their use, but should use additional spermicidal agents or mechanical devices. If one pill is missed or if breakthrough bleeding occurs, the dosage should be doubled. If two pills are missed in sequence, some other form of contraception should be used for the remainder of that cycle. If no bleeding occurs by 7 days after the last pill, a new cycle of medication should be started as though bleeding had occurred. If two or more amenorrheic cycles occur in succession, the pill should be stopped and the possibility of pregnancy investigated.

The pill should be taken from the fifth to the twenty-eighth day of the cycle and begun again on the fifth day after the onset of bleeding, or on the fifth day of amenorrhea if no bleeding has occurred during that cycle. It is advisable to take the pill at the same time each day. If one pill is forgotten, it should be taken as soon as possible after the regular time and the next pill at the regular time. If two pills in succession are forgotten, two pills should be taken as soon as possible after remembering and two pills at the regular time on the next day. Another form of contraception should be used for the remainder of that cycle. If three pills in succession are missed, a different procedure is advised. No additional pills should be taken. The patient is advised to wait 4 days longer and resume the medication regardless of whether the absence of hormones for 7 days has resulted in uterine bleeding and even if the bleeding is still in progress. During the 7 days when no pills have been taken and during the first 10 days of the new cycle an additional form of contraception is required for maximal safety.

Slight spotting during the cycle, especially during the first 2 months of use, is not necessarily a contraindication to the pill. A tampon may be worn during the time of uterine spotting and a different pill prescribed. If the bleeding is equal in amount to a normal period, the pill should be stopped and a cycle of 21 pills begun on the fifth day, counting Day 1 as the first day of bleeding. If such heavy bleeding occurs twice, the patient should consult her physician. If a period is missed after proper use of 21 pills, it is most unlikely that pregnancy has occurred and the next cycle should be resumed on the eighth day after taking the last pill of the preceding cycle. If two periods in succession are missed, an examination is indicated to rule out pregnancy and possibly to switch medication.

Most of the side effects of the pill are mild, reversible, and related to the dosages of the steroids. The following less common but more serious complications require medical advice: cramps or swelling of the legs, chest pain, hemoptysis, dyspnea, sudden severe headache, dizziness, difficulty with vision or speech, and weakness or numbness of the extremities.

Many drugs in common use may interfere with the action of oral contraceptives. The more important of these drugs include ampicillin, penicillin V, neomycin, phenobarbital, rifampicin, phenytoin, and phenylbutazone. Other drugs that may decrease the effectiveness of oral contraceptives include chloramphenicol, nitrofurantoin, phenacetin, meprobamate, clotrimazole, and kaolin in antidiarrheal preparations. When a patient is taking one of these drugs, it is advisable to prescribe an oral contraceptive with a higher dose of estrogen, such as 50 μg.

The "minipill" contains only a progestin (0.35 mg of norethindrone). Unlike other oral contraceptives it is administered continuously in a daily dosage throughout the year. Its effectiveness is lower than that of the conventional combined pills. The theoretical pregnancy rate is approximately 3 per 100 woman-years, compared with less than 1 for estrogen-progestin combinations. The "minipill" has not achieved great popularity in the United States. The rate of dropout for minipills is higher than that for conventional oral contraceptives, presumably because of a significant incidence of unpredictable bleeding that may not follow any consistent pattern even after prolonged use.

The mode of action of the minipill is not clear, although it is known that it does not necessarily inhibit ovulation. For that reason the risk of ectopic pregnancy is increased. It may prevent the thinning at midcycle of the cervical mucus, preventing penetration by sperm, possibly affecting capacitation of sperm, or rendering the endometrium unfavorable for implantation.

Estrogen-progestin preparations with 20 to 30 µg of estrogen produce fewer estrogen-related complications, but are associated with a high incidence of breakthrough bleeding. Thus, after an initial period of popularity their use has declined.

Intramuscular contraception with long-acting progestins is used widely in many parts of the world (developed and developing), but the Food and Drug Administration continues to withhold its approval of medroxyprogesterone acetate for routine contraception, mainly because of the finding of mammary tumors in beagles that had received large doses of chlormadinone, a related drug. Furthermore, in rhesus monkeys that had received large doses of medroxyprogesterone, endometrial carcinoma was found, although animals that received the dose normally given to women were free of cancer. Medroxyprogesterone acetate, however, in large doses has been used widely for treatment of endometrial carcinoma (p. 218). The drug, given as a monthly injection or possibly even as an injection every 3 months in doses of 150 mg, could provide contraception for mental defectives and other women who cannot be relied upon to take a pill daily. It could also provide a logical alternative to sterilization for those women.

Considerable effort in research and development has been spent on delivery of long-acting contraceptive steroids that need not be taken orally on a daily basis. Finally, in 1991, the first new contraceptive option in 30 years was made available to American women. Norplant consists of six small Silastic-coated capsules that contain levonorgestrel, which is released at a predictable rate of about 30 µg daily. The drug received FDA approval after extensive studies of more than 50,000 women in 46 countries demonstrated its safety and efficacy. The capsules are implanted under local anesthesia subcutaneously on the inside of the woman's nondominant arm. The principal mode of action of the implant appears to be inhibition of ovulation, and the onset of action of the drug is very soon after insertion. The realistic failure rate (pregnancies per 100 women per year) is less than one, the lowest of any currently available contraceptive. This form of contraception has a greater rate of failure in obese women, in whom the hormone is trapped in the adipose tissue. Because this formulation contains only a progestin, it may be suitable for women in whom estrogens are contraindicated. The most frequent side-effect is irregular uterine spotting, but the drug does not appear to influence blood pressure and does not have an unfavorable effect on plasma lipids. The implant may provide effective contraception for 5 years.

Another promising technique is the vaginal ring, made of Silastic containing levonorgestrel and estradiol. The ring, which is worn for 3 weeks out of 4, releases the two hormones into the vagina at a constant rate. A vaginal ring that contains only progestin and is worn continuously is under development.

A third technique is the injection of biodegradable polymeric microspheres containing norethisterone. These microspheres are injected intramuscularly as a suspension. A single dose containing 65 to 100 mg of norethindrone provides contraception for 3 months.

The differing proportions and dosages of the steroids in the conventional contraceptive formulations cause a variety of side effects. Fortunately, the drugs may be switched with ease, maintaining contraceptive effectiveness and minimizing the complications.

Signs of excess estrogen include nausea, edema, leg cramps, vertigo, leukorrhea, growth of myomas, melasma, and uterine cramps. Estrogenic deficiency is manifested by irritability, nervousness, flushes, hot flashes, early and midcyclic bleeding, and decreased uterine bleeding.

Excess of progestins may be manifested by increased appetite and weight gain, fatigue, depression, acne, change in libido, jaundice, and hypomenorrhea. A deficiency of progestins may result in late breakthrough bleeding, heavy flow and clots, and delayed onset of the menses. The wide variety of combinations and dosages of estrogens and progestins usually permits the choice of a pill with minimal side effects and maximal effectiveness.

The "morning-after" pill is basically a large dose of an estrogen that is taken between 24 hours and 72 hours after unprotected intercourse. It is currently recommended in situations such as rape or other emergencies. It often causes nausea and vomiting. Diethylstilbestrol (DES) in doses of 25 mg b.i.d. for 5 days is a convenient estrogen to use as a postcoital contraceptive ("interceptive"), but its relation to reproductive losses in the offspring of mothers who took the drug during pregnancy raises doubts about the advisability of its use in any woman of reproductive age. Although the risk of clear cell adenocarcinoma is very small, the associated nonmalignant changes may affect fertility in daughters and possibly sons of DES-exposed mothers. The changes in the vagina and cervix include hoods, pseudopolyps, rims, and collars (p. 263). An antiemetic medication may be given with the stilbestrol to minimize the nausea and vomiting. The availability of abortion in the event that the patient who takes these drugs is already pregnant reduces the hazard.

Several steroidal estrogens, none of which has yet been shown to be associated with vaginal or cervical carcinomas, also are effective. Suggested regimens include ethinyl estradiol, 2.5 mg twice a day; estrone, 5 mg twice a day; conjugated estrogens, 10 mg twice a day; and several combined estrogen-progestin oral contraceptive pills. The steroids have not yet been approved by the FDA for use as postcoital contraceptives. Pregnancy can be prevented also by the insertion of a copper intrauterine device within 5 days of coitus at midcycle. This method has the advantage of providing continued contraception.

EXPERIMENTAL METHODS

Among the experimental techniques, several antizygotic agents have been tested. These drugs are toxic, however, and the differences between abortifacient and teratogenic dosages are small. Again, perhaps the availability of abortion may lead to wider use of this class of drugs.

Male chemosterilants are also under investigation. These drugs may suppress spermatogenesis but are generally toxic, resulting in a decrease in libido and in production of androgens. Some of these drugs have an antabuse effect.

Gossypol, a potential male contraceptive, appears to work by inhibiting lactate dehydrogenase, which is crucial in aerobic and anaerobic metabolism of sperm and sperm-generating cells. The drug has proved highly effective in China, and its contraceptive effects are apparently reversible. Its adverse effects include hypokalemia, nausea, weakness, gastric discomfort, changes in appetite, and rarely, paralysis. It also inhibits glutathione S-transferase, an enzyme that participates in the detoxification of certain potential carcinogens. It is unlikely that gossypol will be recommended for use as a male contraceptive in the United States.

A promising technique of temporary male contraception involves daily injections of GnRH antagonist and weekly injections of testosterone. The men who received these injections reported no reduction in libido or erectile potency during the study. Sperm counts were suppressed completely until 2 weeks after the treatment was stopped, but they returned to baseline by 14 weeks after treatment.

Preliminary data suggesting that prostaglandins may be effective contraceptives or early abortifacients have not been confirmed. The principal problem with the presently available prostaglandins is their widespread undesirable systemic effects.

A logical approach to contraception is the use of agonists and antagonists of gonadotropin releasing hormones. Unlike the oral contraceptives, these hormones have a highly localized site of action. An inhibitor of the gonadotropin releasing hormone (GnRH), for example, would specifically inhibit ovulation or spermatogenesis. These compounds are effective in nanogram doses. By controlling release of gonadotropins, GnRH plays a role in two critical events in the menstrual cycle: follicular development and production of progesterone by the corpus luteum. Subcutaneous injection of an agonist of luteinizing hormone releasing hormone induces a shortened luteal phase, with suboptimal concentrations of circulating estrogen and progesterone. Administration of these agonists for 3 successive days at the time of onset of the menstrual cycle thus appears to be a practical approach to control of fertility. Use of the analogs may be effective in men by suppressing spermatogenesis without interfering with production of LH and testosterone. It is thus necessary to produce a dissociated response of LH and FSH; current research indicates that dissociation is possible.

The immunologic control of pregnancy has much to commend it theoretically, but has not yet reached the stage of clinical application to human reproduction. Antibodies to the β-subunit of hCG seem to provide a logical means of preventing pregnancy, but the dual problems of reversibility and adverse effects on tissues other than trophoblast remain to be overcome.

Several techniques that are theoretically promising have not yet reached the stage of clinical trials. Research is centering on new substances that are crucial to reproductive function. They include folliculostatin, which suppresses secretion of FSH; oocyte maturation inhibitor, which prevents the first meiotic division of the oocyte; inhibin, a hormone that inhibits secretion of FSH without inhibiting LH; antibodies to estrogen receptors; an androgen-binding protein in the testis; an antigonadotropin of the pineal gland, which presumably blocks LH; and an agent that inhibits production of progesterone by the corpus luteum.

29
CHAPTER
STERILIZATION

Sterilization, a permanent form of contraception, is an important adjunct to traditional contraception and abortion. It is now the most popular form of contraception in the United States, probably because of changing personal and societal values and the aging of the population. In about 1 of every 5 married white couples in the United States between the ages of 20 and 40, a sterilizing procedure has been performed on one of the partners. The pregnancy rate, depending on the technique employed, is between 0.1 and 0.5.

Because of recent changes in attitude, sterilization of the male has become much more acceptable. The possibility of sperm banking may have added further impetus to male sterilization. Men who consent to vasectomy only on the condition that their sperm may be banked are generally ambivalent about the procedure and should be discouraged from undergoing an operation that may be irreversible. In general, ambivalence about any sterilizing procedure in the man or the woman is best managed by deferring permanent forms of contraception.

FEMALE STERILIZATION

The major techniques of female sterilization involve destruction or resection of a portion of the oviduct. The principal techniques of tubal sterilization are immediate postpartum resection, laparoscopic cauterization or occlusion, and vaginal or abdominal tubal procedures in the nonpuerperal state.

There are several advantages to postpartum sterilization: the procedure can be performed in 10 to 20 minutes or less under the same anesthetic that is used for delivery; a small abdominal incision is sufficient; the cost to the patient and the length of hospitalization are not significantly increased; and the likelihood of failure and complications is small. The procedure must, however, be discussed with the patient before labor and the possibility that the child may not be of the desired sex or may not survive must be considered.

Laparoscopic sterilization usually involves induction of a pneumoperitoneum (p. 244) and occlusion or destruction of part of the tube. Its advantages include a short hospitalization (usually in an ambulatory care facility), which varies from 8 to 24 hours, a very small point of entry into the abdomen, and relatively few complications. It is often, however, not quite so effective as sterilization through a formal laparotomy and it may involve injury to neighboring abdominal viscera. Several techniques have been devised to reduce the likelihood of thermal and electrical injuries during laparoscopy: the bipolar method, the Yoon (Falope) ring, and the Hulka clip. The rate of ectopic pregnancy after electrocoagulation is greater than that after other techniques. The reversibility of a technique, furthermore, is usually inversely proportional to its effectiveness. Relative contraindications to laparoscopic sterilization include abdominal scars, adhesions, hernias, and peritonitis.

An alternative to laparoscopy is minilaparotomy. The tubal resection is carried out through a small suprapubic incision. Although the technique is inappropriate for obese women, it requires no elaborate equipment and is therefore more readily applicable to developing countries.

Nonpuerperal sterilization may be performed through the abdominal route (laparotomy) or through the vagina (colpotomy). Formal laparotomy provides excellent access and visualization with a very high rate of success, but it entails a stay in the hospital of three or more days, a relatively high cost, and a sizable abdominal scar. Vaginal tubal ligation or resection is performed through an incision in the posterior cul-de-sac. Its advantages are the absence of an abdominal scar and a shorter hospital stay. Disadvantages include increased difficulty in exposure and identification of the tubes. Postoperative complications including abscesses are somewhat more common than with abdominal procedures. A current or recent pregnancy is a contraindication to the vaginal route. Pelvic adhesions are a relative contraindication.

The major reasons for failure of tubal sterilization are: an early undetected pregnancy at the time of the operation, abnormalities of the tube or technical errors during the procedure, and postoperative opening of the tube.

Hysterectomy, abdominal or vaginal, provides virtually complete protection against subsequent pregnancy. It may be performed in conjunction with a cesarean section. It is a more extensive procedure than a tubal resection and is associated with a longer hospitalization and a higher incidence of postoperative complications such as hemorrhage, infection, and injury to the urinary tract. In addition to terminating fertility, it removes a functionless organ and prevents carcinoma of the corpus or cervix.

Hysterectomy terminates menses, which may be an advantage or a disadvantage, depending on the patient's attitude. Despite the prophylactic value of hysterectomy, it cannot be justified as a routine alternative to tubal sterilization. Federal regulations do not permit payment for hysterectomy for purposes of family planning when the operation is performed in programs funded by the federal government. Even though 10% of women may have gynecologic disease that requires surgical operation after tubal sterilization, the complications of hysterectomy justify the procedure only when there is a reason in addition to termination of childbearing potential, such as myomas or intraepithelial neoplasia of the cervix.

The most serious complications of tubal sterilization are pulmonary emboli and ectopic pregnancy. A principal technique of tubal resection is the Pomeroy operation, in which the tube is not crushed, an absorbable suture is used, and the knuckle of ligated tube is resected. The failure rate of a properly performed Pomeroy sterilization does not exceed 0.5%. The reversibility of male and female sterilization varies. The technical success of vasovasotomy after vasectomy can restore ductal patency in up to 90% of men undergoing vasectomy, but irreversible changes in Sertoli cell-directed spermatogenesis may result after an extended interval following vasectomy. Furthermore, some men develop sperm-specific antibodies as a result of the sterilization, which then may compromise male fertility after an otherwise technically successful repair. The potential reversibility of procedures for sterilization varies substantially, depending on the original surgical technique. In general, the more extensive the destruction of the fallopian tube, particularly when the ampulla or fimbriae are involved, the less likely a satisfactory repair becomes. With microsurgical techniques, pregnancy rates of 40 to 70% can be expected in women who have not undergone extensive destruction of their fallopian tubes. The incidence of subsequent ectopic pregnancy, however, may vary between 2 and 10%, depending on the location of the repair.

In techniques such as the Madlener operation, the tube is crushed and ligated with a nonabsorbable suture and the knuckle is not resected. Because the failure rate of this procedure is considerably higher than that of the Pomeroy operation, the technique of ligation without resection is not recommended.

A somewhat more complicated technique with a very high rate of success is the Irving sterilization. In this operation, the proximal end of the tube is buried in a tunnel within the myometrium and the distal end is often buried between the leaves of the broad ligament.

Hysteroscopy, a promising endoscopic technique, permits transvaginal cauterization of the uterine ostia of the fallopian tubes. A potentially reversible hysteroscopic technique involves delivery of a plug of methylcyanoacrylate (MCA) into the uterine ostia of the oviducts. The rapid polymerization of the compound prevents spillage into the peritoneal cavity. The use of MCA provides sterilization in not more than about 85% of cases and is therefore not likely to be popular in the United States. Metal devices inserted hysteroscopically into the uterine ostia of the oviducts and polymerized silicone plugs are additional methods of potentially reversible sterilization, but they too are currently associated with an unacceptably high rate of failure.

Ablation of the endometrium, by cryosurgery or laser, is an additional technique under current investigation. Potentially reversible methods of female sterilization include the use of fimbrial hoods and drugs such as quinacrine, which can be delivered in the form of pellets or in an intrauterine device. The block caused by quinacrine may be reversed by estrogens.

MALE STERILIZATION

The most popular form of male sterilization is vasectomy. This procedure involves bilateral scrotal incisions, or occasionally a single midline incision, and division of each ductus deferens. Its advantages are rapidity, inexpensiveness, and the possibility of accomplishment in the office with only local anesthesia. There is no demonstrable effect on production of androgens, libido, or sexual performance. Disadvantages are the fear of impotence by the male and the obvious but crucial fact that the female partner may still become pregnant. Several techniques of

reversible male sterilization involving insertion of a removable device into the vas are currently under investigation.

The ejaculate must be shown to be free of spermatozoa on two successive occasions before reliance can be placed on the method for complete contraception. Clearing the male reproductive tract of all spermatozoa that were there before vasectomy may require 15 ejaculations. Granulomas that occasionally follow section of the ductus deferens have rarely caused serious clinical problems. Preliminary reports of autoimmune disease resulting from vasectomy have not been substantiated, although antibodies to sperm are found in over half of all vasectomized men. A small preliminary study showed that vasectomy exacerbates the development of atherosclerosis in monkeys fed a diet high in cholesterol, but no association was found between vasectomy and atherosclerosis in human subjects.

FEDERAL REGULATIONS

The Department of Health and Human Services has promulgated regulations governing nontherapeutic sterilizations that are funded federally. It has imposed a moratorium on sterilization of minors and mentally incompetent men and women. Furthermore, it has required a greatly detailed informed consent that lists complications of sterilization and alternatives to the procedure. It also requires a mandatory 30-day period of delay between the signing of the consent and the performance of the sterilization, except in certain cases of premature labor or surgical operations performed as emergencies. In the case of premature labor, the informed consent must have been given at least 30 days before the expected date of delivery.

Patients whose sterilizations are financed by federal funds must be informed that they are free to withhold or withdraw their consent to the procedure without affecting their rights to future treatment and without loss of any federal benefits to which they are entitled. They must be given a description of other methods of birth control, advice that sterilization should be considered irreversible, and a thorough explanation of the specific procedure for sterilization that is to be performed. They must, furthermore, be given a full description of the benefits of sterilization and of the discomforts and risks (including those of anesthesia) that may be expected during and after the procedure. An interpreter must be provided for patients who do not understand English and suitable provisions made for those who are blind, deaf, or otherwise impaired. Consent for sterilization may not be obtained while the patient is seeking or undergoing an abortion.

30
CHAPTER

INDUCED ABORTION

Although abortion is not recommended as a primary means of family planning or population control in the United States, it serves as a backup for failed contraception. Perhaps, with ready availability of abortion, contraceptives can be developed that are less than 100% effective but are devoid of the complications of the currently available drugs and devices.

Until 1973 abortion was closely regulated by statute in most of the states to the extent that a serious medical problem was required to justify the procedure. Circumstances in which abortion is mandatory to save the life of the mother are most unusual. They may include advanced cardiac disease with prior decompensation, severe renal or vascular disease, and carcinoma of the cervix. Psychiatric indications for abortion and fetal indications such as prevention of the birth of an infant with structural or biochemical defects have been subject to wide differences of interpretation by various states. The most restrictive abortion laws allowed the procedure only to save the life of the mother. Other legislatures allowed the procedure to protect the life or health of the mother. The more liberal laws defined health, according to the interpretation of the World Health Organization, as including mental and social well-being. The abortion issue is still debated hotly, largely along religious lines, as a question of maternal versus fetal rights.

The status of abortion in the United States was changed drastically by the historic decision of the United States Supreme Court on January 22, 1973. That decision, which strengthened women's rights, was influenced by the finding that the fetus has no constitutional rights and that neither biologists, theologians, nor legal scholars could agree when life begins. All state laws must be consistent with the ruling of the Supreme Court, which essentially leaves decisions about abortion in the first trimester of pregnancy to the patient and her doctor without any regulation or interference by the State. For the period from the end of the first trimester to approximately the end of the second trimester, the State, in promoting its interest in the health of the mother, may regulate but not prohibit abortion for the protection of maternal health. For the stage subsequent to viability, at approximately the beginning of the third trimester, the State, in promoting its interest in the potentiality of human life, may regulate or proscribe abortion, except where the physician reasonably believes an abortion based on physiologic or psychologic grounds to be necessary for the preservation of the life or health of the mother. To comply fully with the ruling of the Supreme Court, the State cannot impose the requirement of a husband's signature or parental consent, for example, in first-trimester abortions. In 1977, however, the

Supreme Court ruled that individual states are not required to pay for abortions with Medicaid funds. Although its legal basis is clear, the effect of this decision was to deny to poor women a medical service that is available to the wealthy. In 1986, the Supreme Court, in a 5:4 decision, reaffirmed its 1973 ruling. During the years from 1986 to 1991, however, several challenges by the States and several decisions by the United States Supreme Court have restricted access to abortion by certain groups who are most in need of it. It is likely that the Supreme Court will hear challenges to the 1973 ruling (Roe vs. Wade) during 1993.

More than one quarter of all pregnancies in the United States have been terminated by abortion in recent years. The medical justification, which is not necessarily an ethical justification, for liberalization of the laws relating to abortion is based on the following facts: first-trimester abortion is safer than any alternative available to pregnant women; the death-to-case ratio for legal abortion has been reduced from 6.2 per 100,000 procedures in 1970 to less than 0.5; legal abortion has resulted in more abortions that are performed earlier in pregnancy and are associated with a lower maternal risk; the risk of death increases as pregnancy progresses and is greater in women whose pregnancies are unwanted; legal abortion is responsible for a decline in out-of-wedlock births; the option of legal abortion after amniocentesis has resulted in 10% more pregnancies in the population at high risk of having genetically damaged offspring; and there is a positive correlation between increased legal abortion and an increasing proportion of women using contraceptives.

Techniques of abortion fall into several main categories: dilatation of the cervix followed by sharp curettage or evacuation by suction, instillation of solutions into the amniotic cavity, hysterotomy, and hysterectomy.

Medicinal induction of abortion is not considered in detail here. Oxytocin is not effective in the early stages of pregnancy, and numerous herbal and folk remedies are insufficiently tested to be recommended as routine abortifacients. A long-acting prostaglandin analog, 15-methyl-prostaglandin $F_{2\alpha}$, which may be administered either intravaginally in a suppository or intramus-

cularly by injection, has been used as an early first-trimester abortifacient, although it has achieved greater popularity for cervical softening and effacement later in pregnancy. The combined use of RU-486 (p. 172) and prostaglandin may yet provide the long-desired, readily accessible, medical means of terminating pregnancy safely and effectively.

DILATION AND EVACUATION

The principal technique for evacuating the uterus under 12 weeks' gestational size is curettage, usually by suction. Because it is slightly less dangerous and can be performed on larger uteri, suction is more widely used today than is sharp curettage. Occasionally it is necessary to remove some products of conception by gentle sharp curettage after an attempt at evacuation by suction.

A modification of the suction technique applicable to very early pregnancy involves the insertion of a semirigid plastic catheter, with dimensions approximately equal to those of an ordinary drinking straw, through the virtually undilated cervix. Suction may then be applied and products of conception removed. Such techniques performed at the time of the first missed period or earlier have been termed "menstrual regulation" or "menstrual induction," but they are merely early abortions.

Dilation and curettage or suction require a block or a general anesthetic, but may be performed as an outpatient procedure within a hospital or in a facility with immediate access to a hospital for the management of complications. The time required for the surgical procedure and recovery is short. Disadvantages of the procedure are the occasional perforation of the uterus, which may require laparotomy. Infection, hemorrhage, and the likelihood of perforation increase with the size of the uterus and decrease with the experience of the operator.

INTRAAMNIOTIC SOLUTIONS

Injections of intraamniotic solutions are most effectively performed in a uterus of 16 weeks' gestational size or greater, although these techniques are performed much less commonly today. Until the midseventies, it was considered desirable to perform the abortion before 12 weeks' gestation, when a curettage can be performed with minimal danger, or to wait until 16 weeks, when intraamniotic solutions may be instilled. Successful results are now generally obtained with dilation and evacuation of the uterus larger than 12 weeks' gestational size. The data show that, in well-trained hands, midtrimester abortion (up to 20 gestational weeks) by suction may be safer than intraamniotic solutions. Before injection of intraamniotic solutions, it is necessary that the placenta be located by sonography to avoid fetomaternal hemorrhage. The amniocentesis is then performed, removing 100 to 200 mL of amniotic fluid, which is replaced very slowly by the abortifacient solution. The most commonly used solutions for this purpose are prostaglandins and hypertonic saline (20 to 23% NaCl). The current trend is away from intraamniotic solutions and toward dilation and evacuation, even in uteri larger than 20 weeks' gestational size.

The insertion of laminaria tents (natural or synthetic) into the cervical canal the night before abortion reduces the likelihood of damage to the cervix by forcible instrumental dilation or precipitous delivery through an undilated and uneffaced cervix. Variations in technique include simultaneous intraamniotic instillation of prostaglandin and urea, intraamniotic prostaglandin and intravenous oxytocin, and intraamniotic urea and intravenous oxytocin.

Certain studies suggest that there is no increase in risk of reproductive loss after one legally induced abortion but a twofold to threefold increase in the risk of first-trimester spontaneous abortion after two or more prior induced abortions. Other studies come to the perhaps more logical conclusion that the degree of damage to the reproductive tract with any particular abortion or abortions is more significant than the number of prior abortions.

Abortion through injection of intraamniotic solutions avoids instrumental dilatation of the cervix and laparotomy. Abortion usually follows injection of the solutions by 24 to 36 hours. The procedure is generally considered a failure if abortion has not occurred within 48 hours after injection. In cases of failure, the procedure may be repeated, perhaps with the addition of oxytocin, or a dilation and evacuation may be performed. Injection of hypertonic saline is contraindicated in the presence of cardiovascular or renal disease, and use of any intraamniotic solution is impossible in the presence of ruptured membranes.

The main complications of injection of saline result from inadvertent intravascular or intraperitoneal injection. They include hypernatremia, cardiac arrest, pulmonary edema, hemoglobinuria, encephalopathy, and necrosis of tissue. Additional complications include hemorrhage; infection; retained products of conception, which may require curettage; and coagulopathies, which very likely result from disseminated intravascular coagulation. Because of the high rates of these complications, saline is not used commonly today as an abortifacient. Prostaglandins, which are now the most commonly used agents, often result in incomplete abortions, which may require completion by curettage. In addition, their use occasionally results in delivery of a living fetus. Intraamniotic solutions have become less popular as techniques and instruments for midtrimester abortion have improved and as experience with the procedure has increased.

Ideally, abortions should be prevented by effective contraception; when unwanted pregnancy requires abortion, the procedure should be done as early in pregnancy as possible in the interest of maternal safety.

HYSTEROTOMY AND HYSTERECTOMY

Hysterotomy is rarely performed for abortion today, and then only when the uterus is too large to empty by curettage or suction and when intraamniotic solutions are ineffective or medically contraindicated. Disadvantages of hysterotomy include the prolonged hospitalization and the scars in the abdomen and uterus, which may require subsequent delivery by cesarean section.

Abortion may also be effected through hysterectomy, although the increased morbidity associated with this procedure precludes its wider use. The advantages of the procedure include the removal of a potentially or an actually diseased organ and permanent sterilization. Disadvantages include the increased morbidity associated with hysterectomy in general and with hysterectomy in pregnant patients in particular. The special example of carcinoma of the cervix complicating early pregnancy is best managed by abortion through simultaneous radical hysterectomy and pelvic lymph node dissection or complete radiotherapy.

MEDICAL REQUIREMENTS OF ABORTION

The American College of Obstetricians and Gynecologists has described the ideal circumstances for performance of an elective abortion. Abortion should be regarded as a surgical procedure and its performance should require appropriate surgical, anesthetic, and resuscitative equipment. In addition, the diagnosis and duration of pregnancy should be verified. Laboratory procedures should include blood typing and identification of the Rh-type. Any factors or illness that might have a bearing on the anesthesia and any drug sensitivities should be recorded.

Rh immune globulin (p. 172) is given after abortion to any Rh-negative patient when the father's Rh-type is positive or unknown. Postoperative and contraceptive advice should be available. No physician should be required to perform an abortion and no patient should be forced to undergo the procedure. An informed consent should be obtained and the procedure should be performed only by physicians who are qualified to identify and manage the complications that may arise from the procedure. Attempts should be made to provide facilities where abortions can be performed with maximal safety but with minimal disruption of other hospital functions.

GENERAL GYNECOLOGY

31
CHAPTER

GYNECOLOGIC INFECTIONS

BREAST

Infections of the breast, except those related to pregnancy and lactation, are not customarily treated by gynecologists in most parts of the United States. Postpartum mastitis is a pyogenic cellulitis usually caused by staphylococci or streptococci. The mainstay of treatment is the appropriate antibiotic, as determined by culture and sensitivity tests. Analgesics and heat provide symptomatic relief. Treatment of an abscess is best accomplished by incision and drainage (p. 228). Lack of prompt healing suggests the need for biopsy to rule out the possibility of inflammatory carcinoma.

VULVA

The vulva includes all the structures visible from the lower margin of the pelvis to the perineum: the mons veneris, labia majora, labia minora, clitoris, vestibule, hymen, external urethral orifice, and various glandular and vascular structures (Fig. 31–1). Each labium minus is a thin fold of connective tissue devoid of fat and covered on both surfaces with a keratinized, stratified squamous epithelium. The labia minora have no hair, but a few sweat and sebaceous glands are found on their lateral surfaces. The labia majora are covered by typical skin with pilosebaceous complexes and sweat glands. After puberty they are covered with hair, particularly on the lateral surfaces. A digital process of fat below the surface of the skin creates the typical contour of the adult vulva (p. 16).

The clitoris, its crura, and the bulbs of the vestibule contain erectile tissue. The crura and clitoris are surrounded by a tunica albuginea. The bulbocavernosus and ischiocavernosus muscles covering the bulbs of the vestible crura of the clitoris, respectively, consist of skeletal muscle, as do the other muscles of the superficial and the deep perineal pouches. The greater vestibular glands (Bartholin's glands) are of the tubuloalveolar variety.

The vulva is subject to the same diseases that affect the skin of others parts of the body. Vulvitis often causes pruritus, which leads to scratching and secondary trauma. Vulvitis may be associated with vaginitis; the inflammation is then designated vulvovaginitis.

General dermatologic conditions that may affect the vulva include eczema, herpes, and psoriasis. Vulvar eczema is treated by removal of the irritant, steroid creams, and antihistaminics. The vulva is subject to intertrigo because of the moisture of the labia and inguinal areas. Seborrhea and folliculitis may also involve the vulva. Infestations include pubic pediculosis (phthiriasis

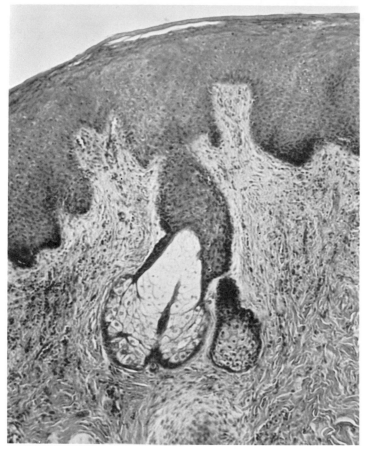

FIG. 31–1. Normal vulva, showing keratinized stratified squamous epithelium and epidermal appendages.

pubis, or "crabs"), fleas (pulicosis), bedbugs (cimicosis), and scabies.

The recommended treatment for pediculosis pubis (lice and nits) is lindane (1%), lotion or cream, applied in a thin layer to the infested and adjacent hairy areas and thoroughly washed off after 8 hours, or lindane (1%) shampoo applied for 4 minutes and thoroughly washed off. Lindane is not recommended for pregnant or lactating women. Alternatively, pyrethrins and piperonyl butoxide may be applied to the infested and adjacent hairy areas and washed off after 10 minutes.

Scabies is also treated with lindane (1%), 1 oz. of lotion or 30 g of cream applied thinly to all areas of the body from the neck down and washed off after 8 hours. Alternative therapies are crotamiton (10%) and sulfur (6%) in petrolatum.

Bartholinitis is often of gonococcal origin but commonly represents a secondary infection with coliform organisms or polymicrobial pathogens. In 15% of cases, *Bacteroides fragilis* may be recovered. Treatment of the acute infection includes antibiotics, analgesics, and heat. An abscess of the Bartholin gland presents as a painful, ovoid, tender mass in the inferior portion of the labia. Treatment is incision and drainage. An abscess may subside to form a cyst (Fig. 31–2), which may be treated by marsupialization (evacuating the contents of the cyst and suturing its edges to those of the external incision), or occasionally excision.

VAGINA

The vagina is lined by nonkeratinized, stratified squamous epithelium (Fig. 31–3). Its lamina propria consists of dense connective tissue. The vagina lacks glands, but the large vessels that supply it dilate during sexual

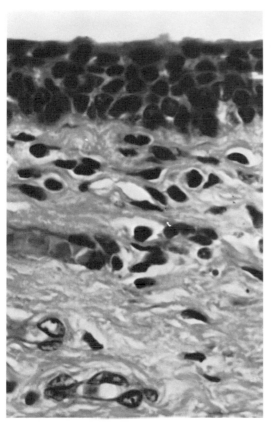

FIG. 31–2. Cyst of Bartholin's duct, lined by transitional epithelium.

excitation and produce the vaginal lubrication that was formerly thought to arise from the cervical and greater vestibular glands. Thickening of the lamina propria creates the anterior and posterior rugal columns with their transverse ridges, as seen in the nullipara. The muscularis is arranged longitudinally and is covered by adventitia except over the posterior fornix, which is coated with peritoneum for about 1 cm.

The vagina also responds to changing levels of hormones. During the estrogenic (proliferative) phase, its epithelium is thick and the mature squamous cells that desquamate have small, pyknotic nuclei. Because progesterone inhibits maturation, the cells sloughed during the secretory phase appear intermediate or immature. In postclimacteric years, when the vagina undergoes atrophy, the desquamated cells are parabasal.

Vaginitis is often secondary to vulvitis or cervicitis. Atrophic vaginitis occurs after natural or surgical menopause as a result of a deficiency of estrogens. It produces an irritating discharge, with pruritus, edema, and often dyspareunia. The pale, thin, smooth vaginal mucosa may be secondarily infected, with resulting purulent or sanguineous discharge. Women who continue regular coitus are less likely to have atrophic vaginitis. Treatment is local application of estrogen cream.

The main causes of adult vaginitis are Trichomonas, Candida, *Gardnerella vaginalis* (bacterial vaginosis), and anaerobic bacteria. Infections may be caused by combinations of these organisms.

TRICHOMONAS

Trichomonas produces a thin, watery, malodorous discharge, which is often described as yellow-green and foamy but may be of different color and consistency. The organism is a flagellated protozoon, which may be identified in a hanging-drop preparation. It is transmitted primarily through sexual contact. The irritating discharge may cause vaginal and vulvar pruritus and pain. The mucosal petechiae, which form the so-called strawberry spots, are not seen regularly. The diagnosis is made by the identification of the motile trichomonads in a suspension of saline. Many leukocytes but few, if any, epithelial cells are found on microscopic examination of the fluid. Manifestations of trichomoniasis are often aggravated after a menstrual period. The best treatment is metronidazole (Flagyl). The drug is effective as a single oral dose of 2 g. An alternative regimen is 250 mg, by mouth, three times a day for 7 days. The male partners of women with trichomoniasis should be treated with the single oral dose of 2 g of the drug. Metronidazole is contraindicated in the first trimester of pregnancy and is best avoided throughout pregnancy. An alternate regimen during pregnancy is clindamycin, 300 mg by mouth, twice a day, for 7 days. Lactating women may be treated with metronidazole, 2 g, by mouth, in a single dose, but breastfeeding should be interrupted for at least 24 hours after therapy.

CANDIDA

Candida (Monilia) may produce a discharge that is thick, white, cheesy, and curdlike, but it may be thin and watery. On micro-

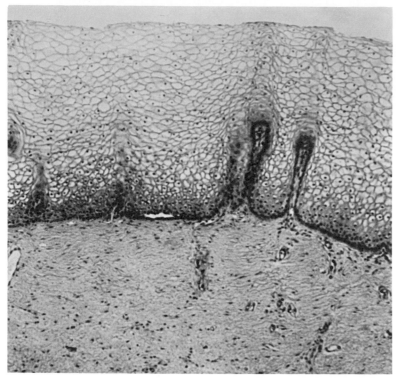

FIG. 31–3. Normal adult vagina, showing nonkeratinized stratified squamous epithelium and absence of cutaneous appendages.

scopic examination or culture the yeastlike buds and hyphae are seen. The infection may produce intense vulvar irritation, burning, and pruritus. Exacerbation of the infection is often noted in pregnancy, in diabetes, and with the use of oral contraceptives or antibiotics. The usual therapy is intravaginal insertion of nystatin (Mycostatin), miconazole nitrate (Monistat), clotrimazole (Gyne-Lotrimin), or a butoconazole (Femstat) in the form of a cream or tablet, daily for 7 days. Intravaginal tablets may be used in conjunction with externally applied creams for vulvar and perianal lesions. Oral ketoconazole is also effective against *Candida albicans* but is contraindicated during pregnancy.

BACTERIAL VAGINOSIS

Bacterial vaginosis, formerly called Gardnerella or Hemophilus vaginitis, produces a nonirritating, odoriferous, thin grayish-white vaginal discharge associated with an elevated vaginal pH (greater than 4.5) and the formation of a fishy odor (amines) when the fluid discharged is alkalinized with 10% potassium hydroxide. The normally acidic environment of the vagina is the result of lactic acid produced by the action of lactobacilli (Döderlein bacilli) on glycogen. The acidic pH of the vagina may protect against many infections. Microscopic examination reveals absence of leukocytes and gram-positive rods (lactobacilli) and presence of small coccobacillary organisms attached to squamous epithelial cells ("clue cells"). Although the etiologic agents that produce the syndrome of vaginosis have not been identified precisely, anaerobic bacteria clearly play a major role. Treatment is metronidazole, 500 mg, by mouth, twice a day for 7 days. An alternative regimen is clindamycin, 300 mg, by mouth, twice a day, for 7 days. Although firm evidence is lacking that clindamycin has an effect on the fetus, it is probably prudent to use ampicillin during pregnancy, despite the greater effectiveness of both metronidazole and clindamycin.

In the investigation of a vaginal discharge, foreign bodies should be sought and removed. Although any severe vaginal infec-

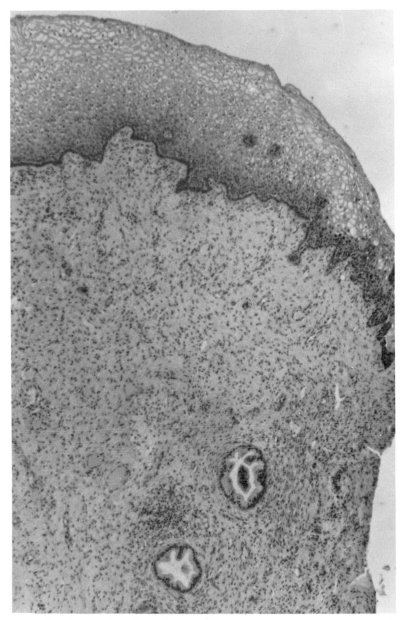

FIG. 31–4. Normal adult cervix, showing nonkeratinized stratified squamous epithelium and glands with mucinous columnar endothelium.

tion may lead to a bloody discharge, carcinoma must be excluded by appropriate diagnostic techniques.

Pediatric vaginitis or vulvovaginitis may be initiated by a foreign body, although nonspecific infection is a more common cause. Predisposing factors are poor hygiene and labial agglutination, which is treated by separation followed by estrogen cream. The organisms frequently involved are *Enterobius vermicularis* (pinworm), gonococci, and coliform bacilli. Pinworms may be identified by examination of a preparation made with scotch tape and are treated with piperazine citrate.

CERVIX

The cervix of the uterus, unlike the corpus, consists primarily of connective tissue rather than muscle. The mucosa of the endocervical canal is composed of a single layer of high columnar cells filled with mucoid material. Many of the epithelial cells are ciliated and the glands are thrown into a complicated system of clefts. The vaginal portion of the cervix is covered by squamous epithelium (Fig. 31–4). The squamocolumnar junction is normally a sharp line near the external os. In older women, the stratified squamous epithelium extends into the cervical canal. When the junction occurs on the portio vaginalis outside the external os, an ectropion results.

Microscopic demonstration of chronic inflammatory cells in the adult human cervix is a normal finding. Gonorrhea produces an acute cervicitis, which may cause a profuse purulent discharge as well as a chronic infection; the frequently associated urethritis causes dysuria and frequency.

Cervicitis may be related to erosion (ulceration of the everted columnar epithelium

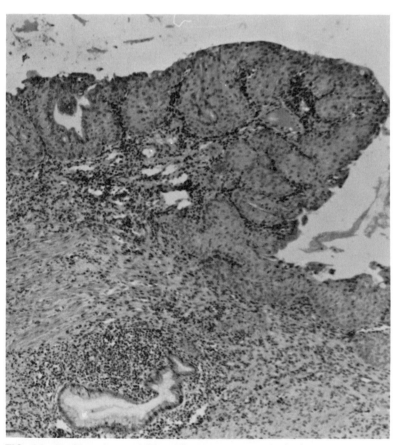

FIG. 31–5. Chronic cervicitis with squamous metaplasia.

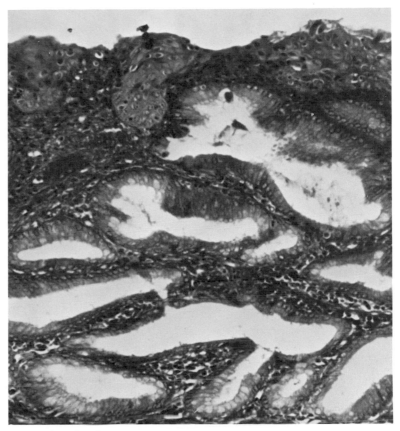

FIG. 31−6. Squamous metaplasia of the cervix, showing columnar epithelium overgrown by squamous epithelium.

of the endocervix and the squamous epithelium of the portio vaginalis) or eversion, or ectropion (rolling out of the endocervical mucosa onto the portio). Epidermidalization (covering or replacement of columnar epithelium by stratified squamous epithelium) and plugging of endocervical glandular ducts may cause retention cysts (nabothian follicles). Chronic cervicitis is the most common cause of leukorrhea (Figs. 31−5 and 31−6), which is an increase in secretions of the endocervical mucus-producing cells, vaginal effusion, and endometrial debris. Less common causes of cervicitis include secondary infection of a cervical chancre, a tuberculous or herpetic lesion, or a condyloma acuminatum.

Before treatment is begun for any cervicitis, a Papanicolaou smear should be obtained. A mucopurulent endocervical exudate suggests cervicitis caused by gonococcal or chlamydial infection. Gonorrheal cervicitis is treated by systemic penicillin or an alternative antibiotic. Because infections with *N. gonorrhoeae* and *C. trachomatis* are frequently concurrent, it is recommended that in addition to penicillin, tetracycline or erythromycin be given to treat the chlamydial component. Other forms of cervicitis may be treated by locally applied antibiotics, cauterization, or removal of infected tissue by cryosurgery or laser.

ENDOMETRIUM

Endometritis usually points to an underlying cause. The principal associated lesions are submucous myomas, endometrial polyps, carcinoma of the endometrium, fragments of retained placenta, or a foreign body. The inflammatory reaction associated with an intrauterine device does not usually produce a clinical endometritis.

32
CHAPTER

SEXUALLY TRANSMITTED DISEASES

SYPHILIS

The primary lesions of sexually transmitted (venereal) diseases are often found on the vulva. The primary lesion of syphilis is a painless chancre, which appears 3 to 4 weeks after exposure. The ulcer has indurated edges with a depressed center. There is edema of the surrounding skin and inguinal adenitis. The initial lesion regresses in about a month. Darkfield examination of the serous exudate from a chancre reveals the spirochete. The serologic test for syphilis is usually not positive until several weeks after the appearance of the primary lesion. Serologic tests for syphilis (STS) include the VDRL, which may be falsely positive in several systemic disorders.

Greater specificity may be obtained by use of the fluorescent treponemal antibody absorption (FTAA) test or the *Treponema pallidum* immobilization (TPI) test. The secondary lesions of syphilis include condylomata lata and mucous patches. The condyloma latum is a slightly raised, flat, ovoid structure that appears in clusters. It must be distinguished from condyloma acuminatum (see p. 196). Condyloma latum produces an exudate, the darkfield examination of which is positive, as are serologic tests for syphilis at this stage. The tertiary lesion, or gumma, is an uncommon finding today. The treatment of choice for primary syphilis is 2.4 million units of benzathine penicillin in a single intramuscular injection.

The treatment of choice for early syphilis (primary, secondary, or latent syphilis of less than 1 year's duration) is benzathine penicillin G (2.4 million units intramuscularly in one dose) because it provides effective treatment in a single visit.

Syphilis of more than 1 year's duration, except neurosyphilis (latent syphilis of indeterminate or more than 1 year's duration, cardiovascular, or late benign syphilis) should be treated with benzathine penicillin G, 2.4 million units, intramuscularly, once a week for 3 successive weeks (7.2 million units total). Patients who are allergic to penicillin should be treated with tetracycline or erythromycin, 500 mg., by mouth, four times a day for 30 days. Neurosyphilis requires treatment with 12 to 24 million units of aqueous crystalline penicillin G, intravenously, daily for 10 days, followed by benzathine penicillin G, 2.4 million units, intramuscularly, weekly, for 3 doses; or aqueous procaine penicillin G, 2.4 million units, intramuscularly, daily with probenecid, 500 mg, by mouth, four times a day, both for 10 days, followed by benzathine penicillin G, 2.4 million units, intramuscularly, weekly for 3 doses.

For patients who are allergic to penicillin, tetracycline hydrochloride (500 mg four times a day by mouth for 15 days) or erythromycin stearate, ethylsuccinate, or base (500 mg four times a day by mouth for 15 days) may be used. Another recommended regimen is ceftriaxone, 250 mg, intramuscularly, once a day, for 10 days. These antibiotics appear to be effective but have been evaluated less extensively than penicillin.

All pregnant women should have a nontreponemal serologic test for syphilis, such as the VDRL or RPR, at the time of the first prenatal visit. The treponemal tests such as the FTA-ABS should not be used for routine screening. In women suspected of being at high risk for syphilis, a second nontreponemal test should be performed during the third trimester and the cord blood should be tested for antibody to syphilis. Seroreactive patients should be evaluated promptly, by history and physical examination as well as by a quantitative nontreponemal test and a confirmatory treponemal test. Both of these tests should be repeated within 4 weeks. If there is clinical or serologic evidence of syphilis, the patient should be treated. Patients for whom there is documentation of adequate treatment for syphilis need not be retreated unless there is clinical or serologic evidence of reinfection, such as darkfield-positive lesions or a fourfold rise in titer of a quantitative nontreponemal test.

Patients at all stages of pregnancy who are not allergic to penicillin should be treated with the same doses of the drug as are used for nonpregnant patients. For patients who are allergic to penicillin, erythromycin (stearate, ethylsuccinate, or base) should be used in the doses recommended for nonpregnant patients. Although these dosages of erythromycin appear safe for mother and fetus, their efficacies are not proven. Tetracyclines are not recommended for syphilitic infections in pregnant women because of potential adverse effects on mother and fetus.

Congenital syphilis may occur if the mother has syphilis during pregnancy. If the mother has received adequate penicillin during pregnancy, the risk to the infant is minimal, but all infants should be examined carefully at birth and at frequent intervals thereafter until nontreponemal serologic tests are negative. Infants should be treated with penicillin at birth if maternal treatment was inadequate or unknown or with drugs other than penicillin, or if adequate follow-up of the infant cannot be ensured.

CHANCROID

Chancroid produces a lesion known as a soft chancre, which unlike the hard chancre of syphilis is very painful. It occurs ten times more frequently in men than in women. The causative organism is the *Hemophilus ducreyi,* a gram-negative coccobacillus, which may be found in a smear or scraping of the primary lesion. A pustule appears 3 to 10 days after exposure. The primary lesion is a progressive ulcer of the vulva. Because it is difficult to culture this organism, material from the lesion must be placed in a sterile tube containing the patient's own blood and sent to the laboratory without delay. Treatment is erythromycin, 500 mg, by mouth, four times a day for 7 days, or ceftriaxone 250 mg, intramuscularly, in a single dose. Alternative regimens include trimethoprim-sulfamethoxazole (160/800 mg), by mouth, twice a day, for a minimum of 7 days; or (in the nonpregnant state) ciprofloxacin, 500 mg, by mouth, in a single dose; or amoxicillin, 500 mg, plus clavulanic acid, 125 mg by mouth, three times daily, for 7 days. Treatment should be continued until ulcers and lymph nodes have healed.

LYMPHOGRANULOMA VENEREUM

Lymphogranuloma venereum, or LGV, is a sexually transmitted disease caused by immunotypes L_1, L_2, or L_3 of *Chlamydia trachomatis,* an obligate intracellular organism that is now classified as a bacterium rather than a virus. The short period of incubation of the infection results in a lesion 1 to 3 weeks after exposure. The primary infection is accompanied by fever and malaise. A suppurative inguinal adenitis (a bubo that may drain) appears 2 to 3 weeks later. Vulvar edema may progress to elephantiasis.

Complications include draining sinuses and pseudoepitheliomatous hyperplasia of the affected skin. The lymphatics of the genital, inguinal, and anal areas are involved, and rectal strictures may form. The Frei test becomes positive 2 to 6 weeks after the initial lesion and may remain positive for life. Because the complement fixation test has greater sensitivity, it has replaced the Frei test. Since squamous cell carcinoma may complicate this lesion, biopsy should be performed before treatment is initiated. Strictures of the large bowel and fistulas may require surgical intervention. The treatment of choice is doxycycline, 100 mg, twice a day for 21 days. Alternative regimens are tetracycline, 500 mg, 4 times a day, for 21 days; or erythromycin, 500 mg, 4 times a day, for 21 days; or sulfisoxazole, 500 mg, 4 times a day, for 21 days.

GRANULOMA INGUINALE

Granuloma inguinale (donovanosis) is a tropical disease that is common in the Caribbean but rare in the United States. The primary lesion is a papule, which may undergo extensive ulceration and necrosis. Unlike lymphogranuloma venereum, this disease does not produce suppurative lymphadenopathy. The pathognomonic, finding is the Donovan body, an inclusion in the mononuclear cells. *Calymmatobacterium granulomatis* the etiologic agent, is a bipolar heavily encapsulated, gram-negative bacterium. Biopsy may be required to rule out carcinoma. The treatments of choice, listed in order of preference, are: doxycycline, 100 mg, orally twice a day, for 21 days; or tetracycline, 500 mg, orally, four times a day, for 21 days; or streptomycin, 500 mg, intramuscularly, twice a day, for at least 21 days; or chloramphenicol, 500 mg, orally three times a day, for at least 21 days; or gentamicin, 40 mg, intramuscularly, twice a day, for at least 21 days. Penicillins are not effective.

CONDYLOMA ACUMINATUM

Condylomata acuminata (venereal warts) appear in the form of multiple papillary warty growth on the vulva, vagina, perineum, cervix, and external urethral meatus (Fig. 32–1). They are caused by a small, slowly growing DNA virus (human papillomavirus) belonging to the papovavirus group. Types 6 and 11 cause genital and anal warts. Types 16, 18, and 31 are associated with genital dysplasia and carcinoma.

This subject is discussed further in Chapter 43. HPV produces a profuse, irritating vaginal discharge, often associated with *Trichomonas vaginalis*. Unlike the condyloma latum, condyloma acuminatum has a narrow base. The diagnosis is made by biopsy. Darkfield examination for spirochetes, culture for the gonococcus, and a Papanicolaou smear should be done at the same time. External and perianal warts may be treated with 10 to 25% podophyllin in tincture of benzoin or trichloroacetic acid (TCA) in a strength of 80 to 90%. Normal surrounding tissue should be protected and the solution washed off in 1 to 4 hours. Podophyllin should not be used during pregnancy. Alternative treatments are cryotherapy and electrocautery for lesions of moderate size, and surgical excision with the scalpel or ablation with the laser for larger condylomata. Colposcopically directed laser therapy is used successfully for cervicovaginal lesions and recalcitrant vulvar and perineal lesions.

Lymphoblastoid interferon has been used successfully on an experimental basis to treat resistant condylomas. Vaginal-cervical condylomas may be treated with 5-fluorouracil or colposcopically directed laser vaporization. Infants delivered through a vagina involved in condylomata may develop lesions in the larynx.

HERPES GENITALIS

Infection with genital herpes simplex virus, a DNA virus (*Herpesvirus hominis, Herpes genitalis*, or *H. progenitalis*) causes a chronic and recurring infection for which there is no known cure. The organism is found in smegma and cervical secretion and is sexually transmitted. The isolates are Type II in 85% of cases and Type I in 15%. In addition to the vulvitis and vaginitis, the infection produces a cervicitis in 75% of cases. The primary lesion is a group of vesicles with surrounding erythema and edema.

For the treatment of initial genital herpes, one 200 mg capsule of acyclovir is prescribed five times daily, while the patient is awake, for a total of 5 capsules daily for 7 to 10 days, initiated within 6 days of the onset of lesions. Acyclovir does not prevent recurrences and has not been tested in pregnant and lactating women. Patients should ab-

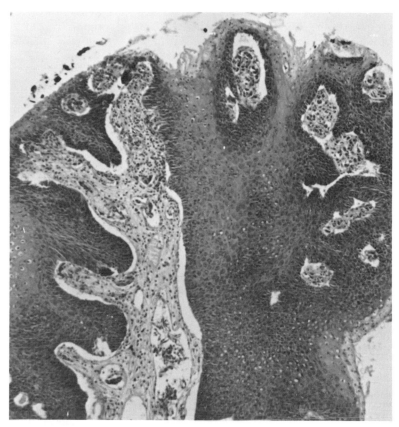

FIG. 32–1. Condyloma acuminatum of the vulva, showing hyperplastic stratified squamous epithelium with hyperkeratosis and parakeratosis and vascular core of connective tissue.

stain from sexual contact when the lesions are present. The risk of transmission of the herpes virus during asymptomatic periods is unknown. Use of acyclovir for recurrent disease may decrease the severity of the recurrence. The intermittent therapy involves use of one 200 mg capsule 2 to 5 times daily while the patient is awake or 400 mg, twice daily. This therapy reduces frequency of active recurrence by at least 75% among patients with frequent recurrences.

For severe recurrent disease, therapy must be started at the beginning of the prodrome or within 2 days of the onset of lesions with acyclovir, 200 mg, by mouth, 5 times a day, for 5 days; or acyclovir, 800 mg, by mouth, twice a day.

Although there is no proof of the etiologic relation between herpetic infection and cervical dysplasia and carcinoma, women with a history of this disease should have annual Papanicolaou smears. As early as possible in pregnancy, women should advise their obstetricians of a history of herpetic infection so that appropriate management of labor and route of delivery may be planned. The differential diagnosis of herpes genitalis includes herpes zoster and erythema multiforme.

CHLAMYDIA TRACHOMATIS

Infections caused by *Chlamydia trachomatis*, an obligate intracellular parasite, are the most prevalent sexually transmitted diseases in the United States today. Chlamydial organisms may be isolated from 10 to 30% of sexually active adolescent girls and approximately 5% of women in college. Infections caused by the various serotypes of *Chlamydia trachomatis* include hyperendemic blinding trachoma and lymphogranuloma venereum (LGV), which are uncommon in the United States; and the prevalent inclusion conjunctivitis; nongonococcal urethritis, cervicitis, endometritis, proctitis, and epididymitis; and pneumonia of the newborn.

Populations of pregnant women have a prevalence of *Chlamydia trachomatis* of 10 to 20%, as compared with 1 to 2% for gonorrhea. Infants born through a vagina infected with *C. trachomatis* may contract conjunctivitis or pneumonia. A positive diagnosis of chlamydial infection requires culture or detection by means of a fluorescein-labeled monoclonal antibody. Screening for both chlamydial and gonococcal infections may be accomplished by solid-phase enzymatic immunoassays (chlamydiazyme and gonozyme, respectively). Oral contraceptives, which have been alleged to offer some protection against gonococcal pelvic inflammatory disease, do not offer similar protection against chlamydial infection.

For culture-proven infections caused by non-LGV strains of *C. trachomatis* the following recommendations have been made by the CDC. Similar treatment is appropriate for nongonococcal urethritis caused by *Ureaplasma urealyticum.* Uncomplicated urethral, endocervical, or rectal infections in adults are best treated with doxycycline, 100 mg, by mouth, twice a day, for 7 days; or tetracycline, 500 mg, by mouth, 4 times a day, for 7 days. For patients in whom tetracyclines are contraindicated or not tolerated, erythromycin base or stearate, 500 mg, by mouth, four times a day for 7 days; or erythromycin ethylsuccinate, 800 mg, by mouth, 4 times a day for 7 days, may be used. For pregnant women with chlamydial infections, the preferred regimen is erythromycin, 500 mg, by mouth, four times a day on an empty stomach for at least 7 days or, for women who cannot tolerate this regimen, a decreased dose of 250 mg, by mouth, four times a day for at least 14 days.

GONORRHEA

Gonorrhea remains a major bacterial disease in the United States. Acute gonorrhea may represent an initial infection or an exacerbation of a chronic infection. The signs and symptoms in the woman occur 3 to 5 days after exposure, but the primary infection may go unnoticed, rendering her an asymptomatic carrier. The gonococcus causes a purulent, malodorous discharge from the urethra, Skene's glands, cervix, and anus. All of these sites and the throat should be cultured in the attempt to make the diagnosis.

The infection is suspected when the gram-negative intracellular diplococci are demonstrated on smear and is confirmed by culture. Thayer-Martin agar plates are often used for culture of gonococci. A change from opaque to transparent colonies is associated with greater virulence.

Uncomplicated urethral, endocervical, or rectal infections may be treated with ceftriaxone, 250 mg, intramuscularly once, with doxycycline, 100 mg, by mouth, twice a day, for 7 days; or with tetracycline, 500 mg, by mouth, 4 times a day, for 7 days. An alternative regimen is spectinomycin, 2 g, intramuscularly, in a single dose. For patients in whom tetracyclines are contraindicated or not tolerated, the single-dose regimen may be followed by erythromycin base or stearate, 500 mg, by mouth, 4 times a day, for 7 days; or erythromycin ethylsuccinate, 800 mg, by mouth, 4 times a day, for 7 days. Pharyngeal infections should be treated with ceftriaxone, 250 mg, in a single dose. Patients who cannot be treated with ceftriaxone should receive ciprofloxacin, 500 mg, by mouth, in a single dose. Pregnant women should be treated with ceftriaxone, 250 mg, intramuscularly, in a single dose, together with 500 mg of erythromycin base or 800 mg of erythromycin ethylsuccinate. Pregnant women who are allergic to β-lactams should be treated with one intramuscular dose of 2 g of spectinomycin.

The treatment of gonococcal infections of the upper genital tract is discussed in Chapter 33.

ENTERIC INFECTIONS

Many organisms produce enteric diseases that are sexually transmissible. The important agents are Shigella (a bacterium), hepatitis A virus, *Giardia lamblia* (a protozoon), and *Entamoeba histolytica.* They are spread most readily by oral-anal contact. Treatment depends on the etiologic agent.

HEPATITIS B INFECTION

This disease is caused by the hepatitis B virus (HBV), a DNA virus with multiple antigenic components. The disease may be transmitted sexually or hematogenously. Both hepatitis B immune globulin (HBIG) and hepatitis B vaccine protect against infection with hepatitis B virus.

MOLLUSCUM CONTAGIOSUM

This disease is caused by the molluscum contagiosum virus, the largest DNA virus of the poxvirus group. It produces papules that are 1 to 5 mm in diameter with umbilicated centers. They are most common on the trunk and anogenital region and are generally asymptomatic. Microscopic examination of the lesions reveals the pathognomonic inclusion bodies. The lesions may resolve spontaneously or may be removed by curettage after cryoanesthesia. Podophyllin, trichloroacetic acid, and liquid nitrogen have been used successfully. To prevent recurrence, it is necessary to extirpate every lesion.

ACQUIRED IMMUNODEFICIENCY SYNDROME

The etiologic agent of this deadly syndrome is HIV-1, a retrovirus. Although the earliest reported cases of acquired immunodeficiency syndrome (AIDS) in the United States occurred in homosexual men and users of intravenous drugs, the proportion heterosexually transmitted and involving women and their neonates is increasing. As of March 31, 1991, 175,000 cases of the syndrome had been reported in the United States with a mortality rate of slightly over 50%. In addition, there are 6 to 8 times that number of HIV-positive but asymptomatic carriers (1 to 1.5 million). Counseling and testing should be offered to all women who have evidence of HIV infection; who have used intravenous drugs for nonmedical purposes; who were born in countries where heterosexual transmission is thought to play an important role in the spread of the virus, such as Haiti or Central Africa; who have

been prostitutes; or who have been sexual partners of users of intravenous drugs, bisexual men, men with hemophilia, men born in high-risk countries, or men who otherwise have evidence of infection with HIV.

If the woman tests positive for AIDS she should be advised to delay pregnancy until more is known about the perinatal transmission of the virus. Infected women who are already pregnant may need additional medical services to reduce the risk of contracting opportunistic infections and should be advised against breastfeeding. Abortion may be offered to the infected woman to prevent perinatal transmission.

Women account for approximately 7% of all AIDS patients but for an ever-increasing proportion of HIV-positive subjects. In 1991, 90,000 to 125,000 women were HIV-positive. The HIV retrovirus utilizes reverse transcriptase to invade its human host through contact with blood or body fluids by means of infected monocytes. The favored target organ is the CD4 lymphocyte (T-lymphocyte helper cell) as opposed to the CD8 lymphocyte (T-lymphocyte suppressor cell). The effect of infection with the HIV is to destroy CD4 cells and therefore lower the CD4/CD8 (helper/suppressor) ratio.

The normal range of CD4/CD8 is 1.7 to 2.3 and for a healthy gravida it is 0.9 to 1.9. In patients with AIDS, the ratio is below 0.8. When CD4 counts fall to below 500/μL, treatment with Zidovudine (ZVD), formerly called azidothymidine (AZT), must be considered. This drug blocks the action of reverse transcriptase in translating the code of RNA into that of DNA. When the CD4 count falls to or below 200/μL, therapy with ZVD must be initiated.

The window from exposure to the virus to HIV-positivity may vary from 6 weeks to 18 months. The interval between HIV exposure to the virus and clinical symptoms, however, may be as long as 10 years or more. The rate of survival of patients with frank AIDS is still abysmal. The 5-year survival is less than 15%, and no 10-year survivors have been reported thus far.

Because HIV-infected monocytes attack CD4 lymphocytes preferentially, experimental therapeutic trials involve development of a soluble (false) CD4 receptor and attempts to immunize patients so that they form antibodies to the GT 120 envelope, the portion of the virus that links selectively onto the CD4 target cell.

When a pregnant woman is HIV-positive, there is approximately a 50% chance (with a range of 13 to 60%) that the HIV will be transmitted to the fetus and neonate. The virus may undergo antepartum, intrapartum, and postpartum transmission in the breast milk. Cesarean section is not recommended as prophylaxis against neonatal HIV infection. Intrapartum management entails use of external monitors and avoidance of scalp electrodes, intrauterine pressure catheters, and fetal scalp blood sampling. Postpartum breastfeeding should be avoided.

The risk of becoming HIV-positive from a single needle stick is 1 to 4 per 1000, compared with a risk of 6 to 30 per 1000 for hepatitis B. Diagnosis of the clinical syndrome of AIDS requires an illness predictive of cellular immune deficiency, such as Kaposi's sarcoma (KS) or *Pneumocystis carinii* pneumonia (PCP).

33
CHAPTER
SALPINGITIS AND ITS SEQUELAE

PELVIC INFLAMMATORY DISEASE

Pelvic inflammatory disease (PID), acute or chronic, is most commonly polymicrobial. The principal etiologic organisms are listed on p. 205. Less common infections are pyogenic and granulomatous. Gonococcal and chlamydial pelvic inflammatory diseases are ascending infections that spread along mucous membranes from the vulva to the adnexa.

In the adult, gonococcal infection skips from Skene's glands, the urethra, and Bartholin's glands to the cervix, because the stratified squamous epithelium of the adult is rather resistant to the infection. In infants, however, gonococcal vaginitis may be a rapidly progressive and highly contagious infection. Since the endometrium usually resists chlamydial and gonorrheal infection, the disease skips from the cervix to involve the tube, the main site of serious PID.

The oviduct (uterine tube, or fallopian tube) is lined by a low columnar epithelium, comprising both secretory and ciliated cells. The mucosa is thrown into a series of complicated branching folds that are oriented in a longitudinal direction (Figs. 33–1 and 33–2). These folds are most complex in the infundibulum, slightly lower and less complex in the ampulla, still lower in the isthmus, and least complex in the intramu-

ral (interstitial) part of the oviduct. The lamina propria is typical connective tissue and a submucosa is lacking. The muscularis, which consists of an inner circular and an outer longitudinal coat, is poorly developed.

If untreated, the course of tubal infection is as follows: acute, subacute, and chronic salpingitis (Figs. 33–3 and 33–4), which may progress to a pyosalpinx as the fimbriated end is blocked. Resorption of the pus converts the pyosalpinx to a hydrosalpinx (Fig. 33–5). In advanced infection, the ovary, which may be adherent to the tube, is involved in a perioophoritis. In the final stages of the disease, a tubo-ovarian abscess may form, in which a pus-filled cavity is surrounded by a common wall of tubal and ovarian tissue.

When the diagnosis of gonorrhea is made or suspected, a serologic test for syphilis should be performed at the same time and repeated several weeks later.

In patients with acute PID, temperature, leukocyte count, and sedimentation rate are nearly always all elevated. A marked rise in temperature requires a blood culture. Radiologic examination of the abdomen may be required to rule out ileus or mechanical intestinal obstruction. In PID, the pain and tenderness are usually located lower than in an acute abdomen of other cause and the gastrointestinal signs and symp-

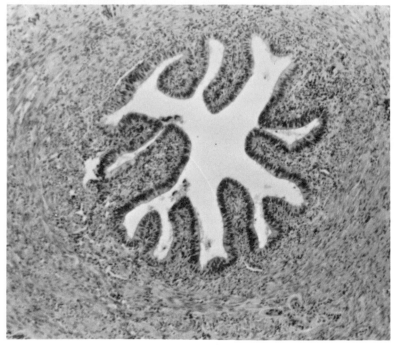

FIG. 33-1. Cornual end of fallopian tube, showing simple rugal pattern.

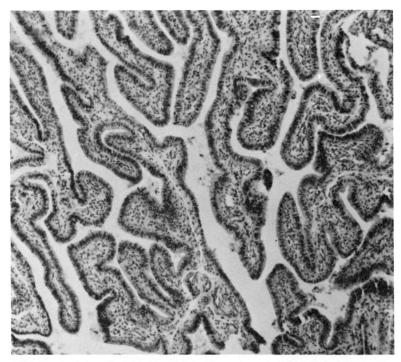

FIG. 33-2. Infundibular end of fallopian tube, showing complex rugal pattern.

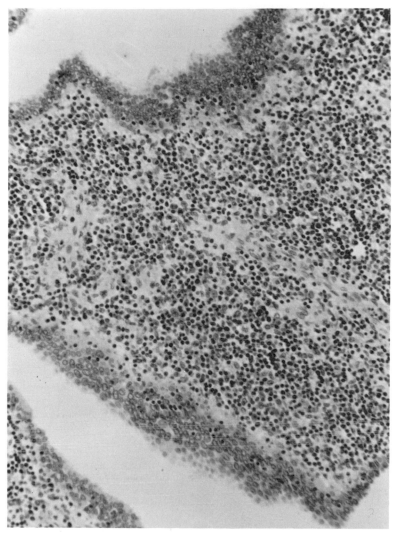

FIG. 33–3. Chronic salpingitis, showing lamina propria infiltrated by numerous lymphocytes and plasma cells.

toms are less prominent. Tachycardia, rigidity, and rebound are nonspecific, but an adnexal mass and pain on motion of the cervix suggest PID, which in gonococcal salpingitis is often exacerbated during the menses.

The differential diagnosis of salpingitis includes all causes of the acute abdomen. With salpingitis, the pain is more likely bilateral and there is less nausea and vomiting than with appendicitis, for example. With ectopic pregnancy, the leukocyte count and temperature are lower and the patient usually shows some signs of pregnancy (p. 95). When the peritonitis is caused by salpingitis, the patient frequently appears less ill than when the acute abdomen is a result of appendicitis or pancreatitis, for example.

In the diagnosis of the acute abdomen, it is most important to distinguish PID from the other causes, since acute salpingitis (like acute pyelonephritis) is a nonsurgical disease, which responds to antibiotic therapy, as opposed to ectopic pregnancy, appendicitis, and torsion of an adnexal mass, for example. If doubt about a "surgical abdomen" persists, laparoscopy, or if necessary, laparotomy must be performed. If the diagnosis proves wrong and acute salpingitis is

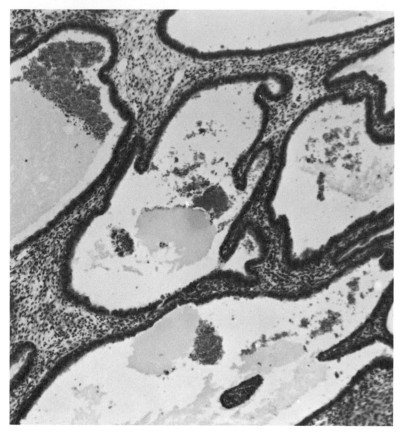

FIG. 33–4. Chronic follicular salpingitis.

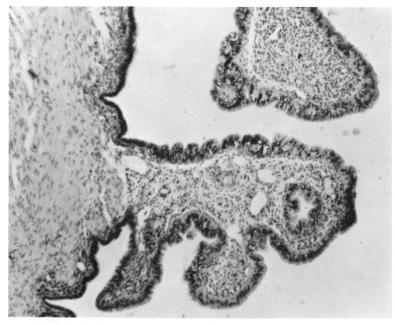

FIG. 33–5. Hydrosalpinx, showing blunted rugae projecting into distended lumen.

found, the abdomen should be closed without further procedures.

Because of the rapid spread of PID, it is appropriate to treat infection of the lower genitourinary tract before confirmation of the diagnosis is obtained. A standard treatment for gonorrhea of the lower genitourinary tract is ceftriaxone, a third-generation cephalosporin, 250 mg, intramuscularly, in a single dose, together with either doxycycline, 100 mg, orally, twice a day, for 7 days; or with tetracycline, 500 mg, orally, 4 times a day, for 7 days. For patients unable to take the ceftriaxone, alternative treatments include spectinomycin, 2 g, intramuscularly, in a single dose, together with doxycycline, 100 mg, orally, twice a day, for 7 days. If the infection is proved not to be caused by a penicillinase-producing (not penicillin-resistant) organism, ampicillin, 3.5 g, or amoxicillin, 3 g, by mouth, with probenecid, 1 g, may be substituted along with doxycycline or tetracycline.

For patients who cannot tolerate doxycycline or for whom it is contraindicated (as in pregnancy), erythromycin, 500 mg, orally, 4 times a day, for 10 to 14 days, may be used. Patients who cannot tolerate ceftriaxone can be treated with ciprofloxacin (a 4-fluoroquinolone), 500 mg, orally, in a single dose. Pregnant patients, for whom ciprofloxacin is contraindicated, should be treated with ceftriaxone and erythromycin. Pregnant patients who are allergic to β-lactams should be treated with spectinomycin, 2 g, intramuscularly, in a single dose. Approximately 10 to 20% of women with acute gonococcal infections of the lower genital tract develop PID and are at risk for its sequelae. The oral regimen is ineffective against anorectal and pharyngeal gonococcal infections, and both the oral semisynthetic penicillins and intramuscular aqueous procaine penicillin are ineffective against chlamydial infections, which may coexist with gonorrhea in as many as 45% of cases. A combined regimen that may be effective against gonorrheal and chlamydial infections is the aforementioned dose of amoxicillin or ampicillin together with tetracycline, 500 mg, by mouth, four times a day for 7 days, or doxycycline, 100 mg, by mouth, twice a day for 7 days.

Ceftriaxone, 250 mg, intramuscularly, in a single dose is the preferred therapy for pharyngeal gonococcal infection, which is not treated effectively by amoxicillin, ampicillin, or spectinomycin. Patients with proven penicillinase-producing *Neisseria gonorrhoeae* (PPNG) infection should receive 2 g of spectinomycin, intramuscularly, in a single injection. Tetracycline may be added to treat coexistent chlamydial infection.

All pregnant women should have endocervical cultures for gonococci and chlamydia during their first prenatal visits (p. 67). A second culture late in the third trimester should be obtained from women at high risk of gonococcal infection. The treatment of choice is ceftriaxone, 250 mg, intramuscularly, in a single dose, together with erythromycin base, 500 mg, or erythromycin ethylsuccinate, 800 mg. Women allergic to penicillin or probenecid should be treated with spectinomycin, 2 g, intramuscularly. Erythromycin in the doses previously recommended may be added to treat coexistent chlamydial infection. Tetracycline should not be used in pregnant women because of possible adverse effects on the fetus.

Acute PID refers to the endometritis, salpingitis, parametritis, and peritonitis caused by the ascending spread of microorganisms from the vagina and endocervix. The principal etiologic agents are *Neisseria gonorrhoeae, Chlamydia trachomatis,* anaerobic bacteria including *Bacteroides sp.* and gram-positive cocci, facultative aerobic gram-negative rods such as *Escherichia coli* and genital mycoplasmas. The most appropriate treatment includes agents active against the broadest range of these pathogens. The CDC recommends hospitalization of patients with acute pelvic inflammatory disease in the following circumstances: when the diagnosis is uncertain, when surgical emergencies such as appendicitis and ectopic pregnancy cannot be excluded, when a pelvic abscess is suspected, when severe illness precludes management as an outpatient, when the patient is pregnant, when the patient cannot follow or tolerate the regimen as an outpatient, when the patient has failed to respond to therapy as an outpatient, and when clinical follow-up after 48 to 72 hours after the start of antibiotic treatment cannot be arranged.

A useful clinical staging of acute salpingitis has been proposed. Stage I is acute salpingitis without peritonitis. It is divided into monomicrobial and polymicrobial with or without *N. gonorrhoeae*. Stage II is acute salpingitis with peritonitis (including all patients with intrauterine devices). Stage III is acute salpingitis with evidence of tubal occlusion or tubo-ovarian complex. Stage IV is ruptured tubo-ovarian complex.

No treatment of choice has been determined and no single agent is effective against the entire spectrum of pathogens, but several antimicrobial combinations are recommended because of their activity against the major pathogens in vitro. Doxycycline, 100 mg, intravenously, twice a day together with cefoxitin, 2 g, intravenously, four times a day, should be continued for at least 4 days and at least 48 hours after fever subsides. Alternatives to cefoxitin are cefotetan, intravenously, 2 g, every 4 hours, or another cephalosporin such as ceftizoxime, cefotaxime, or ceftriaxone. Doxycycline should be continued in doses of 100 mg, by mouth, twice a day after discharge from the hospital to complete 10 to 14 days of therapy. The combination of doxycycline and cefoxitin provides optimal coverage for *N. gonorrhoeae*, including PPNG, *C. trachomatis*, and most anaerobes.

Another regimen is clindamycin, 900 mg, intravenously, every 8 hours, together with gentamicin or tobramycin, 2 mg/kg, intravenously, followed by 1.5 mg/kg, intravenously, three times a day in patients with normal renal function. The drugs should be continued intravenously for at least 4 days and at least 48 hours after fever subsides. Clindamycin may be continued in a dose of 450 mg, by mouth, five times a day after discharge from the hospital to complete 10 to 14 days of therapy as an alternative to doxycycline. The combination of clindamycin with gentamicin or tobramycin provides optimal activity against anaerobes and facultative gram-negative rods, but may not provide optimal activity against *C. trachomatis* and *N. gonorrhoeae*.

When the patient is not hospitalized, use of one of the following regimens is recommended: cefoxitin, 2 g, intramuscularly along with probenecid, 1 g, by mouth, or ceftriaxone, 250 mg, intramuscularly, or an equivalent cephalosporin (without probenecid). Each of the aforementioned drugs is to be followed by doxycycline, 100 mg, by mouth, twice a day for 10 to 14 days, or tetracycline, 500 mg, by mouth, four times a day for 10 to 14 days. Tetracycline is less active than doxycycline against certain anaerobes. Cefoxitin or an equivalently effective cephalosporin together with doxycycline or tetracycline provides activity against *N. gonorrhoeae,* including PPNG, and *C. trachomatis.*

Sexual partners of patients with PID should be examined for STD and treated promptly with a regimen effective against uncomplicated gonococcal and chlamydial infections. All women treated as outpatients should be reevaluated clinically in 48 to 72 hours and admitted if a favorable response is not detected.

Chronic PID is often suspected on the basis of a history of repetitive acute infections. If the disease is untreated, the tubes are ultimately occluded and the mucosa and fimbriae are destroyed. The patient is thus rendered infertile. When antibiotic therapy is inadequate to eradicate the inflammation, a follicular salpingitis may result. This lesion predisposes to ectopic pregnancy (p. 94). In exacerbations of pelvic inflammatory disease and in the chronic form, polymicrobial infections with anaerobic organisms are found.

The signs and symptoms of chronic PID are referable primarily to the adnexal disease. Exacerbation of the infection leads to adhesions, more or less constant pelvic pain, and dyspareunia. A palpable mass and recurring spikes of temperature suggest a tubo-ovarian abscess or a pelvic abscess.

The important surgical decision in chronic PID is whether or when to operate rather than what procedure to perform, for in many cases total abdominal hysterectomy with bilateral salpingo-oophorectomy is the operation of choice for the advanced lesion. The decision to operate therefore depends upon the symptoms and the degree of incapacitation. With the advent of in-vitro fertilization and embryo transfer, patients with advanced PID have been managed with antibiotics and conservative surgical procedures, with retention of the uterus.

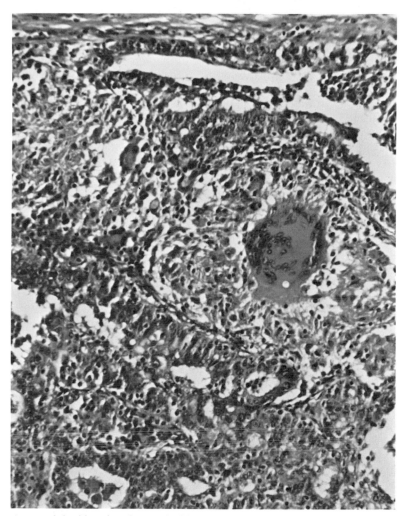

FIG. 33–6. Tuberculous salpingitis, showing typical Langhans giant cell and microtubercle.

The possibility that an adnexal mass is an ovarian neoplasm must be excluded by the appropriate diagnostic method. The differential diagnosis of chronic PID also includes ectopic pregnancy and endometriosis.

The sudden disappearance of a mass accompanied by softening of the abdomen suggests rupture of a tubo-ovarian abscess. This emergency usually is best treated by total hysterectomy and bilateral salpingo-oophorectomy and administration of broad-spectrum antibiotics. An abscess that points in the cul-de-sac occasionally may be drained by colpotomy, but a true tubo-ovarian abscess cannot be approached safely through that route. PID is occasionally ac-companied by septic shock. The management is the same as that of septic shock of other causes (p. 98).

Particularly in the young patient, conservative surgical procedures are often attempted. Rarely, however, can a tube seriously damaged by gonococcal salpingitis be reconstructed sufficiently to ensure fertility, especially if the fimbriae are destroyed.

Active gonococcal infection in the mother may lead to gonococcal ophthalmia in the newborn. For prophylaxis, erythromycin ointment (0.5%), tetracycline ophthalmic ointment (1%), or silver nitrate (10% solution) is placed in the conjunctival sacs of all newborn infants as a routine.

Pyogenic infections caused by streptococci and staphylococci were formerly more common complications of abortion and delivery. Unlike gonorrhea, they spread by lymphatic and hematogenous routes. The infection extends directly through the endometrium and the myometrium into the parametria and broad ligaments, causing a pelvic cellulitis and involving the tube from the outside. In these infections also, the involved organs are occasionally invaded secondarily by coliform organisms and anaerobes. The pyogenic salpingitides usually respond to large doses of penicillin.

GRANULOMATOUS SALPINGITIS

The granulomatous salpingitides are exemplified by tuberculosis, which still accounts for a small percentage of all PID in the United States. The infection is almost always secondary to pulmonary tuberculosis. Tuberculosis PID is a hematogenous infection that involves the tube as the primary site in the pelvis. The abdominal end of the tube may remain open, although the fimbriae are often destroyed and peristalsis is abolished. Histologically the highly proliferative lesions may superficially resemble carcinoma (Fig. 33–6). Peritoneal tuberculosis may be accompanied by ascites.

The infection involves primarily women between the ages of 20 and 40 and is characterized by malaise, a low-grade fever, and nagging abdominal pain. Menstrual disorders and infertility are common. Tuberculosis should be suspected in a case of salpingitis that does not respond to penicillin and in PID in virgins. A granuloma on endometrial biopsy directs suspicion to the lesion, and the presence of acid-fast bacilli on a Ziehl-Neelsen stained preparation of the tissue is confirmatory. Final diagnosis is made by inoculation into guinea pigs.

When surgical extirpation was the mainstay of treatment, postoperative complications such as fistulas were common. Antituberculous drugs are now the treatment of choice. The drugs are usually continued for 9 to 18 months, with surgical treatment reserved for an adnexal mass (to rule out carcinoma of the ovary) and for unresponsive pain or fever.

The primary drugs used for treatment of pelvic tuberculosis are rifampicin, ethambutol, and isoniazid (INH). Streptomycin and paraaminosalicyclic acid (PAS) are used less commonly today.

An unusual form of chronic salpingitis is salpingitis isthmica nodosa, which causes fibrosis of the tubal wall with nodular thickenings and obstruction at the cornual end (Fig. 33–7). The cause of this lesion is poorly understood. It may not be of infectious origin at all but rather a disorder allied to adenomyosis of the uterus (endosalpingiosis).

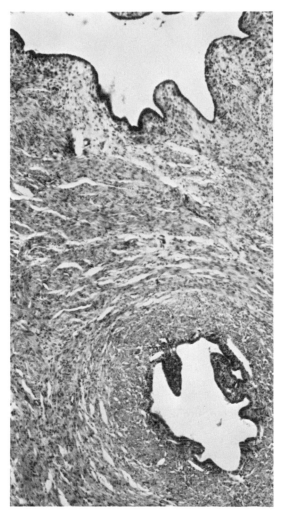

FIG. 33–7. Salpinigitis isthmica nodosa, showing central lumen and cleft-like glandular spaces in myosalpinx.

34
CHAPTER

PELVIC RELAXATION AND UROGYNECOLOGY

PELVIC RELAXATION

Pelvic relaxation refers to a group of anatomic, sometimes symptomatic, defects including uterine prolapse (descensus), relaxation of the anterior vaginal wall (urethrocele and cystocele), relaxation of the posterior wall (rectocele), herniation of the peritoneum of the cul-de-sac (enterocele), and laceration of the perineum. These disorders usually are related to childbirth or aging and are rarely congenital. Prolapse of the vagina may occur after hysterectomy.

The principal weakness is in the endopelvic fascia and the muscular levator sling. Attenuation of the vesicovaginal (anterior) portion of the endopelvic fascia, between bladder and anterior vaginal wall, results in prolapse of the bladder into the anterior vaginal wall (cystocele). Weakening of the connective tissue between the urethra and vagina produces a urethrocele. Weakening of the rectovaginal (posterior) portion of the endopelvic fascia causes bulging of the anterior wall of the rectum into the vagina (rectocele).

Laceration or attenuation of the condensed pericervical areolar tissue (endopelvic fascia), laceration of the perineum, and injury to the levator sling usually result from obstetric injuries or the atrophy of aging. Attenuation of the cardinal and uterosacral ligaments contributes to the relaxation. Herniation of small bowel through the hiatus between the uterosacral ligaments produces an enterocele, which is a true hernia. The components of pelvic relaxation occur in various degrees and combinations. The best prevention is good obstetric care.

The syndrome of pelvic relaxation is related in part to the anatomic changes associated with the bipedal condition. Women with pelvic relaxation are more likely than the general population to develop hemorrhoids, hernias, and varicose veins. Racial factors also play a role in susceptibility to pelvic relaxation. Black women, for example, are less likely than white women to develop uterine prolapse.

The greater prevalence of pelvic relaxation in many foreign countries as compared with the United States, however, is more likely related to differences in obstetric practice. Prophylactic obstetric measures include the appropriate use of outlet forceps and episiotomy, shortening of the second stage, and anatomic repair of lacerations. These maneuvers may protect the perivaginal connective tissues and the muscles of the pelvic floor.

The relative roles of the pelvic musculature and the connective tissue ligaments in the prevention of pelvic relaxation remain somewhat controversial. The levator ani, which consists of the pubococcygeus, iliococcygeus, and ischiococcygeus, forms the deep support. The perineal muscles form a second line of defense; they comprise the ischiocavernosus, bulbocavernosus, and superficial and deep transverse perineal muscles, together with the urogenital diaphragm and external anal sphincter. The broad ligament and the round ligaments provide no support, but the condensed connective tissue in the cardinal and uterosacral ligaments helps to maintain the uterus in its normal position.

The signs and symptoms of pelvic relaxation depend on the combination and degree of anatomic defects. Uterine prolapse usually produces merely a sagging sensation in the pelvis. Severe degrees of prolapse are associated with other symptomatic components of pelvic relaxation.

In first-degree prolapse, the uterus descends, but the cervix remains within the vagina. In second-degree prolapse, the cervix appears partially or totally outside the vaginal orifice. In third-degree prolapse (procidentia), the entire uterus is outside the vaginal orifice. In a prolapsed uterus, the cervix is often hypertrophied and ulcerated but is not more frequently subject to carcinoma than is the normally situated cervix.

A cystocele may reach large size without becoming symptomatic. Problems referable to a cystocele include frequency of urination, a sensation of pelvic pressure, and a predisposition to recurrent urinary tract infections. The cystocele does not, however, produce stress incontinence (the involuntary loss of urine upon increase in intraabdominal pressure).

A rectocele causes a sensation of a mass in the vagina and difficulty in evacuating the rectum without placing a hand in the vagina to reduce the bulge. The enterocele is subject to all the complications of hernias elsewhere in the body. Strangulation of bowel within an enterocele sac is unusual, however. The relaxed perineum may lead to unsatisfactory intercourse.

The most serious complaint in patients with pelvic relaxation is stress incontinence, which results from a urethrocele, or more accurately, a funneling of the bladder neck.

Differential diagnosis of pelvic relaxation usually presents few problems. A prolapsed uterus must be differentiated from a normally situated uterus with an elongated cervix. An enterocele must be differentiated from a high rectocele, a urethrocele from a suburethral diverticulum, and a cystocele from a large midline mesonephric ductal cyst.

The treatment of pelvic relaxation depends on correction of the fascial and muscular defects. The cystocele is repaired by plication of the anterior portion of the endopelvic fascia (anterior colporrhaphy). Care must be taken to avoid overcorrection, thereby obliterating the posterior urethrovesical angle and producing stress incontinence. An extensive anterior colporrhaphy should be accompanied by a plication of the bladder neck (Kelly plication) to maintain the urethrovesical angle.

The rectocele is repaired by plication of the posterior portion of the endopelvic fascia (posterior colporrhaphy). In complete pelvic repairs, it is desirable to perform only minimal posterior colporrhaphy in a young woman in order to preserve sexual function. A relaxed perineum may be reconstructed to provide normal support by the operation known as perineorrhaphy. An enterocele is repaired by excision of the hernial sac and obliteration of the hiatus between the uterosacral ligaments. The vagina may be suspended to the sacrospinous ligaments. This operation maintains a functional vagina, whereas colpocleisis does not.

Retroversion, except possibly the adherent variety found in endometriosis, is a normal variant of uterine position. It does not require surgical therapy.

The abdominal approach to correction of pelvic relaxation is anatomically illogical and therapeutically unsuccessful. The principal treatment of uterine prolapse is vaginal hysterectomy. This procedure in itself, however, does not correct the often accompanying cystocele and rectocele or the stress incontinence. These problems are managed by colporrhaphy and Kelly plication. The advantages of vaginal hysterectomy are the prevention of pregnancy, which could break down a previously successful repair, and after the menopause, removal of a functionless organ, which could be the site of benign or malignant disease. The operative procedures mentioned here are described further in Chapter 38.

Before vaginal hysterectomy and repair of a cystocele, local infections of the vagina, cervix, and bladder should be eradicated.

For minor degrees of pelvic relaxation, exercises to strengthen the perineal muscles may be helpful.

Pessaries are used infrequently today, except for temporary replacement of a prolapsed uterus during preoperative healing of an infected cervix. They may be used also as a therapeutic test to ascertain whether repositioning of the uterus will relieve the patient's symptoms. Pessaries are used for definitive treatment only in the aged patient or the woman who is too sick or unwilling to tolerate a surgical procedure. Pessaries are associated with increased incidences of discharge, ulceration, and rarely, vaginal carcinoma, unless they are periodically removed and cleaned and unless the atrophic vagina is treated with exogenous estrogen.

UROGYNECOLOGY

Stress incontinence of urine is the most troublesome result of pelvic relaxation. Urinary incontinence is defined as the involuntary loss of urine that may occur continuously or intermittently during the day or night. It may be associated with pain, urgency, frequency, and hematuria, and may become sufficiently serious to render the patient a social invalid. Of women aged 35 to 64 years, up to 10% may have some type of urinary incontinence.

Continence of urine depends on maintenance of normal detrusor function and normal support by the muscles of the pelvic floor. Normal voiding begins with increase in intravesical pressure, followed by contraction of the detrusor, and finally, relaxation of the internal sphincter and pelvic floor. Urinary incontinence may occur as a result of interference with any of these steps.

The four main types of urinary incontinence are stress, urge, overflow, and total. Stress incontinence usually manifests itself when a small volume of urine leaks from the urethra upon increase in intraabdominal pressure, as with coughing or sneezing. Normally the posterior urethrovesical angle is 90 to 100 degrees; in stress incontinence it is usually blunted. The basic anatomic defect is weakness of the musculofascial supports of the bladder and upper urethra. As a result, the bladder is constantly in the state of prevoiding, or first-stage voiding.

Urge incontinence results from detrusor instability, or detrusor dyssynergia, with involuntary and uninhibited contractions of the detrusor and resulting loss of urine. With classical detrusor instability, large volumes of urine may be voided uncontrollably. Infections of the urinary tract and atrophic or infectious vaginitis can be contributing factors. They can be diagnosed easily and treated effectively with the appropriate medication (antibiotics or estrogen).

Overflow incontinence results from overdistension of the bladder. In this condition a small volume of urine escapes from a constantly filled bladder. Underlying causes include neuropathies, as with diabetes mellitus, syphilis, multiple sclerosis, and spinal injuries.

Total incontinence results most often from a urinary tract fistula, which causes more or less constant loss of urine. The "lead pipe" urethra, which is often a result of radiation fibrosis, may cause total incontinence when loss of the normal urethrovesical angle coexists.

Fistulas reflect the close anatomic relation of the female reproductive tract and the urinary tract. The obstetric causes of fistulas have decreased relatively as a result of technical improvements and the avoidance of difficult vaginal deliveries and long labors. The gynecologic causes, however, have increased relatively as a result of more extensive and radical surgical procedures and radiotherapy.

Accurate diagnosis of urinary incontinence, which is essential to successful therapy, first requires a careful history of the signs and symptoms, including frequency, urgency, nocturia, patterns of voiding and loss, number of pads used, pain, hematuria, hesitancy in voiding, number of times voiding occurs, duration of the problem, and prior medical and surgical treatments.

Pelvic and neurologic examinations must be performed carefully and urine cultures obtained. Rigidity, tenderness, pain, prolapse, and associated lesions should be noted meticulously. With her bladder full, the patient is asked to cough while in the lithotomy position. Stress incontinence is suggested if only small spurts of urine are produced on coughing. If incontinence is not demonstrated in the lithotomy position, the test should be repeated with the patient standing. In a Bonney test (using fingers) or a Marshall-Marchetti test (using an Allis clamp), the urethrovesical angle is supported to see whether leakage of urine can be controlled. These tests may sometimes predict the success of surgical treatment of the incontinence, but they are not entirely reliable because they may occlude the urethra and suggest an overly optimistic surgical prognosis.

The Q-tip test assesses the mobility and descent of the urethrovesical junction when the patient strains. A lubricated Q-tip is inserted into the urethra to the level of the urethrovesical angle with the patient in the lithotomy position. The resting angle between the Q-tip and the horizontal is measured. The patient then bears down and the new angle is measured. If the difference between the angles at rest and during straining is greater than 30 degrees, the urethra may be excessively mobile, possibly because of detachment from its normal anatomic site.

Bedside cystometric examinations provide information about total capacity, residuals after voiding, first-urge sensation, and full-bladder sensation, and may demonstrate incontinence. Further urodynamic evaluation of the lower urinary tract (with multiple simultaneous measurements of pressure and flow) is particularly useful in patients with complicated or confusing histories or after of prior therapy.

Urethroscopy and cystometrograms provide objective evidence of intrinsic lesions of the urinary tract and of the relations of the bladder neck and urethra to the vagina and symphysis pubis. Intravenous pyelography may be required to rule out an ectopic ureter and other lesions higher in the urinary tract.

Although perineal exercises and estrogen therapy for patients with estrogenic deficiency may be helpful in the management of patients with mild stress incontinence, more severe degrees of the disorder usually require surgical treatment. A Kelly plication is often the first procedure employed, whereas retropubic suspension of the vesical neck through the abdominal route is frequently required for more severe lesions. The rate of cure after 5 years may be as high as 80% with either procedure, if properly chosen and performed.

When conventional vaginal and abdominal operations are unsuccessful, one of the many "sling" operations may be effective.

In these procedures a sling of rectus fascia, fascia lata, or synthetic material is passed under the urethra through the space of Retzius and reattached to the anterior abdominal wall. Other operative procedures include implantation of an artificial sphincter and urinary diversion. Reduction in weight and treatment of a chronic cough may improve the results of surgical management of stress incontinence.

Vesicovaginal fistulas may result from unrecognized injury during hysterectomy or colporrhaphy. If not repaired immediately, these fistulas are most successfully closed, usually by the vaginal route, after a delay of 4 to 6 months. Other causes are injury from radiation and direct involvement by carcinoma.

A vesicovaginal fistula may be demonstrated by the appearance of dye in the vagina after instillation of methylene blue into the bladder. A ureterovaginal fistula may result from a radical or difficult total hysterectomy in which the ureter is ligated or cut. This fistula may be demonstrated by the appearance of dye in the vagina after intravenous injection of indigo carmine or by pyelography. A urethrovaginal fistula in the distal third of the urethra is unlikely to result in urinary incontinence and ordinarily requires no treatment. Vesicovaginal and ureterovaginal fistulas may coexist.

The surgical principles of repair of a vesicovaginal fistula are as follows: adequate dissection and mobilization of the involved organs without injury to adjacent structures; excision of the scarred, epithelialized fistulous tract; separate closure in layers of the vesical and vaginal walls without tension on the suture lines; minimization of infection by good hemostasis, use of fine sutures, obliteration of dead space, and administration of appropriate antibiotics; and postoperative drainage of the bladder.

Vaginal fistulas may involve the bowel as well as the urinary tract. A rectovaginal fistula may result from unrecognized obstetric injuries, gynecologic operations, radiation therapy, or direct growth of a carcinoma. A small rectovaginal fistula may result only in incontinence of gas, whereas a larger fistula usually causes fecal incontinence as well. The principles of closure are similar to those of vesicovaginal fistulas.

35
CHAPTER

ADENOMYOSIS AND ENDOMETRIOSIS

Adenomyosis and endometriosis are frequently discussed together although they are etiologically different disorders, which require different treatments.

Adenomyosis is a condition in which endometrial tissue penetrates the myometrium by direct extension from the lining of the uterine cavity. The circumscribed lesion is termed an adenomyoma and the diffuse form, adenomyosis (Fig. 35–1).

Endometriosis is a disorder in which endometrial tissue occurs outside its normal intrauterine location not connected with the endometrial surface. It also may be a circumscribed (endometrioma) or diffuse (endometriosis) lesion.

ADENOMYOSIS

Diagnosis of adenomyosis can be made only by examination of the excised tissue and requires the finding of endometrial glands and stroma a specified distance from the base of the endometrium. The distance varies, according to different authorities, from one high-power to two low-power fields. One low-power field, however, is a commonly accepted definition.

Adenomyosis comprises endometrial tissue surrounded by myometrium. In special circumstances, gland or stroma may predominate or stroma may occur exclusively. Since the tissue is composed largely of basal endometrium, it is not fully responsive to the endocrine changes of the endometrial cycle or to exogenously administered hormones.

Adenomyosis, unlike endometriosis, is most common in multiparas in the fourth to sixth decades. It may be associated with myomas and endometrial polyps and hyperplasia and occasionally with endometriosis and carcinoma of the endometrium. Grossly, the myometrium is irregularly thickened on cut surface.

The characteristic symptoms and signs of adenomyosis are progressive dysmenorrhea, menorrhagia, and an enlarging tender uterus. Additional findings include dyspareunia and a premenstrual syndrome that resembles pelvic congestion (p. 357). The diagnosis is often made incidentally at the time of laparotomy. The differential diagnosis includes carcinoma of the corpus, endometrial polyps, and myomas. The gross pathologic differential diagnosis includes sarcoma and myoma. Unlike the myoma, neither the adenomyoma nor the sarcoma has a pseudocapsule that allows easy enucleation from the surrounding myometrium.

A special form of the lesion is stromal adenomyosis, or endometrial stromatosis. This disease may clinically resemble a low-grade endometrial sarcoma.

The etiologic factors in adenomyosis are unknown, although an estrogenic imbalance may be influential.

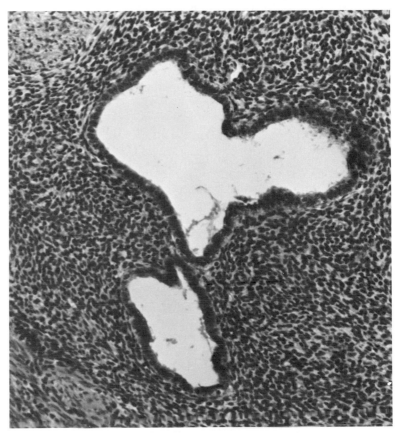

FIG. 35–1. Adenomyosis, showing endometrial gland and stroma.

The prevalence of the disease is difficult to assess, although it is commonly found in uteri removed for other causes. Since hormonal treatment is generally unsatisfactory, the symptomatic lesion most often is treated by hysterectomy. In women near the menopause, after malignant disease has been excluded, temporization may be logical, for the lesion regresses with cessation of ovarian function.

ENDOMETRIOSIS

The prevalence of endometriosis is difficult to ascertain because it also is often discovered as an incidental finding at laparotomy. Endometriosis, unlike adenomyosis, is most commonly found in nulliparas between the ages of 25 and 40. The widespread use of laparoscopy has resulted in the detection of many more examples of endometriosis recently. It is said to occur more commonly in white, middle-class, high-income patients who marry late. These differences most likely reflect socioeconomic rather than racial factors. Private patients, furthermore, are more likely to register minor complaints, thereby creating the impression of a greater prevalence of the disease in that group.

Endometriosis is rarely, if ever, found in the prepuberal or postmenopausal period and often, but not always, seems to be improved during pregnancy. Early childbearing plays a role in preventing endometriosis.

Several etiologic concepts remain debatable. One hypothesis favors retrograde menstruation, with the resulting implantation of endometrial tissue on the ovaries and peritoneum. A retroverted uterus, which is found commonly in patients with endometriosis, may predispose to retrograde menses. A second etiologic hypothesis is coelomic metaplasia, by which coelomic derivatives are transformed into tissues of endometrial type. A third concept, which combines retrograde menses with metaplasia, is induction, by means of which a chemical substance from sloughed endometrial tissue leads to transformation of other tissues to the endometrial type. Hematogenous and lymphatic spread probably plays only a small role in the histogenesis of endometriosis. Hereditary factors may play an etiologic role in some cases.

Several studies suggest that the peritoneal fluid in women with endometriosis contains higher than normal levels of thromboxane B_2 and 6-keto-prostaglandin $F_{2\alpha}$. Thus, the relation between endometriosis and infertility may be based in part on the action of prostaglandins on oviductal function. Current research, furthermore, suggests an increase in activated macrophages in the peritoneal fluid and an autoimmune response to endometrium in patients with endometriosis. None of these explanations, however, is currently accepted by all authorities in the field.

Endometriosis usually comprises both gland and stroma, although one or the other element may be predominant and stroma may be present alone occasionally. The gross lesions may resemble "powder burns" on the peritoneum and serosal surfaces. Large hemorrhagic cysts of the ovary containing dark blood are referred to as "chocolate cysts," although not all such hemorrhagic ovarian cysts are the result of endometriosis.

When the wall of a hemorrhagic cyst contains hemosiderin but the epithelium of origin is unidentifiable, the diagnosis should be hemorrhagic cyst rather than endometrial cyst.

Rupture of an endometrial cyst may lead to extensive adhesions, denser that those of pelvic inflammatory disease. Intraperitoneal bleeding or pain resulting from rupture of an endometrioma may create a surgical emergency. The resulting adhesions may cause fixed retroversion of the uterus, involvement of adjacent organs, and strictures of the bowel. In extreme cases, a "frozen pelvis" may result.

The structures involved in endometriosis, in order of frequency, are the ovary (Fig. 35–2), the posterior cul-de-sac, the uterosacral ligaments, the rectovaginal septum, the oviducts, the rectosigmoid, and the bladder. Distant organs are involved rarely. Endometriosis of the lymph nodes, pleura, and extremities is difficult to explain on the basis of the common histogenetic theories.

Carcinoma may develop in ovarian endometriosis, but unless a clear transition from normal endometrium to malignant tissue is seen within the ovary, the origin of the tumor from endometriosis cannot be proved.

The endometriotic tissue is usually responsive to the hormones of the menstrual cycle and to externally supplied hormones. This endocrine dependence explains the progress of the disease as well as the response to treatment.

The accuracy of preoperative diagnosis of endometriosis is relatively low. The lesion is often found incidentally in patients operated upon for other reasons. The number of false-positive and false-negative diagnoses is reduced by preoperative laparoscopy. Definitive diagnosis is made only after histologic examination of a biopsy specimen.

Endometriosis characteristically presents with acquired dysmenorrhea, acute and chronic pelvic pain, and abnormal uterine bleeding. Infertility may become a major problem. The dysmenorrhea, which usually begins after age 25, is progressive. As the disease continues, pain and bleeding occur in increasingly greater portions of the menstrual cycle. Dyspareunia may result from involvement of the uterosacral ligaments and implants in the cul-de-sac and fornices. The abnormal bleeding may result from ovarian dysfunction, which together with dense adhesions may lead to infertility, but there is no good correlation between the severity of the symptoms and the anatomic extent of the disease.

Less common manifestations of endometriosis include pain, bleeding with bowel movements or tenesmus (as a result of involvement of the rectovaginal septum and rectum), and dysuria and cyclic hematuria (as a result of involvement of the bladder). A less specific but more common manifestation is dull pain radiating to the thighs.

A careful rectovaginal examination is essential for the clinical diagnosis of endometriosis. Highly suggestive findings include nodules in the cul-de-sac, the posterior fornix, the anterior fornix, and the uterosacral ligaments; fixed retroversion of the

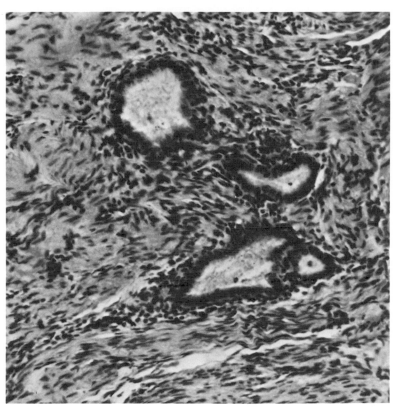

FIG. 35–2. Endometriosis of the ovary, showing endometrial glands and stroma.

uterus; obliteration of the cul-de-sac by dense adhesions and tender, enlarged, or fixed ovaries. Differential diagnosis includes chronic pelvic inflammatory disease and ovarian neoplasms. Additional diseases to be considered are carcinoma of the rectum or sigmoid, diverticulitis, and tuberculosis.

With endometriosis, a greater degree of fixation of organs is found than with other diseases that are considered in differential diagnosis. Laboratory data are not diagnostic, but a normal white count points to endometriosis rather than pelvic inflammatory disease.

Pelvic examination under anesthesia may differentiate endometriosis from the pelvic congestion syndrome, because in endometriosis the thickening and nodularity of the uterosacral ligaments, for example, do not decrease or disappear. The diagnostic workup, depending on signs and symptoms, may include barium enema, cystoscopy, and intravenous pyelography.

Treatment of endometriosis is influenced by the patient's age and parity. The three methods of management are supportive, hormonal, and surgical. Supportive therapy entails careful observation, reassurance, and analgesics. A trial of pregnancy, where feasible, is sometimes recommended, for it may be curative. Observation is contraindicated in the presence of an undiagnosed adnexal mass.

Surgical and hormonal techniques of management of endometriosis are complementary. Prolonged hormonal therapy, which is time-consuming and expensive, should be reserved for patients who have a histologic diagnosis of endometriosis.

Surgical intervention in endometriosis may be limited to laparoscopy for staging and biopsy of suspect lesions, electrocauterization of lesions, or utilization of the carbon dioxide laser for vaporization. Laparoscopy is particularly well suited to the evaluation of patients with the possible diagnosis of endometriosis, for it permits staging of the extent of the disease as well as treatment by electrocautery, laser, or conventional sharp surgical dissection.

No single therapeutic modality (expectant, hormonal, or surgical) is clearly superior in all cases of mild or moderate endometriosis. Formal laparotomy is indicated, however, in the face of failure of medical management, persistent infertility for more than 1 year after hormonal therapy, and presence of adnexal masses greater than 5 cm in diameter. Laparotomy is often the treatment of choice also in patients in whom the desire for or the possibility of pregnancy is no longer a factor in management.

Total abdominal hysterectomy and bilateral salpingo-oophorectomy are often curative even when not all of the implants are removed. It is unwise to attempt excision of every implant when adjacent organs would be jeopardized thereby. The laser may be used to advantage in removal of small foci of endometriosis that are in intimate relation to easily damaged structures. Hysterectomy without removal of the adnexa may be performed in a young patient who has completed her family. After hysterectomy and removal of the adnexa and implants, it is possible to provide hormonal supplementation, because there is no longer a proliferating endometrial mucosa to generate additional endometriotic implants, and stimulation of other coelomic epithelial derivatives is only a remote possibility.

In connection with conservative operations, uterine suspension and presacral neurectomy may be performed for symptomatic relief. Further decrease in pain may be achieved by interruption of the nerve tracts in the uterosacral ligaments.

In many patients, the hormonal therapy of endometriosis is often the treatment of choice. It may be adjunctive to conservative operations and is indicated in patients who refuse operations. Estrogens, androgens, and progestins have all been used to interrupt the ovarian cycle and control endometriosis. Danazol has been used both preoperatively and in cases of residual endometriosis, postoperatively. Gonadotropin-releasing hormone (GnRH) analogies are the latest hormonal method of treatment.

Almost any estrogen may be employed successfully. Androgens are also effective but they carry the danger of masculinization. Methyltestosterone in doses of 5 mg every day for 3 to 6 months, however, rarely produces permanent side effects.

The mainstays of current hormonal therapy are GnRH analogues and Danazol. Large doses of the steroids used in oral contraceptives are prescribed less frequently today than in the past few decades. The progestins produce a pseudopregnancy, characterized by atrophy of the endometrial glands and decidual transformation of the stroma.

Almost any of the currently used oral contraceptives may be employed for treatment of endometriosis, but good results have been achieved over long periods of time with norethynodrel and ethinyl estradiol. The initial dose of 10 mg/day is gradually increased at 2-week intervals to a maximum of 20 to 40 mg/day. Such therapy continued for 9 months has resulted in cures or remissions in 80% of cases of endometriosis.

Estrogen-progestin therapy is commonly complicated by nausea, edema, irregular uterine bleeding, and possible growth of myomas. The hormones have also been used preoperatively to "soften" the adhesions in a patient about to undergo surgical treatment. This form of therapy is being replaced gradually by Danazol and GnRH agonists.

Danazol, a 17-α-ethinyl derivative of testosterone, is an orally effective agent that inhibits the anterior pituitary. It is anabolic and weakly androgenic. Its main side effect is weight gain. The drug is required in doses of up to 800 mg/day for 6 months, during which time amenorrhea is maintained. The considerable expense of this form of therapy is a major drawback. Unlike the progestational agents, which stimulate parts of the endometrium and produce a pseudopregnancy, danazol does not stimulate the target organ but produces a pseudomenopause. It is not contraindicated in patients who are susceptible to thrombophlebitis.

Progestins alone, either by mouth or intramuscular injection, also have been used successfully. Medroxyprogesterone acetate (Depo-Provera) is currently approved by the FDA for use in endometriosis but not routine contraception. The injection may be given every 2 weeks in doses of 50 or 100 mg. If breakthrough bleeding occurs, the progestin is supplemented with estrogen by injection or by mouth.

Radiotherapy, which was formerly used to effect castration, plays no role in the modern management of endometriosis.

The gonadotropin-releasing hormone agonists are an expensive but effective means of temporary suppression if not complete eradication of endometriosis. They may be administered by nasal spray and are approved by the FDA for this route and indication. Treatment with these drugs is associated with climacteric but not androgenic side-effects.

36
CHAPTER
THE AGING WOMAN

As women are living longer into the post-menopausal years, they form an increasingly large share of the gynecologist's practice. Their problems and concerns extend far beyond those of the menopause and its treatment (Chapter 55). Geriatric gynecology therefore deserves far greater attention than it has received in the past.

Menopause, the absence of menstruation for 6 to 12 months, is a natural phenomenon that occurs, on the average, at about age 50. Menses may cease at age 40 to 45 or continue until age 55 in normal women. Premature menopause may occur at any age. The actual menopause is preceded by an interval during which ovulation and menstruation occur irregularly and subjective symptoms may develop. This is the climacteric phase of life. Perimenopause refers to the portion of the climacteric phase that immediately precedes menopause. The postmenopausal period is the phase of life after the menses cease. Menopause may be precipitated by removal or destruction of the ovaries at any age (surgical or artificial menopause).

Menopause is the result of the gradual decrease in secretion of ovarian estrogen as a result of progressive diminution in the number of functional ovarian follicles. The menses cease when insufficient estradiol is secreted to stimulate endometrial growth.

Ovulation occurs sporadically during the climacteric and eventually ceases, but estrogen secretion continues for some time thereafter. Although there is minimal ovarian secretion of estrogen after the menopause, the ovarian stromal cells continue to secrete testosterone, which is aromatized to estradiol in fat, muscle, liver, and other tissues. Adrenal and ovarian androstenedione is converted to estrone in those tissues. The amount of estrogenic hormone produced in the early postmenopausal years may be sufficient to prevent symptoms and the atrophy of estrogen-dependent tissues. Production of estrogen gradually decreases as the ovaries and adrenals age.

As secretion of estrogen and progesterone decrease, the negative feedback to the hypothalamus and anterior pituitary is reduced and the circulating concentrations of FSH and LH rise and fall in an irregular manner. The hormonal pattern after the menopause includes low estrogen, low to absent progesterone, and elevated FSH and LH.

The principal results of the postmenopausal estrogen-deficiency state are atrophy of the reproductive structures that were stimulated formerly by estrogen, changes in the physiologic functions of other organ systems, and the appearance of often distressing symptoms and signs.

SYMPTOMS

At least three quarters of women experience unpleasant symptoms during the climacteric and postmenopausal phases of life. The most typical symptom is the "hot flash." A characteristic flush is preceded by a sensation of intense heat and flushing of the skin, principally that of the head, face, neck, chest, and back, followed by profuse diaphoresis. Flushes may last a few seconds to several minutes. They may occur many times during the day and quite characteristically disturb sleep. If not treated, they gradually diminish in severity and disappear, except during periods of stress, in about 2 years. In a few women, the flushes are severe and disabling; other women have none.

Although the exact cause of hot flashes has not been identified, they are related undoubtedly to neuroendocrine changes in the hypothalamus and anterior pituitary. The actual flush is preceded by vasodilatation, a slight increase in core temperature, and increased pulse rate.

CHANGES IN REPRODUCTIVE TISSUES

The first evidences of estrogen deficiency during the climacteric are ovulatory failure and changes in the menstrual cycle. Although menstruation may stop abruptly, a more usual pattern is a gradual diminution in the amount and duration of bleeding, a change in the length of menstrual cycles, and missed menses. These changes are caused by irregular ovulation and gradually diminishing secretion of estrogen. Vulvar, vaginal, and uterine atrophy occurs as estrogen is withdrawn. These changes usually are not pronounced until several years after the actual menopause. The vaginal epithelium becomes thin and the rugae flatten. The tissue is easily injured and may become infected, causing atrophic vaginitis. The cervix becomes shorter and eventually may be flush with the vaginal vault. The uterus becomes smaller and the ovaries atrophy.

Urinary incontinence may occur because of atrophy of the estrogen-dependent tissues in the urethra and posterior bladder wall (Chapter 34). The breasts also undergo atrophy.

CHANGES IN OTHER ORGANS

Growth of bone is dependent on estrogen, and during the postmenopausal phase bony resorption exceeds bony growth. Loss of bone progresses in untreated women at a rate of 1.5 to 2% a year. Trabecular bone loss begins earlier and progresses more rapidly than does cortical loss. Osteoporosis occurs more often in white and Oriental women than in black women and is exacerbated by smoking, inactivity, and use of adrenal corticosteroids. The principal complications of osteoporosis are fractures of vertebrae, long bones, and the femoral neck. All of these fractures occur more often in women than in men in the same age groups. Bone loss can be prevented and retarded by estrogen. Calcium alone or calcium combined with exercise has a limited beneficial effect.

The relationship between estrogen and myocardial infarction has become more evident in recent years. Estrogen offers protection against heart attacks, which are relatively infrequent during reproductive years but increase after the menopause. Estrogen replacement therapy may help reduce the incidence of myocardial infarctions.

PSYCHOSOCIAL PROBLEMS IN AGING WOMEN

Until relatively recently, physicians were concerned primarily with the menopause itself, paying little attention to the other physiologic changes and the psychosocial needs of postmenopausal women. Women now live 30 to 35 years after menopause on the average. The fastest growing segment of our population consists of those over age 85. By 2010, about 5% of the total population will be over 85, and most of them will be women.

Because life expectancy for men is several years shorter than that of women, more women, about 69%, over age 75 are widowed, whereas only 22% of men at the same age are widowers. Lack of a partner limits social contacts, and income may be inadequate to support a woman's usual activities. She may be unable to afford an adequate diet or may have no interest in preparing nutritious meals only for herself. Many elderly women have inadequate health insurance and cannot afford to pay for medical care.

Because each woman has individual characteristics and emotional responses, there is no standard response to aging. Most women welcome the freedom from menstruation and fear of pregnancy, even though menopause is clear evidence of aging and the end of reproductive life. Women who equate menstruation with youth may be devastated by menopause.

Depression is common in elderly women, but basic personality changes little throughout adult lives. Reactive depression may be precipitated by events that occur simultaneously with menopause, but it is not a direct result of declining ovarian function. Some of the stresses result from a decrease in domestic responsibilities in women who have no way of replacing them with other activities. Children have left home and husbands may be preoccupied with business or other activities. This situation produces the "empty nest syndrome."

The most frequent symptoms associated with depression are feelings of sadness and despair, loss of interest in usual activities, bouts of crying, emotional lability, disturbances of sleep, and changes in eating habits. Because this form of depression often begins at or about the time of menopause, it is easy, but usually incorrect, to attribute it to low levels of reproductive hormones. Hormonal therapy alone does not reverse depression.

Changes in thyroid and parathyroid functions, which are common in postmenopausal women and which may cause symptoms similar to those of depression, are frequently overlooked. About one third of patients with hyperparathyroidism, for example, are over age 60 and 70% are women.

Many women anticipate decreased sexuality and sexual activity with aging, and some have bizarre ideas of what to expect. For the most part, their fears are unwarranted, for most women continue to enjoy sexual activity. Those who consider coitus to be a duty to a demanding partner and menstruation as evidence of youth may lose libido completely.

Sexual activity does decrease during the postmenopausal years, but often because of changes in the male partner. Unless women understand these normal changes, they may interpret them to be loss of interest in them as sexual persons. In elderly men, erection usually becomes less firm and may be lost during coitus, or it may be impossible to achieve ejaculation, and the force and quantity of the ejaculate decrease. Many elderly couples continue to have satisfying sex lives either with coitus or other forms of sexual stimulation.

Abuse of people over age 75, particularly women, exceeds that of any other group except children. Physical injury and emotional harassment are the two most common forms of abuse. Abuse can be suspected by detection of unexplained injury, significant family stresses, or deepening depression. Women are often unwilling to report abuse, particularly from their partners or children, but with understanding questioning they may become willing to discuss it.

Many of the reactions that are attributed to aging are effects of medications. About 75% of drug reactions in elderly persons are dose-related. Physiologic changes may interfere with metabolism of drugs, which may accumulate in the body. As a rule, treatment with a new drug should be initiated at one third to one half the standard dose and gradually increased to an effective amount.

TREATMENT OF AGING WOMEN

Counseling in preparation for the menopause and advancing years should begin well ahead of the actual events. A simple description of the reason for menopause and the normal changes in bodily functions and sexuality to be expected may allay many fears. Initial preventive measures against osteoporosis can be initiated at about age 35, when bone loss begins.

Periodic examinations should be directed toward detecting the conditions that are likely to occur in elderly women. They include cardiovascular diseases and cancers of the lung, breast, and colon, in addition to diseases of the reproductive organs.

Although hormone replacement is advantageous in aging women, it is of little help in managing long-standing depression and has limited use in improving sexual responses other than those caused by atrophic changes in the reproductive organs.

The principal benefits of hormone replacement are control of true estrogen-deficiency symptoms, maintenance of reproductive tissues in a healthy state, and reduction of risk of cardiovascular diseases and osteoporosis. The amount of estrogen sufficient to relieve symptoms usually accomplishes the other aforementioned objectives.

Because unopposed estrogen increases the risk of endometrial carcinoma, a progestin, which reduces that risk, is given simultaneously. The usual dose of conjugated equine estrogens is 0.625 mg daily with medroxyprogesterone acetate 10 mg daily for 12 to 14 days each month. Bleeding after the progesterone is common, but it gradually diminishes and eventually stops. Both conjugated estrogens, 0.625 mg, and medroxyprogesterone acetate, 2.5 mg, can be given daily on a continuous basis. This regimen may be accompanied by irregular spotting, which gradually diminishes and stops in 4 to 6 months. Bleeding is less of a problem when combined daily treatment is first given after menopause than when it is started during the perimenopausal phase.

Most women need education and counseling about the problems that accompany aging. Such help is provided best by a gynecologist who is interested in making the woman's life more comfortable and enjoyable as well as in detecting and curing diseases.

THE BREAST

37
CHAPTER

DISEASES OF THE BREAST

The American Cancer Society predicts that there will be about 175,000 new cases of mammary carcinoma in the United States in 1991 and that they will result in 44,500 deaths. One of nine newborn girls is destined to have mammary carcinoma and one of 14 will die of it. Breast cancer accounts for 27% of all cancer in women and 19% of deaths from cancer.

The obstetrician-gynecologist should understand thoroughly the diagnosis and the management of diseases of the breast. A careful and complete examination of the breasts should precede each pelvic examination (p. 30). It is especially important in the evaluation of the pregnant patient (p. 40).

Development and Anatomy

At birth, the breasts consist almost entirely of ducts. With the rise in the level of estrogen at puberty, growth of the breasts occurs along with pigmentation of the areolae and enlargement of the ductal system. After the onset of ovulation and increased production of progesterone, the alveolar components appear. The alveolae, which are small sacs that lead into lactiferous ducts, are quite small and inconspicuous in the nonpregnant, nonlactating breast. The ducts, which are much larger, are embedded in a matrix of fibrous tissue and fat. Ten to 100 alveolae form a single lobule in the lactating gland. The collection of many lobules forms one lobe, which is drained by a single lactiferous duct. Each breast comprises approximately 15 to 20 lactiferous ducts and therefore 15 to 20 lobes. Each duct terminates in a sinus as it reaches the nipple. The lobes are surrounded by fat containing blood vessels, nerves, and lymphatics.

The breast contains lymphatic channels that drain radially as well as deeply into the underlying lymphatics. The most important pathways are those to the axilla, in which the nodes are divided into three levels. Level 1 nodes are those lateral to the border of the pectoralis minor muscle. Level 2 nodes comprise those deep to the pectoralis minor muscle, and level 3, those medial to the muscle (Fig. 37–1). The nodes between the pectoralis minor and major muscles are known as interpectoral, or Rotter's, nodes. The internal mammary chain of nodes is particularly important for lesions that lie in the medial portion of the breast. These nodes drain the upper anterior surface of the diaphragm, the superior portion of the liver through the falciform ligament, and the upper portion of the rectus abdominis muscle as well as the medial quadrants of the mammary gland. Thus, retrograde spread of neoplastic cells from breast to liver may occur when anterograde drainage of lymph is blocked.

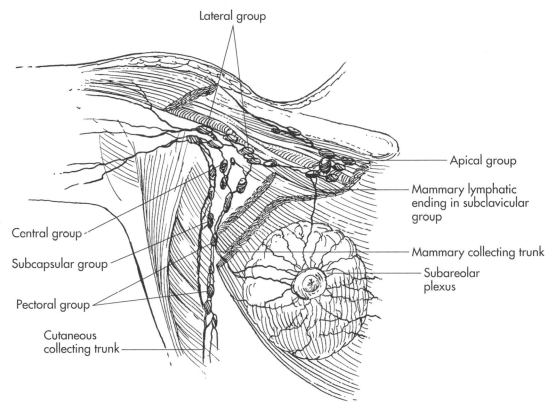

FIG. 37–1. Lymphatics of the mammary gland and the axillary nodes. (Poirier and Charpy.)

CHANGES IN PREGNANCY

During pregnancy, increasing amounts of estrogen, progesterone, and placental lactogen stimulate growth of functional mammary tissue (p. 91). Plasma prolactin increases from the nonpregnant level of 10 ng/mL to 200 ng/mL at term. The parallel increase in estradiol and prolactin suggests that estradiol may be related to the increase in prolactin. Although estrogen may initiate secretion of prolactin, high levels of the steroid apparently block its physiologic effect. Secretion of prolactin is controlled also by the prolactin inhibiting factor (p. 92). A decrease in the level of estrogen after delivery suppresses the prolactin inhibiting factor. Suckling markedly increases the level of prolactin and leads to lactation. Engorgement of the breast occurs approximately 3 days after delivery, when levels of estrogen and progesterone fall markedly. Suckling stimulates release of prolactin and oxytocin. Myoepithelial cells contract in response to oxytocin and empty the alveolar lumina. Levels of prolactin return to nonpregnant values about 4 weeks after delivery but increase to a value 10 to 20 times that of the nonpregnant state during suckling. By 4 months post partum the response of prolactin to suckling is lost; thereafter suckling remains the only stimulus required for lactation. Cessation of suckling terminates lactation and the release of oxytocin. Formation of milk is depressed by the effect of local pressure. Termination of suckling initiates release of prolactin-inhibiting factor (?dopamine) and a decrease in the level of prolactin.

The breasts secrete antibodies that are taken up and may be concentrated selectively from the serum. Certain antibodies probably are formed within the breast. In some species ingestion of colostral antibodies from mothers sensitized to fetal isoantigens may be deleterious to the newborn. Colostrum contains distinctive ingredients that are potentially autoantigenic for both the secretor and the recipient. Both colostrum and milk contain large numbers of living leukocytes, which may confer immunologic benefits upon the fetus. IgA, the predominant immunoglobulin in milk, probably serves an important protective function in the gastrointestinal tract of the infant. Breast milk contains IgA antibodies against *Escherichia coli*. This finding is consistent with the clinical evidence that breast-fed babies are less susceptible to enteric infection than are bottle-fed babies. The superiority of human milk over cow's milk in protecting the newborn against infection is related to the higher content of IgA antibodies against bacteria that are pathogenic in man.

DISORDERS OF THE BREAST

Indications of mammary disease include a dominant mass, marked increase in size or firmness of one breast, retraction (dimpling) of the skin, erythema or edema of the skin, spontaneous discharge from the nipple, changes in the epithelium of the nipple, and mammographic evidence of abnormalities (p. 30).

A careful history must include the date of consultation and the reason for the consultation. The duration of the signs and symptoms should be carefully recorded. The menstrual history must include the dates of menarche, last menstrual period, and menopause. The familial history must elicit information about mammary cancer in maternal relatives. The history in first-degree relatives is most important in ascertaining risk, particularly if the disease occurred in the mother or sisters premenopausally; thus, the date of onset of cancer of the breast in any family member is important. The history of intake of drugs, including the use of oral contraceptives, estrogen replacement therapy, tranquilizers, and antihypertensive medications is essential.

Mammary cancer is neither painful nor tender; nor does it undergo changes with the menstrual cycle. Benign lesions are more often painful and tender and likely to undergo cyclic changes. Bloody or serosanguineous discharge from the nipple suggests cancer, whereas clear or greenish fluid is more often associated with benign lesions. A history of trauma and the finding of a firm tender area suggest fat necrosis, which may be confused with carcinoma.

A satisfactory examination of the breast requires at least 5 minutes if the teaching of self-examination is included. The axilla is palpated with support of the patient's arm by the examiner's opposite hand. Axillary examination, even if well performed, is accurate in only 50% of patients. Approximately 40% of patients carefully examined and thought to have a disease-free axilla will be found to have nodes containing tumor at the time of axillary dissection. It is important, however, to detect clinically evident metastatic disease before recommending treatment because extensive axillary involvement will alter therapy.

A single dominant hard mass suggests cancer, whereas multiple indistinct nodules suggest fibrocystic disease. Bilateral venous engorgement, deviation of the nipples, and areolar excoriation are usually associated with benign lesions, whereas the corresponding unilateral alterations may be associated with cancer. Dimpling of the skin connotes cancer, although superficial thrombophlebitis (Mondor's disease) may produce a similar change in the lateral portion of the breast. Fixation of the lesion to the chest wall and gross enlargement of regional nodes are characteristic of cancer.

Physical examination is best recorded using a diagram that indicates the location, size, and mobility of the lesion as well as nodal involvement and cutaneous changes. Diagnostic recommendations such as biopsy and mammography should be recorded with an indication that the patient will be notified of the results. The final therapeutic plan must be recorded as well.

The patient should be taught the technique of self-examination of the breast before she leaves the examining room. The value of self-examination has recently been questioned as has the assumption that it is easily learned. Lesions often are still discovered accidentally during the interval between examinations. Nevertheless, women who perform monthly self-examination of the breast usually present with earlier stages of mammary cancer than do those who do not perform these examinations. Gynecologists should not only teach the technique of self-examination of the breast to all their patients but should ascertain that these women are performing the examination properly. A model of the breast with simulated lesions may be an educational aid to the patient.

Benign lesions include abnormalities of development, physiologic alterations, inflammations and infections, and nonmalignant neoplasms. Abnormalities of development include accessory mammary tissue and supernumerary nipples. Because the milk ridge that forms in the embryo extends from the axilla to the groin, accessory mammary tissue (including ducts, alveolae, and nipples) may develop anywhere along this line. Macromastia, micromastia, and amastia (absence of the mammary gland) have been reported.

Physiologic alterations such as inappropriate lactation, or galactorrhea, with or without amenorrhea, may result from decreases in gonadotropin releasing hormone (GnRH) and prolactin inhibiting factor, with an excess of prolactin. The patient should be questioned carefully about stimulation of the breast and ingestion of medications. Levels of gonadotropins and serum prolactin should be measured. The higher the prolactin level, the more likely is a pituitary tumor to be the cause (p. 332).

Discharge from the nipple may be related to tranquilizers (particularly the phenothiazines), oral contraceptives, and manual stimulation. The discharge may be unilateral or bilateral, and spontaneous or provoked. Clear or milky discharge is usually associated with physiologic alterations or manual stimulation. Serosanguineous or bloody discharge more often indicates a benign intraductal papilloma, although it may be associated with a malignant lesion; bilateral clear or milky discharge with or without amenorrhea may be associated with a pituitary lesion. The fluid from patients with unilateral serosanguineous or bloody discharge should be examined by means of a Papanicolaou smear. In cases of grossly bloody drainage, a mammogram is indicated. Usually the quadrant involved can be identified by careful palpation and probing under anesthesia. Excision of the involved duct is recommended for biopsy.

Mastodynia, or pain in the breast, particularly if it occurs premenstrually, is a common complaint among women of childbearing age, although it may occur in the perimenopausal years as well. In the absence of a palpable lesion, the condition is best treated with reassurance, analgesics, and the use of a properly fitted brassiere. Diuretics, hormones including androgens, and restriction of salt are seldom effective. Recently danazol, 100 to 400 mg/day, has been used for this complaint. It is very effective when used in patients with fibrocystic disease, but long-term effects of this expensive drug have not been evaluated. Undesirable side effects of hirsutism, deepening of the voice, and menstrual irregularity limit its use.

FIBROCYSTIC DISEASE

Almost all women have minor degrees of fibrocystic change. These lesions are usually bilateral and multiple. The mammary pain and tenderness associated with them increase premenstrually. Early changes may be found in girls and women in their teens and twenties and include tenderness in the axillary tail. In later stages, the breast becomes multinodular and on palpation has a characteristic "bean bag" feel. Occasionally a dominant mass may be present. In the late stages, cysts, which may rapidly increase in size, are circumscribed, generally tender, and mobile. The fluid aspirated is usually clear or yellow. In cysts of longer duration, the fluid may be dark brown or black. The prevalence of these cysts is greatest between the ages of 30 and 50 and may result from unopposed stimulation by estrogen. The risk of mammary carcinoma is increased in patients with dysplastic changes but not in those with solitary or multiple cysts without dysplasia.

INFECTIONS

Mondor's disease is a superficial thrombophlebitis of the breast. On physical examination, a vertical grove is present in the lateral portion of the breast and a tender cord is palpable. If there is any question about the possibility of carcinoma, appropriate diagnostic studies including mammography and biopsy should be performed. This self-limited disease requires only analgesics for treatment. The tenderness usually diminishes over a period of three to four weeks.

Ductal ectasia or plasma cell mastitis may be manifested by discharge from the nipple. The fluid, which is variably colored and sticky, arises from multiple ducts in both breasts. Palpable swellings are noted under the areolae. Chronic inflammation produces a fibrosis that causes thickening of the walls of the ducts and occasionally retraction of the nipple. At this stage, a hard retroareolar mass may be found. It may be necessary to excise the entire ductal system to achieve cure and exclude carcinoma.

Postpartum mastitis (p. 187) causes tenderness and induration. Occasionally there is a slight elevation in temperature. Management includes effective periodic emptying of milk from the breast and occasionally the use of antibiotics. The inflammation may progress to the formation of an abscess, which requires drainage and antibiotics. If prompt resolution of the process does not occur, biopsy to exclude carcinoma is mandatory.

FAT NECROSIS

Fat necrosis is a lesion that mimics carcinoma. Most patients are obese, give a history of trauma, and complain of pain. A mass and tenderness are frequently present. In about 25% of the cases, ecchymosis and erythema of the skin are seen; in almost all cases a mass can be palpated. Retraction and axillary adenopathy are occasionally associated. The treatment is local excision.

Sebaceous cysts are common in the skin over the breasts. They are superficial and circumscribed. These cysts, when infected, may be associated with induration, inflammation, and formation of an abscess, and thus may be confused with carcinoma. The treatment is local excision.

FIBROADENOMA

Fibroadenoma (Fig. 37–2) is a common benign neoplasm of the breast. It appears predominantly in young women and presents as a firm, painless, mobile mass. It may occasionally attain large size, especially in adolescents. These lesions tend to be multiple but are bilateral in only 10 to 20% of cases. The majority are discovered accidentally and, unlike fibrocystic disease, they do not change during the menstrual cycle. They may grow rapidly during adolescence, pregnancy, and other times of endocrine upheaval. If a neoplasm increases rapidly in size, phyllodes tumors must be considered.

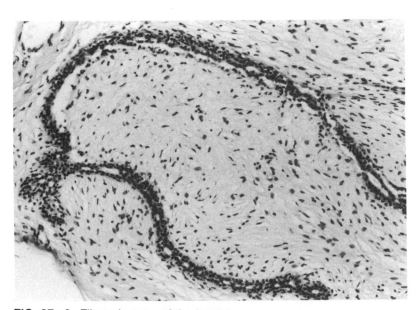

FIG. 37–2. Fibroadenoma of the breast.

INTRADUCTAL PAPILLOMA

The predominant sign of a solitary intraductal papilloma (Fig. 37–3) is discharge from the nipple. Patients with intraductal papillomas tend to be older than patients with other benign neoplasms. Most of the patients present with spontaneous, often bloody discharge from the nipple. The duct should be probed under anesthesia and the tissue surrounding the probe should be excised for biopsy to rule out carcinoma.

Physical examination may reveal a dominant mass that is either cystic or solid, and benign or malignant. If the lesion feels solid and the patient is under 25 years of age, observation for a period of 4 to 6 weeks or excisional biopsy, depending on the size of the mass, is recommended. If the mass is still present after the period of observation, excisional biopsy is mandatory. If the patient is over 25, mammography and excisional biopsy are recommended. If the mass is cystic, an attempt should be made first to aspirate the fluid with a 20-gauge needle prior to biopsy. If no residual mass is palpated immediately after aspiration, reexamination in one month and monthly self-examinations of the breast are recommended. If the mass persists after aspiration or if the fluid is bloody, the patient should have a mammogram and biopsy. If there is a residual mass on the first reexamination, mammography and biopsy are mandatory.

Outpatient biopsy is uncomplicated and cost-effective. Occult lesions noted only on mammogram are difficult to identify by biopsy under local anesthesia. In such cases, the operation is best performed in a standard operating room after localization by needle in the radiology department. A circumareolar incision is preferred, but incision should be placed so that mastectomy, if necessary, will include the incision made for biopsy.

Outpatient biopsy for definitive diagnosis is an acceptable procedure even with lesions that appear clinically malignant. Delay of definitive treatment for 1 or 2 weeks does not appear to influence survival adversely, but the operation must be performed with minimal manipulation of the mammary tissue, meticulous hemostasis, and asepsis. When the lesion is excised, a sample of at least 500 mg of tissue should be submitted fresh for hormone-binding studies.

CARCINOMA OF THE BREAST

Systematic controlled screening for mammary carcinoma began in 1963. It utilized mammography and clinical examination. This technique of screening was shown to be of unequivocal value only in women between the ages of 50 to 59. The value of the screening was less impressive in women in other age groups.

Despite increasing enthusiasm for screening programs, many scientists and clinicians have expressed concern about the risk of radiation from mammography. The current recommendation is that a baseline mammogram be done at the age of 40 and repeated at 2-year intervals until age 50, at which time mammograms should be done annually. The risks associated with screening include anxiety, unnecessary operations, false security, and carcinogenesis.

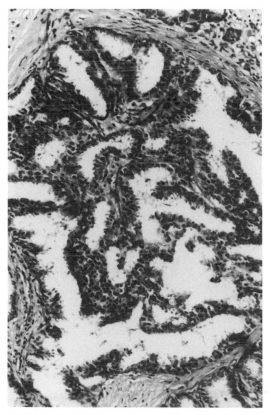

FIG. 37–3. Intraductal papilloma of the breast.

The theoretic risk of developing mammary cancer after irradiation is six cancers per 10 million person-years per rad after a 10-year latent period. It is now possible to perform acceptable mammography with an absorbed dose to the midplane of the breast that is considerably less than 0.5 rad.

In patients treated for cancer of one breast, mammography of the opposite side should be performed annually. In the presence of a lesion that looks or feels malignant on clinical examination, biopsy is indicated even though mammography suggests a normal breast or a benign tumor, for as many as 20% of palpable cancers may not be detected by mammography.

Thermography measures infrared radiation emitted by the skin. Although this technique is innocuous, its specificity is low and it is not recommended. Ultrasonography is helpful in distinguishing solid from cystic lesions.

Carcinoma of the breast (Fig. 37–4) is slightly more prevalent in white women and usually occurs after the age of 35. Most of these cancers begin after age 50 and only 1.5% occur under age 30. Major factors that

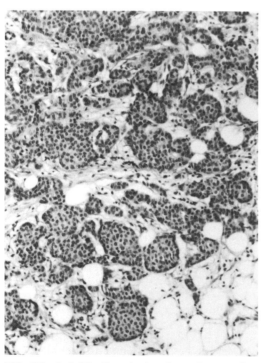

FIG. 37–4. Infiltrating duct cell carcinoma of the breast.

determine risk of mammary cancer are previous cancer of one breast, age, age of menarche, age at first term pregnancy, age at menopause, and weight.

The woman with prior cancer of one breast is at risk for cancer in the opposite breast. The risk is about 1% per year. Most women who manifest cancer of the breast in the late postmenopausal years do not live long enough to develop another cancer in the opposite breast.

Women with an earlier menarche are at greater risk for mammary carcinoma. Parity is associated with a decreased risk particularly if the mother is young at the time of her first delivery. Women whose natural menopause occurs before the age of 45 have only half the likelihood of subsequent carcinoma of the breast when compared with those whose menopause occurs after the age of 55. Artificial menopause similarly reduces the risk of mammary cancer. Women who have had their ovaries removed before age 35 have a 70% reduction in the occurrence of carcinoma of the breast.

The relation between weight and mammary cancer, particularly in the postmenopausal woman, is strong. For women under 50, there is little or no increased risk, but in those between the ages of 60 and 69, an increase in weight from 60 to 70 kilograms or more increases the risk by about 80%.

Genetic, viral, and endocrine factors have been implicated in the pathogenesis of carcinoma of the breast. Relatives of women who had mammary cancer, particularly if bilateral, in the premenopausal years, are at particular risk. The pattern of inheritance in most patients, however, is not clear and environmental factors have been implicated. Viruses have been suspected, but there is no proof that they are etiologic in mammary carcinoma. The most popular hypothesis relates to increased estrogens, either exogenous or endogenous, which usually arise from increase in peripheral conversion of androgens. Estrone is the most important estrogen after the menopause. Recent evidence suggests that although estrone binds to the receptor with less affinity than does estradiol, both induce specific estrogenic effects. The primary site of the peripheral conversion of androgens to estrone is fat. The major factor related to increase in susceptibility to carcinoma of the breast over which control can be exerted is therefore obesity.

Because many patients with cancer of the breast present with metastatic disease, previously held concepts of therapy must be reassessed in the light that this carcinoma may be a systemic disease. Evaluation of the patient with mammary cancer includes a complete physical examination and roentgenogram of the chest. Isotopic scanning of liver and bone and films for metastatic disease are obtained when indicated by signs and symptoms, and in the presence of lesions greater than five cm in diameter. Scans of bone and liver are not obtained routinely.

The TNM system provides for the preoperative and postoperative staging of the primary lesion. T refers to the primary tumor, N to the regional nodes, and M to distant metastases. T0 means no evidence of primary disease; TIS means carcinoma in situ; T1 refers to a tumor less than 2 cm in diameter; T2 refers to a tumor between 2 and 5 cm; T3 refers to a tumor greater than five cm in diameter; and T4 implies a tumor of any size with fixation to skin or chest wall or a tumor with edema, ulceration, or inflammation.

N0 refers to lack of palpable axillary lymph nodes; N1 refers to palpable and mobile lymph nodes with or without metastatic cancer; and N2 refers to palpable nodes that contain tumor and are fixed to each other or to other structures. N3 refers to palpable supraclavicular nodes that contain tumor. M0 and M1, respectively, refer to the absence or presence of distant metastases.

Clinical staging combines the various possibilities of the TNM classification into four stages. Table 37–1 shows the various combinations of TNM possibilities and staging.

For most patients a two-step plan of diagnosis and therapy is recommended. The biopsy is obtained as a first step and if cancer is found, estrogen- and progesterone-binding receptor studies are performed. After permanent sections are reviewed, the options for treatment are discussed with the patient. There is no evidence that a delay of 1 or 2 weeks between diagnosis and definitive therapy adversely affects prognosis.

Prior to 1970, radical mastectomy was the standard operation in the United States for the primary treatment of mammary cancer. It is still the standard against which the results of all other procedures must be judged. With radical mastectomy, the pectoral muscles are removed and a complete axillary dissection performed. In about 20% of cases significant morbidity or functional impairment follows this operation.

Total mastectomy with axillary dissection (modified radical mastectomy) has supplanted the radical operation as the operation of choice of most surgeons for curable carcinoma of the breast.

Total removal of the breast with axillary dissection is common to both radical and modified radical procedures, although complete axillary dissection is technically more difficult if the muscles of the chest wall are not removed. If both pectorales (major and minor) are preserved, complete dissection of level 3 nodes is difficult. If the pectoralis minor is removed, access to the axilla is facilitated. Preservation of the bulk of the pectoralis major decreases deformity of the chest wall and leads to greater strength and mobility of the arm. Furthermore, preservation of the musculature of the chest wall permits more effective reconstructive procedures. The modified radical mastectomy is as effective as the classical radical operation in the surgical treatment of curable mammary cancer.

Radiation combined with conservative surgery (lumpectomy) achieves better cosmetic results. Complete excision of the tumor is important for adequate local control and cosmetic appearance with radiation therapy. It must be emphasized that lumpectomy without radiation is inadequate therapy of mammary cancer. After complete removal of the macroscopic mass of tumor (lumpectomy), 5000 rads may be adequate to control microscopic disease. Additional therapy ("boost") to the area of excision can be provided with a variety of techniques. Primary radiotherapy should be

TABLE 37–1. STAGING ACCORDING TO THE TNM CLASSIFICATION

	Stage 1	Stage II		Stage III		Stage IV	
T	1	1	2	3	any	any	any
N	0	1	0,1	0,1	2	N₃	any
M	0	0	0	0	0	0,1	1

reserved for patients whose lesions are small in comparison with the size of the breast and who have T1 and T2 lesions. Sampling of axillary nodes by limited or formal axillary nodal dissection is important for prognosis and for identification of women who may benefit from adjuvant chemotherapy.

The 5-year survival for mammary cancer that is diagnosed in the early localized stages has risen from 78% in 1943 to over 85% at present. If the disease is confined to the breast in its noninvasive form, rates of cure approaching 100% can be achieved. If cancer is invasive but confined to the breast, the 5-year survival rate is 85%. When nodes are involved, the survival rate drops to 45%.

Age by itself is not a prognostic factor for women with carcinoma. Young women frequently present themselves with cancer at an advanced stage. The most important prognostic factors are the stage of cancer, which includes size of the tumor, the presence or absence of lymph node metastases, and the presence or absence of estrogen and progesterone receptors in the tumor. The combination of axillary lymph node metastases and the absence of hormone receptors portends a poor outcome. In general, the greater the number of axillary node metastases, the worse the prognosis. Delay in diagnosis may allow a carcinoma to grow and metastasize, but certain carcinomas grow more rapidly than others. The reasons for the differences in biologic behavior of various breast cancers remain obscure. More than 80% of patients who do not die of other causes are found to die of or with their mammary cancer if they are followed for 25 years or more.

Several varieties of breast cancer require specific mention. One variety of breast cancer in younger women is of particular importance. Inflammatory carcinoma is associated with a particularly dismal prognosis. Its appearance is most suggestive of infection and thus the possibility of carcinoma frequently is not considered until late. The diagnosis is made histologically by the identification of tumor cells in the subdermal lymphatics, and hence the axillary nodes invariably contain metastatic cancer.

Paget's disease of the nipple is characterized by a weeping eczematoid lesion of the nipple and is invariably associated with ductal carcinoma of the breast. A periareolar mass may or may not be present, and the diagnosis is made by biopsy of the nipple or underlying mass. Treatment is usually modified radical mastectomy because of the central location of the carcinoma. The prognosis is better for patients without a mass than for those with a mass.

Carcinoma of the breast occurs uncommonly in pregnant women and is said to be particularly aggressive. Diagnosis is frequently delayed because of failure to consider the possibility of carcinoma, and the lesion is not diagnosed until it has reached an advanced stage. Hence, the outlook is poor for such patients, but whether the tumor is particularly aggressive or simply the diagnosis is delayed is not clear.

With optimal combinations of surgical therapy and radiation, approximately 5% of patients with mammary cancer have a local recurrence. More than 70% of all patients with carcinoma of the breast, however, die of or with active mammary cancer in the 30-year period after initial diagnosis (before metastasis) and treatment of microscopic metastases.

Adjuvant chemotherapy is most effective in premenopausal patients with significant axillary involvement. No single agent, however, can be considered the standard drug of choice. Patients with T1 and T2 lesions with no histologic evidence of nodal involvement do not require adjuvant treatment.

Tumors positive for estrogen receptors respond to hormonal therapy with a prolonged interval between diagnosis of cancer and recurrence. If the estrogen receptor (ER) analysis is positive (greater than 10 femtomoles/mg protein), the likelihood of response is greater than 50%. If the ER is negative (less than 10 femtomoles/mg protein), the rate of response is less than 8%. A high content of receptor (greater than 100 femtomoles/mg protein) is associated with a rate of response greater than 80%. The estrogen receptor assay should be used in conjunction with other clinical factors that predict response to hormonal therapy. These factors include postmenopausal status, prior response to hormonal therapy, and metastatic or recurrent disease predominantly in skin or lymph nodes. The relation of the estrogen receptor assay to clinical response to cytotoxic chemotherapy remains controversial.

Treatment of recurrent or metastatic mammary cancer comprises hormonal manipulation that is based on analysis of endocrine receptors, the menopausal or postmenopausal status of the patient, and the location of the metastatic disease. Antiestrogens may be indicated in the patients with cancers containing estrogen receptors. If the analysis of estrogen receptors is negative or if there is rapidly advancing visceral disease, chemotherapy should be started. If there is no response to antiestrogens, chemotherapy should be instituted. For the postmenopausal patient with cancer-containing estrogen receptors, antiestrogens may be employed. If endocrine therapy fails, the patient should receive chemotherapy. Combined chemotherapy given either weekly or cyclically seems to achieve the highest rate of response, the greatest complete response, the longest duration of remission, and the greatest increase in survival. Single drugs appear to be less effective than a combination of drugs, which usually includes cyclophosphamide, methotrexate, and 5-fluorouracil. The National Institutes of Health recently recommended that treatment with tamoxifen be the standard for follow-up in women over age 50 whose mammary cancers involve lymph nodes and whose tumors are positive for hormone receptors.

For certain patients, a simultaneous or delayed reconstructive procedure after mastectomy is an important part of their rehabilitation. Several techniques are available and the quality of the results is variable. More complex procedures generally provide better results, but the risks are significantly greater. Although anatomic results are imperfect, the psychologic benefits are significant. As knowledge of mammary carcinoma is disseminated more widely in the lay press, women are more likely to perform self-examination of the breast and to consult their physicians earlier.

The diagnosis and treatment of mammary cancer often require the talents of the surgeon, gynecologist, diagnostic radiologist, medical oncologist, radiotherapist, and plastic surgeon, in addition to the psychologic support than can be provided by professionals in the fields of psychiatry, nursing, and social work.

GYNECOLOGIC PROCEDURES

38
CHAPTER

COMMONLY PERFORMED PROCEDURES

THE PAPANICOLAOU SMEAR

Because cytologic examination of the cervix should routinely accompany physical examination of the adult woman, the method of obtaining the smear was described under physical examination.

Of the several methods of reporting the results of the examination of the cells exfoliated from the female genital tract, none has received unqualified acceptance by pathologists and gynecologists. The simplest but insufficiently specific scheme uses the terms negative, suspicious, and positive for malignant cells (Figs. 38–1 and 38–2). The nomenclature that groups the smears into five classes is not used widely in the United States at present. In that system, Class I is negative; Class II is atypical but benign; Class III is atypical and suspicious; Class IV and V are positive, with Class V unequivocally malignant. The cytologic terms ideally should be consistent with the findings on confirmatory biopsy. The Papanicolaou smear is a screening test only, albeit an important one, upon which therapy is never based without histopathologic confirmation.

The term cervical intraepithelial neoplasia is used to encompass dysplasia and carcinoma in situ (intraepithelial carcinoma). Cervical intraepithelial neoplasia (CIN)I corresponds roughly to mild dysplasia; CIN II corresponds to moderate dysplasia; and CIN III to severe dysplasia and carcinoma in situ. The Bethesda System, based on a conference in 1988, uses the term squamous intraepithelial lesion (SIL) to replace the terms dysplasia and CIN. Low-grade SIL includes the changes of human papillomavirus (HPV) along with CIN I. High-grade SIL includes lesions that were designated formerly CIN II, CIN III, and CIS (carcinoma in situ). Because some gynecologists object to grouping HPV lesions with CIN I and because of other objections to the current terminology, a second Bethesda conference was convened in 1991 to attempt a closer approach to a consensus.

A single Papanicolaou test has a rate of false negativity of about 30%. The false negatives are divided into those caused by faulty sampling and others caused by faulty interpretation. As annual smears are repeated, the likelihood of false negatives and therefore undiagnosed carcinoma becomes increasingly small. The Bethesda System of reporting requires a statement about the adequacy of the specimen, a general categorization of the diagnosis (within normal limits or other), and a descriptive diagnosis.

The descriptive diagnoses include reference to the major microorganisms that cause infection of the female genital tract: fungi such as *Candida species*, bacteria such as *Gardnerella species*, *Actinomyces species*, and

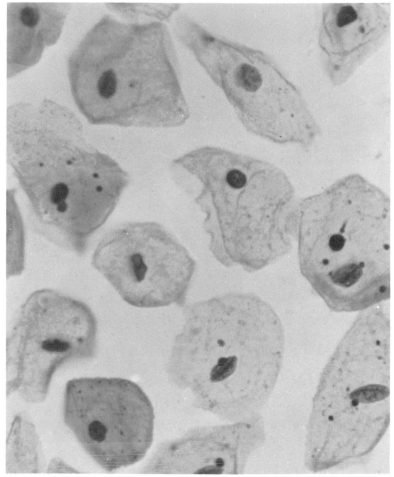

FIG. 38–1. Negative Papanicolaou smear, showing superficial squamous cells with normal nuclei and abundant cytoplasm.

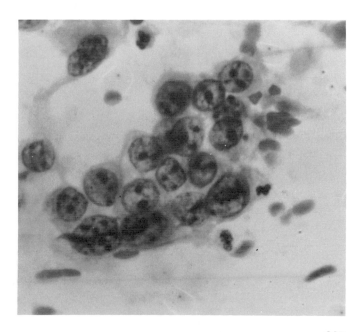

FIG. 38–2. Positive Papanicolaou smear, showing malignant cells with nuclei containing clumps of chromatin and increased nucleocytoplasmic ratio.

cellular changes suggestive of *Chlamydia species*, protozoa such as *Trichomonas vaginalis;* and cellular changes associated with viruses such as *Cytomegalovirus* and *Herpes simplex.* Reference to human papillomavirus is made in the section on abnormalities of squamous epithelial cells.

Reactive and reparative changes include those associated with inflammation and miscellaneous changes such as those related to ionizing radiation, chemotherapy, the effects of drugs such as diethylstilbestrol, and miscellaneous nonneoplastic alterations.

Epithelial cellular abnormalities include the category of atypical squamous cells of undetermined significance. In this category, a specific recommendation for further study and follow-up is made. The category of squamous intraepithelial lesion is divided into low-grade and high-grade. When this diagnosis is made, a comment about cellular changes consistent with human papillomavirus (HIV) is made if applicable. Low-grade squamous intraepithelial lesions (SIL) include cellular changes associated with HPV and mild (slight) dysplasia/cervical intraepithelial neoplasia grade I (CIN I). High-grade SIL includes moderate dysplasia/ CIN II, severe dysplasia/ CIN III, and carcinoma in situ/ CIN III. The report includes mention of frank squamous carcinoma cells and of any glandular cells, including their site of origin and their atypical features.

The report in the Bethesda System should mention whether endocervical cells are present to indicate the adequacy of the smear in a premenopausal woman with a cervix. In this system the term atypia refers specifically to those cytologic findings that are of undetermined significance. The term should not be used as a diagnosis for otherwise defined inflammatory preneoplastic or neoplastic cellular changes. A description of the cytologic changes in the older terminology of dysplasia and CIN may be appended to the Bethesda classification. A separate statement about cellular changes associated with HPV may be included but the Bethesda System does not use the terms koilocytic atypia or dyskaryosis.

Further discussion of cytology and colposcopy is included in Chapter 43, on carcinoma of the cervix and its precursors.

SCHILLER TEST

In this test, the squamous epithelia of cervix and vagina are painted with a solution of iodine and potassium iodide (Lugol's solution). Abnormal epithelia of various kinds including cancer do not take the mahogany stain because they contain little or no glycogen. This test is not diagnostic of a malignant lesion, but may help to direct the biopsy to a particular site. The Schiller test has been supplanted largely by colposcopically directed biopsy of suspicious lesions of the cervix. It may be used to detect non-staining areas of the vagina when colposcopic examination of the cervix fails to identify the source of abnormal cells seen in the Papanicolaou smear.

TOLUIDINE BLUE STAINING

The toluidine blue test helps to identify abnormal areas of squamous epithelium. After the suspicious areas are painted with 1% toluidine blue, they are allowed to dry and are sponged with a 1% solution of acetic acid. The normal epithelium is decolorized. The abnormal areas, which retain the deep blue stain, may then by subjected to biopsy. The test is used primarily for vulvar lesions.

PUNCH AND FOUR-QUADRANT BIOPSIES

This office procedure involves the removal of single or multiple pieces of tissue for histologic examination. In gynecology it is performed mainly for lesions of the cervix, vagina, and vulva. Cervical punch biopsy does not require anesthesia but those performed on the vagina and vulva do.

Four-quadrant cervical punch biopsy has been supplanted largely by colposcopically directed biopsy. It involves biopsy of the cervix at the 3, 6, 9, and 12 o'clock positions around the external os. The squamocolumnar junction should be included in as many specimens as possible. Biopsy at the 6 o'clock position is often performed first to avoid contamination of the operative field by bleeding from above.

COLPOSCOPY AND CERVICOGRAPHY

The first step in evaluation of the patient with an abnormal Papanicolaou smear is usually colposcopy. This is a diagnostic technique used to detect intraepithelial or invasive lesions of the cervix and lower genital tract. The examination is carried out with use of a microscope at magnifications of 6 to 40 times (Fig. 38–3). The essence of the procedure is to detect abnormal white epithelium and atypical vasculature and to direct biopsy to the most severely abnormal area. Colposcopy should be accompanied by endocervical curettage to detect lesions in the canal that may be the source of the abnormal cells found on the Papanicolaou smear. Satisfactory (complete or inclusive) colposcopy requires visualization of the entire squamocolumnar junction (transformation zone). The accuracy of a directed biopsy should be about 90%. If the sites of biopsy continue to bleed, hemostasis is usually achieved easily, except perhaps in pregnancy, by application of Monsel's solution (ferric subsulfate) or silver nitrate.

The rationale for colposcopy is given in the following paragraphs. The normal cervical epithelium is columnar in the canal and squamous on the portio (ectocervix). Under the influence of estrogen, the columnar epithelium is everted onto the portio (ectropion, or eversion). As a result, the position of the squamocolumnar junction is shifted. Columnar epithelium of the cervix is relatively fragile. When it is exposed to the lower pH of the vagina, stromal reserve cells are induced to multiply and hypertrophy, resulting in squamous metaplasia. This process occurs prominently during three phases of a woman's life: the neonatal period, menarche, and first pregnancy. The area in which new squamous epithelium forms is called the transformation zone. If a mutagenic virus such as the human papillomavirus (HPV) is present during transformation, the viral DNA may be incorporated into host DNA, resulting in malignant change, with chromosomal aneuploidy, cervical intraepithelial neoplasia, or invasive cancer.

When the cervix is bathed with saline and visualized through a colposcope, a neoplastic organ may appear redder because its

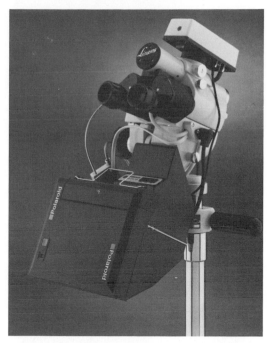

FIG. 38–3. The Leisegang colposcope with photographic attachment.

stroma contains more blood vessels than does normal cervix, presumably as an effect of tumor angiogenesis factor. Acetic acid is then applied to the cervix (or to the vagina or vulva, when appropriate). Ordinary household vinegar (about 5% acetic acid) is quite suitable for this purpose. The acid creates a hyperosmolar environment, which extracts water from the cytoplasm. The effect on normal epithelium is small, because its component cells have abundant cytoplasm and small nuclei. Neoplastic epithelium, however, contains cells with large nuclei and relatively scant cytoplasm. When acetic acid is applied to cells with an abnormal nuclear/cytoplasmic ratio, withdrawal of cytoplasmic water accentuates the ratio. Light energy from the colposcope is absorbed by these dense nuclei and less energy is reflected back to the colposcopist's eye, with the result that the tissue appears white. High-grade intraepithelial lesions contain more abnormal nuclei than do low-grade lesions and therefore appear whiter on colposcopy. Lesions that are white only after application of acetic acid are called "acetowhite lesions" (Fig. 38–4). Those that are

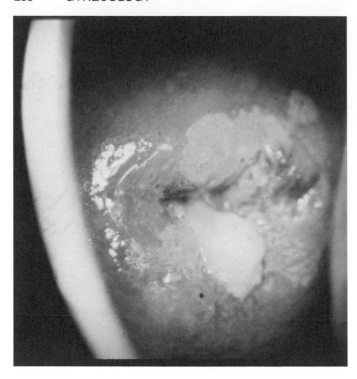

FIG. 38−4. Colpophotograph showing acetowhite epithelium.

white prior to application of the acid are included in the general category of "leuko-plakia."

As the number of neoplastic cells increases, tumor angiogenesis factor induces neovascularization of the lesion and vessels may be seen penetrating the acetowhite areas. Individual vessels appear as small red spots to form the pattern known as puncta-tion (Fig. 38−5). These punctate vessels may form collateral vessels, which create an appearance referred to as a mosaic (Fig. 38−6).

In carcinoma in situ or microinvasive carcinoma, tumor angiogenesis factor in-duces punctate vessels to bend at the surface of the abnormal epithelium and course along the cervix. When seen through the colposcope, these vessels resemble commas or spaghetti and are termed atypical vessels (Fig. 38−7). As the neoplastic process be-comes more severe, these atypical vessels enlarge and the superficial epithelium may become fragile and ulcerate (Figs. 38−8 and 38−9). Damage to these enlarged vessels and the fragile epithelium may lead to postcoital bleeding, which is characteristic of carcinoma of the cervix (Chapter 43).

Patients with high-grade and low-grade squamous lesions detected by Papanicolaou smear should have colposcopy with biopsy of suspicious areas. Some clinicians perform colposcopy on all women who have even inflammatory or reactive cytologic findings to avoid missing intraepithelial lesions. Be-cause the likelihood of high-grade cervical intraepithelial neoplasia is very low in pa-tients with only inflammatory or reparative changes and low even in those with smears that suggest low-grade squamous intraepi-thelial lesions, the necessity for routine colposcopy in those groups has been ques-tioned.

Cervicography, introduced in 1981, is a relatively new diagnostic technique. It uses a camera with telephoto lens and ring flash to photograph the cervix after application of 3% or 5% acetic acid (Fig. 38−10). The photograph is sent for review by an expert colposcopist, in the way that a cytologic smear is sent for examination by an expert pathologist. As a screening test for cervical intraepithelial neoplasia, cervicography is five times more sensitive than cytology alone (Fig. 38−11). As a diagnostic method in patients with atypical cytologic findings,

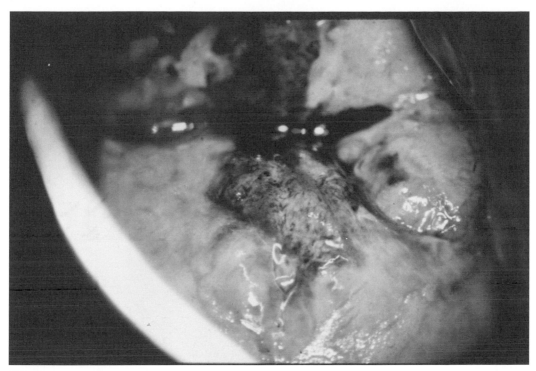

FIG. 38−5. Colpophotograph showing punctation.

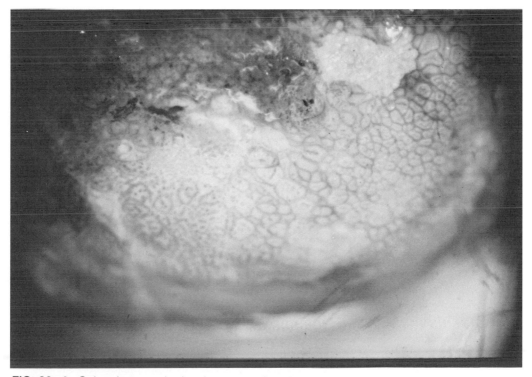

FIG. 38−6. Colpophotograph showing a mosaic pattern.

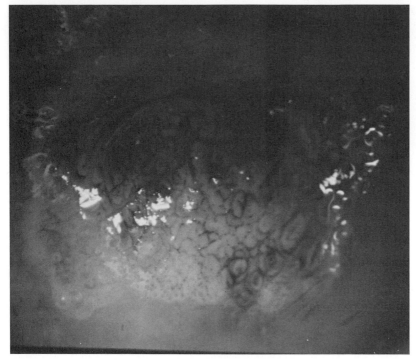

FIG. 38–7. Colpophotograph showing atypical vessels.

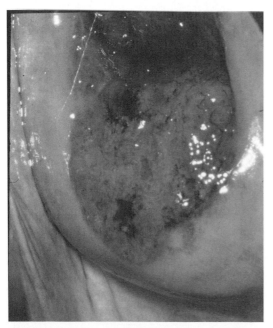

FIG. 38–8. Colpophotograph, showing microinvasive carcinoma with atypical vessels and erosion.

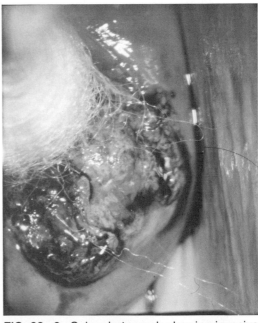

FIG. 38–9. Colpophotograph showing invasive carcinoma.

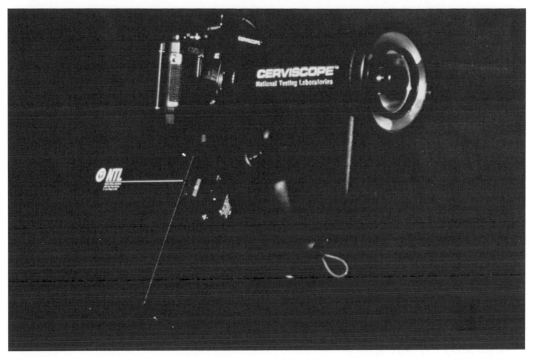

FIG. 38–10. Cerviscope, manufactured by National Testing Laboratories, St. Louis, Missouri.

cervicography is much more sensitive than cytology. Cervicography is a promising new method, which, when combined with cytology, may be used for triage of patients with inflammatory and reparative cytologic smears and perhaps low-grade squamous intraepithelial lesions.

CAUTERIZATION, CRYOSURGERY, AND ELECTROSURGERY

Cauterization is the induction of cellular necrosis by means of chemical or physical agents. In gynecology, it is usually performed upon the cervix. The traditional hot cautery is not employed commonly today. Cryosurgery is the technique of freezing by means of special probes cooled with either liquid nitrogen, Freon gas, or carbon dioxide. Temperatures as low as $-87°$ C are used to destroy tissue. It is used most often in gynecology for destruction of condylomata acuminata or low-grade dysplasias of the cervix. The vaginal discharge that usually follows the procedure is a disadvantage. The comparative merits of and indications for cryosurgery and laser therapy are discussed

in the following section and in Chapters 42 and 43. The loop electrosurgical excision procedure (LEEP) uses a thin wire loop electrode attached to an insulated handle and pencil-type wand, with which cervical intraepithelial neoplasia can be removed. Criteria for use of the loop are identical with those for cryotherapy or laser ablation: the endocervical margin must be visualized in its entirety, there must be no colposcopic suspicion of invasion, and the Papanicolaou smear must be consistent with the colposcopic findings.

THE LASER

The first laser, introduced into medical practice in the 1960s, was the helium: neon instrument, followed, in turn, by the carbon dioxide, the neodymium:yttrium-aluminum-garnet (Nd:YAG), the argon, and most recently, the potassium-titanyl-phosphate (KTP) lasers. CO_2 and Nd:YAG operate in the infrared portion of the spectrum (10,600 and 1064 nm, respectively), whereas the KTP and Argon lasers operate in the blue-green portion of the visible spectrum (532,

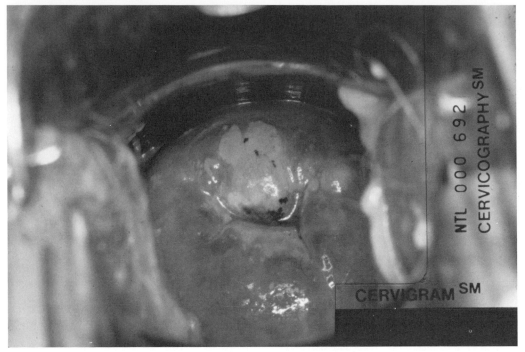

FIG. 38–11. Cervicogram, showing major-grade lesion detected after negative Papanicolaou smear. Courtesy National Testing Laboratories, St. Louis, Missouri.

and 488 and 515 nm, respectively), as shown in Table 38–1.

CO_2 laser vaporization is highly effective treatment for vulvar intraepithelial neoplasia (VIN), with or without condylomata acuminata (Chapter 40). In regions of the vulva that do not bear hair, the laser may need to penetrate only 1 mm. For hairy areas, a depth of penetration of 3 mm is required to eradicate the abnormal tissue. Excellent cosmetic results are obtained by using the laser on the nonhairy portion of the vulva combined with the scalpel, perhaps with aid of a binocular microscope, to remove the lesions in the hairy portions.

TABLE 38–1. PROPERTIES OF GYNECOLOGIC LASERS

Medium	Phase	Wavelength(s) (nm)	Color
CO_2	Gas	10,600	Infrared
He-Ne	Gas	632	Red
Nd:YAG	Solid	1320	Infrared
		1064	Infrared
Argon	Gas	515	Green
		488	Blue
KTP	Gas	532	Green

Acute-phase healing is nearly always complete by the fourteenth day after the procedure and reepithelialization occurs in 3 to 6 weeks. Because vulvar intraepithelial neoplasia has a high rate of recurrence, the laser is highly suitable therapy for this lesion because of the good cosmetic results obtained even after repeated use.

Vaginal intraepithelial neoplasia (VAIN) similarly is amenable to therapy with CO_2 laser vaporization for focal lesions. The depth of penetration should not exceed 1.5 mm. The use of 5-fluorouracil cream (5%) after laser therapy improves the rate of cure. The same combined therapy is effective for treatment of vaginal condylomata acuminata. Reepithelialization and complete healing of the vagina usually require 4 to 6 weeks. Approximately half of all patients with vulvovaginal condylomata have cervical human papillomavirus lesions. These cervical lesions often are vaporized readily with the CO_2 laser to a depth of 6 to 8 mm.

Low-grade cervical intraepithelial lesions of the cervix may be treated with the CO_2 laser with a success rate of over 90%. Cryotherapy with liquid nitrogen at a temperature of $-85°$ C is also effective, but the laser has the advantages of greater control of depth of tissue destruction and the disadvantage of requiring more complicated and expensive equipment. As the degree of dysplasia increases, so does the depth of involvement of the cervical glands. Thus, the laser seems to be superior to cryosurgical ablation for moderate and severe dysplasias of the cervix (Chapter 43). Cervical healing after cryotherapy often leads to inversion of the transition zone and difficulty with subsequent colposcopy, another drawback of cryosurgery as compared with laser therapy. CO_2 laser vaporization is carried to a depth of 6 to 8 mm on the ectocervix and of 12 to 15 mm in endocervical glandular tissue. A new squamocolumnar junction forms after vaporization in the vast majority of patients. With appropriate increase in power (watt/cm^2), the CO_2 laser can be used to perform a conization rather than a vaporization of the cervix. The other lasers mentioned in this section also have been used for conization. Low-grade lesions have a rate of cure of greater than 94% with either cryotherapy or laser surgery. The higher grade lesions have a rate of cure of greater than 90% with the laser but only about 80% for cryotherapy.

Lasers are also used widely in intraabdominal procedures, often with video monitoring (videolaseroscopy), to vaporize endometriotic implants and, in skilled hands, to vaporize ectopic gestations and myomata. Photodynamic therapy involves injection of a substance such as hematoporphyrin derivative (HPD) and subsequent use of the laser, the energy from which will be absorbed by the tissue that takes up the dye.

Such treatment has promise in the management of cancers of the skin, bladder, and other organs.

A comparison of the characteristics of the commonly used lasers is given in Table 38–2.

COLD KNIFE CONE BIOPSY

This is an excision of a cone of cervical tissue for histologic diagnosis. It is required to rule out invasive carcinoma when the Papanicolaou smear is positive and colposcopy has not been performed or has been unsatisfactory. The number of cone biopsies performed has been greatly reduced by the successful use of colposcopy. This procedure is done in the hospital or ambulatory surgical facility. The base of the cone surrounds the external os and the apex is at or near the internal os. The cone thus includes essentially all of the endocervical canal. Clinical situations in which cone biopsy is still required are described in Chapters 42 and 43. The cold-knife conization may be considered the diagnostic standard against which all other procedures must be measured.

DILATION AND CURETTAGE

A therapeutic curettage, as performed for incomplete abortion, serves as both diagnosis and treatment of the condition. A diagnostic curettage is performed to identify a lesion in the endocervix or endometrium. It is best performed fractionally; that is, endocervix and endometrium are curetted in

TABLE 38–2. CHARACTERISTICS OF GYNECOLOGIC LASERS

	CO_2	Argon/KTP	Nd:YAG
Aiming beam	He-Ne	Argon/KTP	He-NE
Delivery system	Articulated rigid mirrors	Fiber	Fiber
Absorption	Water, glass, plastic	Heme, melanin	Proteins
Penetration	0.1 mm	2.0 mm	4–6 mm
Maximum power	100 W	20 W	100 W
Precision cut	+++	+	+
Coagulation	+	++	+++

sequence and the specimens placed in separate containers for orientation and identification of the site of the lesion. For ordinary diagnostic curettage the cervical canal is scraped with a small curette before it is dilated. The size and configuration of the uterine cavity are first ascertained by sounding before the curettage. The endometrium is systematically curetted and polyp forceps are inserted to ensure that large lesions such as polyps have not been missed by the sharp curette.

Complications of dilation and curettage include cervical laceration and uterine perforation. Curettage should therefore be done in a day surgery center or hospital, where accidents may be treated promptly. The procedure is indicated for diagnosis of irregular uterine bleeding except in very young girls. Contraindications include intrauterine pregnancy and acute pelvic inflammatory disease. Suction curettage is the removal of the uterine contents by means of a hollow curette attached to a vacuum pump. Suction curettage usually requires little cervical dilatation. Because it can be performed safely in an outpatient facility, emergency room, or doctor's office, it is gradually replacing sharp curettage as a diagnostic and therapeutic procedure.

ENDOMETRIAL BIOPSY

This procedure involves removal of a small fragment of endometrium by means of a small sharp curette or a suction curette. It is usually performed as part of the investigation of infertility to ascertain ovulation or adequacy of the luteal phase of the endometrial cycle. This procedure and aspiration of endometrial cells by suction are not definitive means of diagnosis of endometrial cancer unless they yield positive findings.

CULDOSCOPY

This is endoscopic visual examination of the female pelvic viscera through the posterior vaginal fornix. It is used most often in the investigation of infertility and endocrine problems. It is performed best in a hospital or day surgery center but does not necessarily require general or regional anesthesia. This technique has been supplanted for most purposes by laparoscopy. Contraindications to culdoscopy are fixed cul-de-sac and adherent uterine retroversion.

LAPAROSCOPY

This an endoscopic procedure performed by introduction of a telescope through a stab incision in the abdominal wall after creation of a pneumoperitoneum. The laparoscope is used for a variety of diagnostic procedures such as the detection of tubal patency, the visualization of adnexa in cases of infertility and endocrine syndromes, and the elucidation of obscure pelvic pain. In addition, it serves many therapeutic purposes such as tubal sterilization. Laparoscopy may be performed using open or closed techniques. Current improvements in the instrument have extended the range of its possible diagnostic and therapeutic uses and increased its safety. Numerous procedures involving the laser, such as lysis of adhesions and ablation of endometriotic implants, may be performed through the laparoscope. Cholecystectomy is often performed laparoscopically and even laparoscopically assisted vaginal hysterectomy is gaining popularity.

CULDOCENTESIS

This procedure is the aspiration of fluid from the rectouterine pouch by puncture of the posterior vaginal fornix. It may be used to identify peritoneal fluid, blood, or pus. It is performed in certain cases of suspected intraabdominal hemorrhage and abscess in the cul-de-sac.

COLPOTOMY

This is an incision of the posterior vaginal fornix into the rectouterine pouch to visualize pelvic structures, perform surgical procedures on the adnexa, and drain pelvic abscesses.

THE RUBIN TEST

This is an office procedure for the investigation of tubal patency. Carbon dioxide is introduced into the cervix and the pressure is monitored with a manometer. If the tubes are patent, a rush is heard by means of a stethoscope over the abdomen when a pressure of between 60 to 90 mm Hg is reached. At that time, the pressure in the manometer drops. Shoulder pain indicates gas under the diaphragm, which provides another criterion of tubal patency. The procedure has been supplanted largely by hysterosalpingography and laparoscopy.

HYSTEROSALPINGOGRAPHY

This is a radiologic procedure for investigation of tubal patency and visualization of congenital anomalies and deformities of the uterine cavity and tube. Both water-soluble and oily contrast media have been employed successfully. The definitive sign of tubal patency is spill of contrast medium into the peritoneal cavity, not merely the presence of contrast medium in the fallopian tube. The radiologically visualized defects may be caused by space-occupying lesions such as polyps and myomas or extrinsic pressure. This examination is now generally performed under fluoroscopy with image intensification and may be combined with laparoscopy for maximal diagnostic information.

HYSTEROSCOPY

Hysteroscopy is an endoscopic technique for visualization of the endometrial cavity. It can be used for diagnosis and, in some countries, sterilization by electrocoagulation of the uterine ostia of the oviducts or placement of plugs in the ostia. It may also be used to remove small myomas and polyps, divide septa, retrieve intrauterine contraceptive devices, and obtain biopsies. Hysteroscopy is replacing "blind" curettage for many diagnostic purposes.

HYSTERECTOMY

Total hysterectomy is removal of the entire corpus and cervix uteri. It may be performed through the abdominal route (abdominal hysterectomy) or through the vagina (vaginal hysterectomy).

Supravaginal hysterectomy, performed through a laparotomy incision, leaves the vaginal portion of the cervix. It is almost synonymous with supracervical hysterectomy, which leaves the entire cervix, or with partial, incomplete, or subtotal hysterectomy. None of these procedures implies removal of the tubes and ovaries, as in complete hysterectomy with bilateral salpingo-oophorectomy. Subtotal hysterectomy is performed today only in emergencies or special circumstances in which continuation of the operation would pose a serious hazard to the patient. The total hysterectomy is preferred because it eliminates the risk of subsequent cervical carcinoma and distressing leukorrhea.

Abdominal hysterectomy is generally preferred for large myomas, ovarian tumors, endometriosis, pelvic inflammatory disease, endometrial cancer, and some cases of carcinoma in situ of the cervix. It is the procedure of choice when exploration of the upper abdomen is required.

Vaginal hysterectomy is indicated for various degrees of uterine prolapse and other forms of pelvic relaxation (often in conjunction with anterior colporrhaphy or operations for the vaginal correction of stress incontinence), small mobile uteri that are bleeding, and certain small myomas. Several conditions may by treated satisfactorily by either vaginal or abdominal hysterectomy.

A major complication of hysterectomy is hemorrhage, immediate or delayed. Formation of a hematoma is manifested by a fall in hematocrit, a rise in temperature, and a palpable mass in the cul-de-sac or parametria. Urologic complications of hysterectomy include pyelonephritis, ligation or transection of the ureter, urinary tract fistulas, and urinary retention. Bowel complications include paralytic ileus, mechanical obstruction, and rectovaginal fistula. Other serious complications are atelectasis and pneumonia, local infection, evisceration, and pulmonary embolism.

Procedures such as endometrial ablation, hormonal management of dysfunctional uterine bleeding and myomas, and restrictions imposed by third-party payers have halted the steady increase in the rate of hysterectomy in the United States. The operation remains, however, indispensable in the management of numerous gynecologic problems.

OTHER MAJOR GYNECOLOGIC OPERATIONS

Radical hysterectomy includes removal of the uterus, upper vagina, and parametria, with mobilization of the ureters. The radical hysterectomy, when performed for invasive carcinoma of the cervix (virtually its sole indication), is usually combined with pelvic lymphadenectomy, which removes en bloc bilaterally the internal iliac, common iliac, obturator, and periaortic lymph nodes.

Exenteration is the complete surgical removal of the pelvic viscera including rectum, bladder, or both, together with all the structures removed during radical hysterectomy and pelvic lymphadenectomy. Its primary indication is persistent or recurrent cervical carcinoma. Anterior exenteration is complete surgical removal of the pelvic viscera anterior to the rectum, including pelvic lymphadenectomy, with urinary diversion. Posterior exenteration is complete removal of the pelvic viscera posterior to the bladder and urethra, including pelvic lymphadenectomy and colostomy. Total pelvic exenteration is complete removal of the pelvic viscera with ureterointestinal anastomosis and colostomy.

Simple vulvectomy, performed for benign disease, is the superficial removal of vulvar structures including skin, mucosa, and superficial fat and connective tissue.

Radical vulvectomy, performed for cancer involving the vulva, is the wide removal of all structures of the vulva together with adjacent skin, a portion of the mons, and subcutaneous fat down to the deep fascia and muscles. It is accompanied by some form of regional lymph node dissection through single or separate incisions.

Anterior colporrhaphy is the repair of a cystocele, or relaxation of the anterior wall of the vagina.

Posterior colporrhaphy is the repair of a rectocele, or relaxation of the posterior wall of the vagina.

Kelly plication is usually accompanied by anterior colporrhaphy. It is a plication of the connective tissue around the bladder neck and urethra for the relief of urinary stress incontinence.

Retropubic suspension of the bladder neck for stress incontinence of urine is performed through the space of Retzius. In one standard operation, sutures attach the periurethral tissue to the posterior surface of the pubic symphysis. Many variations of the procedure based on the same anatomic principles are currently employed, including attachment of the periurethral tissues to Cooper's ligament.

IV

GYNECOLOGIC ONCOLOGY AND RELATED TOPICS

39
CHAPTER

GESTATIONAL TROPHOBLASTIC DISEASE

The subject of trophoblastic growths or diseases has undergone a recent change in terminology. The new terms will be used in this chapter, unless otherwise indicated. The spectrum of trophoblastic disease includes hydatidiform mole (partial and complete), invasive mole (formerly called chorioadenoma destruens), and choriocarcinoma. The so-called placental site trophoblastic tumor falls outside this group and will be discussed separately at the end of this chapter. The systems for clinical staging are shown in Tables 39–1 and 39–2. The FIGO system is not used frequently.

HYDATIDIFORM MOLE

Hydatidiform mole, a developmental anomaly that has characteristic widely distributed hyperplastic and dysplastic trophoblast covering most of the hydropic villi, consists grossly of grapelike vesicles without an embryo. Many moles arise as blighted ova. The edematous molar villi are avascular (Fig. 39–1).

The mole often presents with bleeding in the first half of pregnancy, occasionally with pain, particularly if the uterine growth is rapid. In about half the cases, the uterus is larger than the dates suggest. Abortion of the mole usually occurs at about 5 months'

TABLE 39–1. FIGO STAGING OF GESTATIONAL TROPHOBLASTIC TUMORS

Stage I	Tumor strictly contained in the uterine corpus
Stage II	Tumor extends to the adnexa, outside the uterus, but is limited to the genital structures
Stage III	Tumor extends to the lungs with or without genital tract involvement
Stage IV	Tumor metastatic to any other site(s)

TABLE 39–2. CLINICAL CLASSIFICATION OF GESTATIONAL TROPHOBLASTIC TUMORS

A. Low Risk
 1. HCG <100,000 IU/24-hour urine or <40,000 mIU/mL serum
 2. Symptoms present for less than 4 months
 3. No brain or liver metastases
 4. No prior chemotherapy
 5. Pregnancy event is not term delivery (i.e., mole, ectopic, or spontaneous abortion)
B. High Risk
 1. HCG >100,000 IU/24-hour urine or >40,000 mIU/mL serum
 2. Symptoms present for more than 4 months
 3. Brain or liver metastases
 4. Prior chemotherapeutic failure
 5. Antecedent term pregnancy

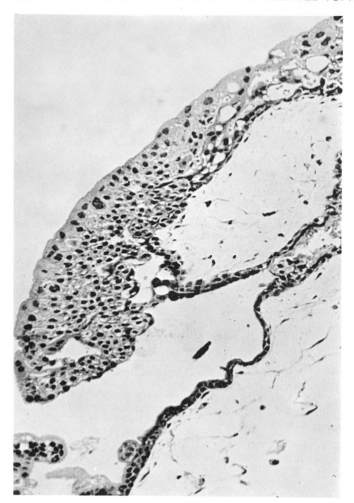

FIG. 39–1. Benign hydatidiform mole, showing avascular villus with hyperplasia of syncytium and cytotrophoblast.

gestation or earlier, and the first indication of the disease is often the passage of vesicles. Severe hyperemesis, preeclampsia before the twenty-eighth week, and anemia are suggestive of the disorder. Since theca lutein cysts are present in about one third of the cases, the finding of adnexal masses may support the diagnosis. These tumors should not be excised because they regress after the trophoblastic tissue has been removed. An unusually high titer of chorionic gonadotropin, especially after the one-hundredth day of pregnancy, helps to confirm the diagnosis of mole. Twins and hydramnios must be excluded.

Diagnosis of mole can be made accurately by ultrasound (Fig. 39–2). As soon as possible after diagnosis, the mole should be evacuated. Oxytocin is used to decrease the size of the uterus while the molar tissue is removed through a large-bore suction catheter. Sharp curettage is permissible only after the size of the uterus is sufficiently reduced to minimize the chance of perforation. Blood should be available during the procedure. In the rare event that the uterus does not respond to oxytocin, hysterotomy may be required. In older multiparas, hysterectomy may be indicated. Because one in about five moles is followed by choriocarcinoma or invasive mole, follow-up by β-hCG titers to detect metastatic or persistent disease is mandatory. Invasive mole and choriocarcinoma are managed with great success by chemotherapy, often beginning with methotrexate or actinomycin D but sometimes requiring more complex regimens.

Benign mole is followed by gestational trophoblastic neoplasia (Figs. 39–3 and 39–4) in about 18.5% of cases. Since intact

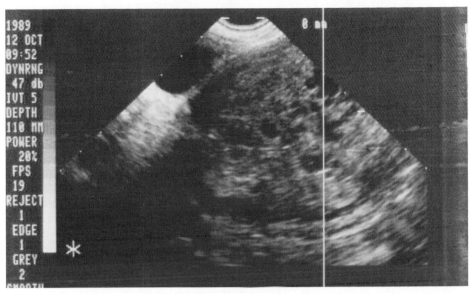

FIG. 39–2. Transvaginal midsagittal view of the uterus, showing ultrasonic appearance of hydatid mole.

hCG produced by persistent trophoblastic neoplastic tissue cannot be differentiated from that produced by a normal conceptus, pregnancy should be interdicted for a year to avoid confusion with persistent trophoblastic disease. Serum β-hCG should be measured weekly. The concentration is normally halved every 10 to 14 days. Patients in whom the serum β-hCG declines at a slower rate, remains at a plateau, or even increases should receive a thorough work-up and chemotherapy. The initial titer of hCG appears to have little bearing on prognosis. Failure of the titer to fall rapidly, however, bespeaks a poorer prognosis. Regression curves for β-hCG after evacuation of a mole are available for use in predicting the course of a particular patient. Deviation from this graph indicates a high likelihood of malignant sequelae and the need for chemotherapy. A simplified scheme of management is presented in Table 39–3. Follow-up should be continued for 1 year. Curettage is repeated and the tissue submitted for histopathologic diagnosis, although the correlation between histologic appearance of the trophoblast and subsequent clinical behavior of the lesion is not good.

Partial moles may occur in conjunction with a normal fetus. The incidence of triploid pregnancy is about 1%, but that of triploid partial moles is much smaller. Partial moles run a less malignant course, with fewer serious sequelae than are seen after a complete mole. Their chromosomal composition is usually triploid (from 40% to 90%), but trisomy, double trisomy, tetraploidy, and normal 46,XX and 46,XY have also been associated with partial moles.

Choriocarcinoma comprises plexiform columns of trophoblast without a villous pattern. Whereas this disease was formerly almost 100% fatal, chemotherapy now effects cures of greater than 80%. About half of all choriocarcinomas follow moles, but the tumor also may be preceded by abortion, term pregnancy, or ectopic gestation.

Moles occur only about once in 1200 to 2000 pregnancies in the United States, but the prevalence is greater in Indonesia, Hong Kong, and other parts of Asia. It is relatively more common at the extremes of reproductive life (particularly after age 30) and in women with a dietary deficiency of carotene, a precursor of vitamin A.

About 2.5% of complete moles are followed by choriocarcinoma and perhaps 16% by the invasive molar form of gestational trophoblastic neoplasia. The classical, or complete, hydatidiform mole has a diploid chromosomal constitution. Cytogenetic studies have shown that all the chromo-

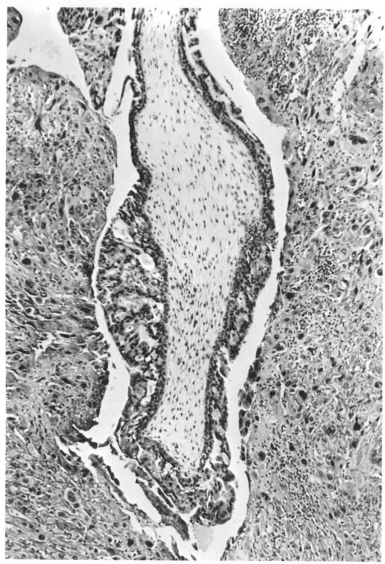

FIG. 39–3. Invasive mole, showing avascular villus with hyperplastic trophoblast penetrating myometrium.

TABLE 39–3. MANAGEMENT OF HYDATIDIFORM MOLE

1. hCG measurements (radioimmunoassay or bioassay) every 1 to 2 weeks until negative two times
   a. Then bimonthly for 1 year
   b. Contraception for 1 year
2. Physical examination including pelvic every 2 weeks until remission
   a. Then every 3 months for 1 year
3. Chest film initially
   a. Repeat only if hCG titer plateaus or rises
4. Chemotherapy started immediately if:
   a. hCG titer rises or plateaus during follow-up
   b. Metastases are detected at any time

somes in these moles are derived from the father. About 90% of complete moles have a 46,XX karyotype and about 10% have a 46,XY pattern. The evidence suggests that the female pronucleus is excluded at syngamy or earlier. The paternal chromosomes then undergo endoreduplication. In the complete mole, trophoblastic dysplasia and hyperplasia and generalized hydatidiform swelling of the villi are conspicuous. The apparently higher rates of incidence of trophoblastic disease in Southeast Asia, as compared with Europe and the United

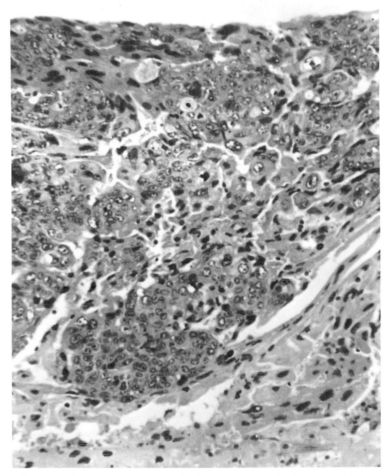

FIG. 39–4. Choriocarcinoma, showing plexiform arrangement of syncytium and malignant cytotrophoblast.

States, for example, may be attributed in part to a smaller proportion of deliveries in hospital and hence a smaller denominator and a higher ratio of molar to total counted pregnancies.

In contrast to complete moles, partial moles are usually triploid (either 69,XXY or 69,XYY) with the extra set of chromosomes most often derived from the father. In addition, partial moles are associated with identifiable embryonic or fetal tissues (alive or dead), variably sized chorionic villi with focal hydatidiform swelling and cavitation, focal trophoblastic hyperplasia, marked scalloping of the chorionic villi, and prominent trophoblastic inclusions in the stroma. Partial moles are much less likely to be followed by metastatic trophoblastic gestational disease than are complete moles.

Although partial mole and complete mole were originally described as two entirely different entities, the distinction has become somewhat clouded. Histologic, flow cytometric, and genomic criteria for differentiation of the two lesions are not always consistent. Thus, histologically identified partial moles, for example, may have a chromosomal composition typical of complete mole and vice versa.

Chromosomal aneuploidy as detected by flow cytometry or image analysis predicts a more virulent tumor with a poorer prognosis. Knowledge of the spread of trophoblastic neoplasia indicates that involvement of the brain or liver is a poor prognostic sign. The World Health Organization (WHO) has developed a clinical scoring system that is correlated well with clinical behavior of the

TABLE 39–4. SCORING SYSTEM FOR TROPHOBLASTIC DISEASE BASED ON PROGNOSTIC FACTORS

	SCORE			
PROGNOSTIC FACTORS	0	1	2	4
Age (years)	Below 39	Above 39		
Antecedent pregnancy	Mole	Abortion	Term	
Interval (months) before start of chemotherapy	Less than 4	4–6	7–12	Greater than 12
HCG (IU/L)	Less than 10^3	10^3–10^4	10^4–10^5	Greater than 10^5
ABO groups		O × A	B	
(female × male)		A × O	AB	
Largest tumor (cm)		3–5	Greater than 5	
Site of metastases	—	Spleen, kidney	G-I tract, liver	Brain
Number of metastases	—	1–4	4–8	More than 8
Prior chemotherapy	—	—	1 drug	2 or more drugs

The total score is obtained by adding the individual risk scores. Score 4 or less = low risk; 5 to 7 = middle risk; 8 or above = high risk.

lesion (Table 39-4). Patients with a score of less than 4 have low-risk metastatic disease and are cured generally with single-agent chemotherapy. Patients with a score of 5 to 7 have moderate-risk disease and require triple chemotherapy to achieve a high rate of cure. High-risk patients have scores of 8 or more and require the most extensive regimens of multiple chemotherapeutic agents to achieve a moderate (75%) rate of survival.

Pregnancy-specific β_1-glycoprotein (SP$_1$) and placental protein 5 (PP5) are found in higher concentrations in hydatidiform mole than in choriocarcinoma, although the β-hCG level is high in both forms of trophoblastic disease. The ratios of free β-hCG to total hCG may be of value in distinguishing the various forms of trophoblastic disease, with a higher free β/total hCG ratio indicating more aggressive disease. Moles are said to occur less commonly in patients with group O blood.

Some authorities prefer to administer methotrexate or actinomycin before evacuation of a benign mole, but most reserve these drugs for proven or suspected metastatic or persistent disease.

GESTATIONAL TROPHOBLASTIC NEOPLASIA

Nonmetastatic gestational trophoblastic neoplasia (GTN) may be treated with methotrexate (30 to 50 mg/m^2) by weekly intramuscular injection. Treatment should be continued until three consecutive weekly hCG titers are negative. Patients who do not respond to this therapy may be salvaged by actinomycin D (0.5 mg/m^2) given daily intravenously for 5 days and repeated every 14 to 21 days. Treatment must be stopped temporarily if the patient develops neutropenia or thrombocytopenia.

Patients with low-risk GTN may be treated with any of the regimens listed in Table 39–5. Treatment should be continued until neutropenia or thrombocytopenia supervenes or until three negative hCG titers are obtained. Patients with moderate-risk GTN are treated generally with methotrexate 15 mg intramuscularly, together with actinomycin D 8 to 10 μg/kg intravenously, and chlorambucil 8 to 10 mg by mouth. All three drugs are given daily for 5 days. A hiatus in treatment of 10 to 14 days is allowed, depending on the status of the bone marrow. Courses are repeated until three consecutive negative hCG titers are obtained. Patients with high-risk GTN may be treated with actinomycin D (300 μg/m^2),

TABLE 39–5. SINGLE-AGENT CHEMOTHERAPY

1. Methotrexate 20–25 mg IM every day for 5 days (repeat every 7 days if possible)
2. Actinomycin D 10–12 μg/kg IV every day for 5 days (repeat every 7 days if possible)
3. Methotrexate 1 mg/kg IM on days 1,3,5, and 7 Folinic acid 0.1 mg/kg IM on days 2,4,6, and 8 (repeat every 7 days if possible)

platinum (100 mg/m^2, and etoposide (VP 16, 100 mg/m^2). This so-called APE regimen has achieved excellent results as primary treatment. If the patients have been subjected to prior unsuccessful chemotherapy or if the APE regimen has not produced a remission or a cure, the modified Bagshawe regimen may be used (Table 39–6).

PLACENTAL SITE TROPHOBLASTIC TUMOR

The placental site trophoblastic tumor histologically is not part of the spectrum of gestational trophoblastic disease that includes partial mole, complete hydatidiform mole, invasive mole, and choriocarcinoma. Instead, it is a lesion composed entirely of one form of trophoblast, the intermediate cell. Formerly called trophoblastic pseudotumor, the lesion is now designated a true tumor, as witnessed by the occasional metastases and death of the affected patients. The lesion must be distinguished from an exaggerated placental site reaction. The tumor, unlike choriocarcinoma, produces relatively little hCG but large amounts of hPL. The benign varieties of the tumor may be cured by simple curettage. For the more aggressive lesions, hysterectomy is indicated, because of the poor response to chemotherapy after the lesion has spread beyond the uterus.

TABLE 39–6. MODIFIED BAGSHAWE REGIMEN

Day	Hour	Treatment
1	0600	Hydroxyurea 500 mg PO
	1200	Hydroxyurea 500 mg PO
	1800	Hydroxyurea 500 mg PO
	1900	Actinomycin D 200 μg IV
	2400	Hydroxyurea 500 mg PO
2	0700	Vincristine 1 mg/m^2 IV
	1900	Methotrexate 100 mg/m^2 IV
		Methotrexate 200 mg/m^2 by infusion
		Actinomycin D 200 μg IV
3	1900	Actinomycin D 200 μg IV
		Cyclophosphamide 500 mg/m^2 IV
		Folinic acid 14 mg IM
4	0100	Folinic acid 14 mg IM
	0700	Folinic acid 14 mg IM
	1300	Folinic acid 14 mg IM
	1900	Folinic acid 14 mg IM
		Actinomycin D 500 μg IV
5	0100	Folinic acid 14 mg IM
	1900	Actinomycin D 500 μg IV
6	No treatment	
7	No treatment	
8	1900	Cyclophosphamide 500 mg/m^2 IV
		Doxorubicin 30 mg/m^2 IV

40
CHAPTER
LESIONS OF THE VULVA

BENIGN LESIONS OF THE VULVA

Benign tumors of the vulva include those of the skin in general and a few special growths. Condyloma acuminatum is viral rather than primarily neoplastic and is discussed extensively elsewhere in this text. Abscesses and cysts of Bartholin's gland are discussed under inflammatory lesions (p. 188). Solid benign epithelial tumors include papillomas, adenomas, and nevi. Sebaceous cysts and hidradenomas are also found on the vulva.

The hidradenoma may be highly cellular and therefore mistaken for an adenocarcinoma, but it is rarely malignant, as shown in Figure 40–1. Benign connective tissue tumors of the vulva include lipomas, fibromas, hemangiomas, and lymphangiomas. Varices of the vulva may be mistaken for neoplasms.

Any suspicious lesion of the vulva, and any lesion that does not respond quickly to conservative treatment, particularly in older women, should be subjected to biopsy.

The International Society for the Study of Vulvar Disease has suggested a logical and succinct classification of the vulvar dystrophies (Table 40–1). Included among the nonneoplastic epithelial disorders are some formerly described as leukoplakia, kraurosis, atrophic dystrophy, hyperplastic vulvitis, leukoplakic vulvitis, and neurodermatitis. Additionally, the following terms are no longer recommended: lichen sclerosus et atrophicus, leukokeratosis, Bowen's disease, erythroplasia of Queyrat, and carcinoma simplex.

Dystrophic lesions are important because they are sometimes precursors of carcinoma of the vulva. "White lesions" of the vulva include a variety of disorders, only some of which are premalignant. The greater the cellular atypia, the more likely is a white lesion to be a precursor of carcinoma.

In squamous cell hyperplasia, there is epithelial hyperplasia, acanthosis, hyperkeratosis, and chronic inflammation (Fig. 40–2). In lichen sclerosus, there is thinning of the squamous epithelium with loss of the rete pegs (Fig. 40–3). The dermis just beneath the squamous epithelium appears acellular and homogeneous. In "mixed dystophy," areas of lichen sclerosus and hyperplastic dystrophy are found in the same lesion. These lesions are now included as a variety of lichen sclerosus. The atypia accompanying any of the dystrophies may be classified as mild, moderate, or severe. Hyperkeratosis and parakeratosis may be found in all grades of atypia. It has been shown that many of these hyperplastic lesions are related to HPV infection (Chapter 43). The new classification of vulvar atypias (vulvar intraepithelial neoplasia) is shown in Table 40–2).

Atrophic lesions of the vulva may cause pruritus, which leads to scratching and secondary infection. Dystrophic lesions with

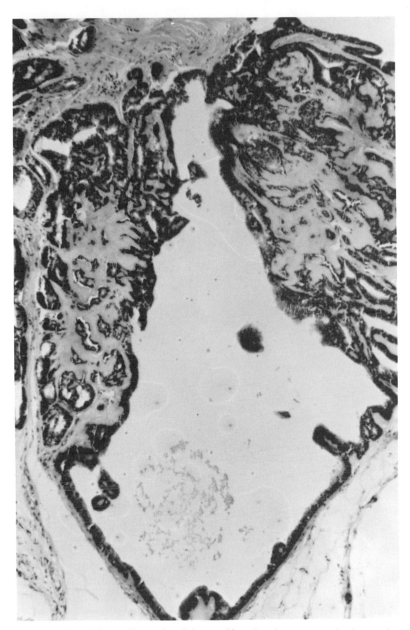

FIG. 40–1. Hidradenoma of the vulva with papillary glandular proliferation but no cytologic atypia.

TABLE 40–1. NONNEOPLASTIC EPITHELIAL DISORDERS OF THE VULVA

1. Lichen sclerosus (lichen sclerosus et atrophicus)
2. Squamous cell hyperplasia (formerly hyperplastic dystrophy)
3. Other dermatoses

cellular atypia may be precursors of vulvar carcinoma. Suspicious lesions should be subjected to biopsy. Widespread dysplastic lesions may be managed best by prophylactic vulvectomy.

MALIGNANT LESIONS OF THE VULVA

Carcinoma of the vulva accounts for about 5% of all gynecologic cancers. The invasive lesion may be preceded by dysplasia and carcinoma in situ.

The typical vulvar carcinoma in situ is of the squamous cell variety. Another intraepithelial form, Paget's disease, which may be of apocrine origin, usually involves postmenopausal women. Pathognomonic Paget

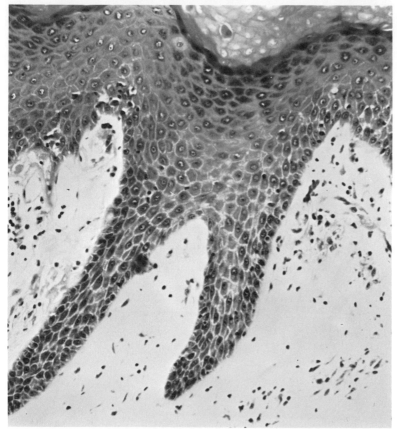

FIG. 40–2. Squamous cell hyperplasia (hyperplastic dystrophy) of the vulva, showing acanthosis, hyperkeratosis, and parakeratosis.

cells with clear, vacuolated cytoplasm are found, initially in the basal layers of the epidermis and later throughout the epithelium (Fig. 40–4). Papanicolaou smears are unreliable for diagnosis of vulvar carcinoma because of the frequently associated hyperkeratosis. Toluidine blue and colposcopy may aid in selecting a site for the biopsy. Because these lesions are often multifocal, multiple biopsies are required to rule out invasion. The preinvasive lesion may be treated safely by simple vulvectomy or vaporization by laser. Paget's disease may recur in the vulva after local excision and may involve anus, cervix, and breasts.

Invasive carcinoma of the vulva is of the squamous cell variety in 95% of cases (Fig. 40–5). It occurs most frequently in postmenopausal women but occasionally is found in younger women as well. About 40% of vulvar carcinomas are preceded by identifiable dysplastic lesions and intraepithelial carcinoma. Etiologic factors include chronic infections (such as lymphogranuloma venereum), human papillomavirus, and poor hygiene.

TABLE 40–2. CLASSIFICATION OF VULVAR INTRAEPITHELIAL NEOPLASIA (VIN)

VIN I	Mild dysplasia	(formerly mild atypia)
VIN II	Moderate dysplasia	(formerly moderate atypia)
VIN III	Severe dysplasia and carcinoma in situ	

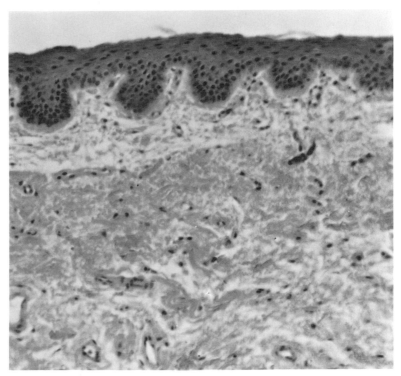

FIG. 40–3. Lichen sclerosus of the vulva, showing atrophic epithelium and homogenization of subepithelial connective tissue.

Vulvar intraepithelial neoplasia, or VIN (see Table 40–2) is the precursor of invasive carcinoma of the vulva. Although the natural history of VIN is not so well understood as that of CIN, etiologic, virologic, and histologic features are similar. As with CIN and invasive carcinoma of the cervix, both VIN and invasive carcinoma of the vulva are associated with smoking, genital warts, and multiple sexual partners. Because VIN is seen in 10 to 20% of patients with CIN, routine colposcopy of the vulva in patients with high-grade CIN is recommended. As with other HPV-related lesions, VIN is being detected with increasing frequency in young women.

Treatment of VIN should be directed toward removal of all abnormal epithelium with a margin of 1 to 2 cm of normal tissue. Because it is impossible to eradicate HPV from surrounding histologically normal tissue, the patients must be counseled accordingly. Therapeutic options for VIN include excisional biopsy under colposcopic guidance; cryosurgery; ablation with the CO_2 laser; wide local excision with scalpel, scis-

sors, or CO_2 laser; and skinning vulvectomy. The choice of treatment depends on the amount of abnormal epithelium to be excised and its location.

The most common sites of carcinoma of the vulva, in order of frequency, are the labium majus, the posterior commissure, the clitoris, and the labium minus. Spread occurs locally and lymphatic drainage is first to inguinal and femoral nodes and later to deep pelvic nodes.

Carcinoma of the vulva may present as a persistent asymptomatic exophytic mass or ulcer or may cause pruritus, a foul-smelling bloody discharge, or pain on urination or defecation. Diagnosis is provided by biopsy, which is the only means of distinguishing an intraepithelial from an early invasive lesion. Use of toluidine blue and colposcopy may aid in directing biopsy to the most abnormal areas. Because treatment of the two lesions varies greatly, multiple biopsies should be performed to rule out invasion. Differential diagnosis includes syphilis and other granulomatous sexually transmitted lesions.

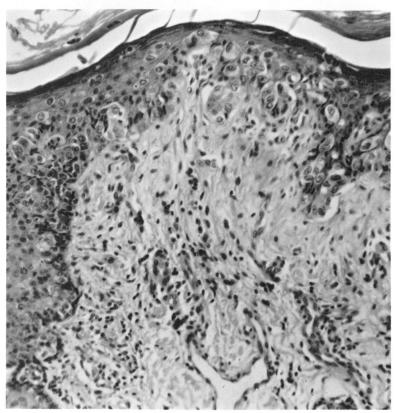

FIG. 40–4. Paget's disease of the vulva, showing typical large, pale cells adjacent to basal layer and in underlying epidermal appendages.

The classification of vulvar intraepithelial neoplasia is shown in Table 40–2. The International Federation of Gynecology and Obstetrics (FIGO) staging for carcinoma of the vulva is shown in Table 40–3. It is now a surgical rather than a clinical staging and is based largely on involvement of inguinal and femoral nodes, a highly important prognostic factor.

Standard surgical treatment of carcinoma of the vulva has long been radical vulvectomy with en bloc removal of inguinal and femoral lymph nodes, but today less extensive treatment is often tailored to the patient's particular lesion.

Patients with Stage I vulvar cancer and low risk of positive nodes may be treated safely with wide local excision (radical hemivulvectomy) and ipsilateral superficial groin node dissection. This procedure is associated with much less morbidity than is traditional radical vulvectomy and appears to be equally effective.

Lymph node metastases in vulvar cancer are related to depth of penetration of the carcinoma, spread to venous or lymphatic capillaries, confluence of tongues of invasive tumor, poor differentiation of the lesion, and width of the primary. Lesions smaller than 2 cm in diameter with 1 mm or less of deep penetration, without confluence, and of grade 1 or 2, practically never spread to lymph nodes. These lesions may be treated safely with wide local excision and ipsilateral groin node dissection. Lesions with greater than 5 mm of deep penetration or with palpable nodes or any other poor prognostic feature should receive standard radical vulvectomy and groin node dissection.

Patients whose lesions fall between the aforementioned low-risk and high-risk groups may be treated with wide local excision and ipsilateral groin dissection, but if positive nodes are found, this intermediate group of patients must have subsequent

TABLE 40–3. FIGO STAGING OF CARCINOMA OF THE VULVA

Rules for Clinical Staging

Stage 0

Tis — Carcinoma in situ; intraepithelial carcinoma

Stage I

T1 N0 M0 — Tumor confined to the vulva and/or perineum—2 cm or less in greatest dimension, nodes are not palpable

Stage II

T2 N0 M0 — Tumor confined to the vulva and/or perineum—more than 2 cm in greatest dimension, nodes are not palpable

Stage III

T3 N0 M0

T3 N1 M0 — Tumor of any size with . . .
1) Adjacent spread to the lower urethra and/or the vagina, or the anus, and/or . . .

T1 N1 M0 — 2) Unilateral regional lymph node metastasis

T2 N1 M0

Stage IVA

T1 N2 M0 — Tumor invades any of the following:

T2 N2 M0 — Upper urethra, bladder mucosa, rectal mucosa, pelvic bone, and/or bilateral regional node metastasis

T3 N2 M0
T4 any N M0

Stage IVB

Any T

Any N, M1 — Any distant metastasis including pelvic lymph nodes

The rules for staging are similar to those for carcinoma of the cervix.

TNM Classification of Carcinoma of the Vulva (FIGO)

T   Primary tumor

Tis — Preinvasive carcinoma (carcinoma in situ)

T1 — Tumor confined to the vulva and/or perineum—$\geqq 2$ cm in greatest dimension

T2 — Tumor confined to the vulva and/or perineum—2 cm in greatest dimension.

T3 — Tumor of any size with adjacent spread to the urethra and/or vagina and/or to the anus

T4 — Tumor of any size infiltrating the bladder mucosa and/or the rectal mucosa, including the upper part of the urethral mucosa and/or fixed to the bone

N   Regional lymph nodes

N0 — No lymph node metastasis

N1 — Unilateral regional lymph node metastasis

N2 — Bilateral regional lymph node metastasis

M   Distant metastasis

M0 — No clinical metastasis

M1 — Distant metastasis (including pelvic lymph node metastasis)

International Federation of Gynecology and Obstetrics. Annual report on the results of treatment in gynecological cancer. Int J Gynecol Obstet 1989; 28:189–190.

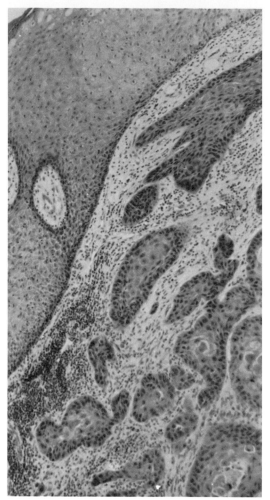

FIG. 40–5. Well differentiated invasive squamous cell carcinoma of the vulva.

radical vulvectomy and bilateral groin node dissection or pelvic radiotherapy.

Megavoltage radiation therapy has become the treatment of choice for patients with positive nodes after radical vulvectomy. It is associated with a higher rate of cure and a lower morbidity than is pelvic lymphadenectomy.

Radiation therapy has been used preoperatively in patients with large Stage III and Stage IV lesions in conjunction with radical vulvectomy and node dissection. In the past these patients were treated with total or partial exenteration. With radiotherapy, these patients may retain function of their bowels and bladders.

Combination therapy consisting of external beam radiotherapy with platinum and 5-fluorouracil is highly effective in reducing the volume of tumor in patients with advanced or recurrent vulvar carcinoma. Many of the patients thus treated have been subjected afterward to surgical therapy and cured.

Basal cell carcinoma may be treated by wide local excision or simple vulvectomy without node dissection.

An adenocarcinoma of the vulva may arise rarely from Bartholin's gland. Secondary carcinomas of the vulva may be metastatic from a primary cancer of the uterus or rectum. Uncommon malignant tumors of the vulva include melanoma (pigmented and unpigmented), lymphoma, and fibrosarcoma.

41
CHAPTER

LESIONS OF THE VAGINA

BENIGN LESIONS OF THE VAGINA

Symptomatic benign lesions of the vagina are uncommon. Inclusion cysts are commonly 1 to 2 cm in diameter. They usually result from burial of tags of squamous epithelium under a suture line after episiotomy or repair of a laceration. Myomas and fibromas are rare lesions that produce no characteristic clinical findings. Cysts of Gartner's duct (mesonephric duct) may form in the upper portion of the vagina. Endometriosis of the vagina may produce dysmenorrhea and dyspareunia (p 216).

Adenosis of the vagina develops from müllerian remnants. Administration of diethylstilbestrol (DES) to the mother during pregnancy has been associated with adenosis and rarely with adenocarcinoma of the vagina in the offspring. For this reason, DES is contraindicated in pregnancy. Children of mothers who have received the drug during pregnancy should be examined carefully to detect vaginal lesions.

Palpation and the Schiller test are the main methods of detecting DES-induced lesions. The likelihood of induction by DES of clear cell carcinoma of the upper vagina and cervix is between 0.14 and 1.4 per thousand, but benign anomalies of the genital tract are far more common. Abnormalities of the female upper genital tract include a T-shaped uterus, a small uterine cavity, fundal constrictions, filling defects, and synechiae. Abnormalities of the lower genital tract include transverse vaginal and cervical ridges (collars, rims, cockscombs, or pseudopolyps). The male progeny of DES-exposed women may also be affected. Abnormalities in the male include cysts of the epididymis, hypoplastic testes, cryptorchidism and microphallus.

The cervix in a DES-affected woman may have a wide transformation zone (p. 266). As the patient matures, the epithelial lesions undergo metaplasia and evolve into grossly more nearly normal cervix and vagina. Follow-up examination of DES-affected women includes cytologic smears of the ectocervix, endocervix, and vagina; colposcopy of cervix and vagina; and careful palpation of the vaginal fornices.

MALIGNANT LESIONS OF THE VAGINA

The most important carcinoma of the vagina is of the squamous cell variety (Fig. 41–1), although it accounts for only 2% of female genital cancers. It usually occurs in women 60 years of age or older. Spread occurs locally and by lymphatics. An intraepithelial form resembling that of the cervix often precedes invasive cancer. A positive Papanicolaou smear after hysterectomy suggests

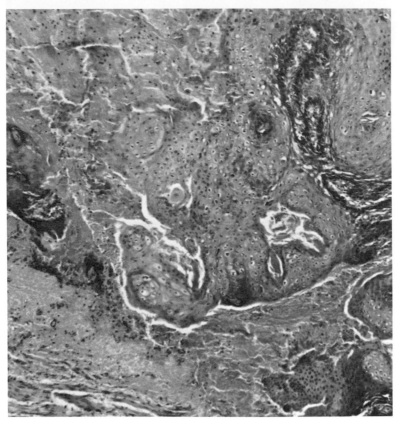

FIG. 41–1. Infiltrating well differentiated squamous cell carcinoma of the vagina.

carcinoma of the vagina. Diagnosis is made by biopsy, usually aided by Schiller's test and colposcopy.

The most common site for vaginal carcinoma is the posterior wall of the upper third of the vagina. The lesion may be exophytic or ulcerative. In advanced stages, the vaginal tube may be fixed to the pelvic wall. Carcinomas of the upper vagina may behave like those of the cervix, whereas those of the lowermost vagina spread like those of the vulva. Death is commonly from uremia.

Staging of carcinoma of the vagina resembles that of the cervix. The new FIGO staging is shown in Table 41–1.

The usual treatment for carcinoma of the vagina is irradiation of the whole pelvis combined with intravaginal radium. Radical surgical therapy may be indicated for selected young patients with Stage I disease. Exenteration may be beneficial in highly

TABLE 41–1. FIGO STAGING OF CARCINOMA OF THE VAGINA*

Stage 0	Carcinoma in situ, intraepithelial carcinoma
Stage I	The carcinoma is limited to the vaginal wall
Stage II	The carcinoma has involved the subvaginal tissue but has not extended to the pelvic wall
Stage III	The carcinoma has extended to the pelvic wall
Stage IV	The carcinoma has extended beyond the true pelvis or has clinically involved the mucosa of the bladder or rectum. Bullous edema as such does not permit a case to be allotted to stage IV
Stage IVA	Spread of the growth to adjacent organs and/or direct extension beyond the true pelvis
Stage IVB	Spread to distant organs

*International Federation of Gynecology and Obstetrics. Annual report on the results of treatment in gynecological cancer. Vol. 20. Stockholm, FIGO, 1988.

selected patients with involvement of the bladder or rectum. For all stages combined, the 5-year survival remains about 35%, although survivals of 65% to 80% have been reported for Stage I lesions. The rates of survival for clear cell adenocarcinoma are higher: for Stage I the rate is 90%, compared with 78% for all stages combined.

Carcinoma in the vagina is more often secondary than primary. The vagina is in-volved by direct spread from the cervix or by metastases from the ovaries, oviducts, cho-riocarcinoma, and occasionally carcinoma of the breast or hypernephroma. The vagina is involved by metastases, direct extension, or recurrence in about 10% of carcinomas of the corpus.

Sarcoma botryoides is a rare, highly ma-lignant, often fatal tumor that involves the vagina and is ordinarily found in infants.

42
CHAPTER

NONMALIGNANT DISEASES OF THE CERVIX

Benign lesions of the cervix include polyps and condylomata acuminata. Polyps, which may be single or multiple, have a core of connective tissue and an epithelial covering (Fig. 42–1). They are usually glandular, arising from the endocervix, but are occasionally squamous, arising from the portio. They range in size from minute to several centimeters in length. They may cause no symptoms or produce irregular bleeding or increased vaginal discharge. They very rarely undergo malignant change. A large polyp may be confused with a prolapsed myoma. The treatment is polypectomy, followed by fractional curettage.

Occasionally hyperplasia of the endocervical epithelium may result from the use of oral contraceptives. This change should not be confused with adenocarcinoma. This form of hyperplasia may produce contact bleeding but will regress after discontinuation of oral contraception.

Benign tumors of the cervix include leiomyomas, hemangiomas, and squamous papillomas. In addition, endometriosis and adenomyosis, as well as cysts and adenomas arising from mesonephric remnants, may involve the cervix. Adenosis and adenocarcinoma of the cervix, as well as of the vagina, have been reported in the children of mothers who received stilbestrol during their pregnancies (p. 263).

Because of the important relation of human papillomavirus to cervical neoplasia, that infection will be discussed in Chapter 43.

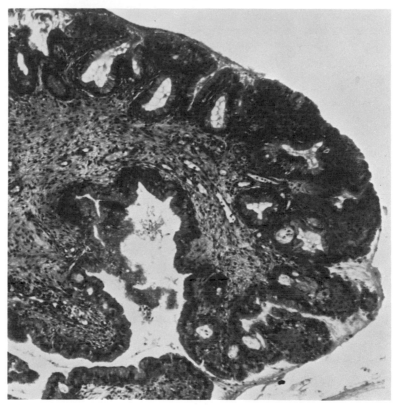

FIG. 42–1. Endocervical polyp, showing covering of mucinous columnar epithelium and connective tissue core with vascular congestion and inflammatory cells.

43
CHAPTER

CERVICAL CANCER AND ITS PRECURSORS

Invasive carcinoma of the cervix accounts for about 30% of all deaths from gynecologic cancer. The estimated number of new cases of invasive cancer of the cervix for 1990 was 12,000 and the number of deaths was 6500. Invasive cancer is usually preceded by an intraepithelial form, which in turn is preceded by various degrees of increasing dysplasia. Cervical intraepithelial neoplasia (CIN) is a term that includes epithelial changes ranging from mild dysplasia to carcinoma in situ (CIS). All forms of cervical intraepithelial neoplasia may regress, but the earlier stages do so more commonly. The etiologic factors in dysplasia, carcinoma in situ, and invasive carcinoma are similar. The disease is more common in lower socioeconomic classes and in women who begin coitus and childbearing early in their lives. It is also more common in prostitutes and other women with multiple sexual partners. Contact with *Herpesvirus hominis* type II is no longer considered an important etiologic factor, but exposure to the human papillomavirus (HPV) is attracting greater attention in the genesis of cervical cancer. The concentration of histones in the semen is positively correlated with the risk of cervical carcinoma. Cigarette smoking has been associated with an increase in both dysplasia and carcinoma of the cervix.

There is a close and probably causative relation between human papillomavirus and both cervical intraepithelial neoplasia and invasive cancer of the cervix. Virtually all women with CIN and invasive cancer demonstrate DNA of HPV by techniques of in situ hybridization. Subclinical, asymptomatic HPV infection is detected on cytologic screening (Fig. 43–1). Careful colposcopic examination demonstrates features of HPV in the vulvas, vaginas, and cervices of most patients with abnormal cytologic smears. Typical koilocytes are seen on histologic examination (Fig. 43–2).

The human papillomavirus is an obligate intranuclear DNA virus with a circular double-stranded genome surrounded by a polyhedral capsid with 20 faces (eicosahedral). Over 60 types of HPV have been isolated to date. The term koilocytic atypia was coined in 1956 to describe the characteristic lesion in cells infected with the HPV virus (see Fig. 43–2).

Accurate detection of HPV varies widely according to method of testing. The immunoperoxidase staining method requires intact viral particles to achieve a positive test. These intact particles are found only in moderately or fully differentiated squamous cells and indicate a "permissive" HPV infection, usually associated with exophytic acuminate warty lesions. Although these lesions are highly infectious, they are involved only rarely in malignant transformation. The HPV genome is usually episomal, existing as a free entity usually located peripher-

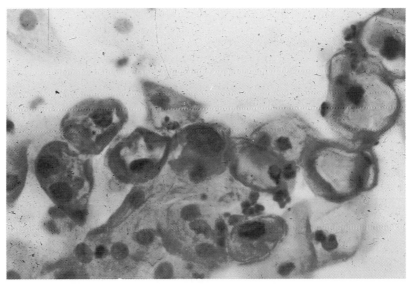

FIG. 43–1. Asymptomatic infection with human papillomavirus, detected on cytologic smear of cervix.

ally within the nucleus. Inasmuch as intact viral particles are found infrequently in clinical situations and their malignant sequelae are rare, the peroxidase test is of little clinical value.

Hybridization tests, based on the ability of a cloned HPV probe to link and form a stable duplex with HPV genetic material, offer reliable and reproducible evidence of HPV genetic material. These tests can identify complete viral particles or small fragments of the virus.

The Southern blot was developed in 1975. The test is based on the separation according to size of DNA fragments in electrophoretic gels. After transfer to nitrocellulose filters, exposure to probes of known HPV type is accomplished. Each type produces a characteristic pattern. This highly accurate technique can detect small amounts of viral DNA. Because it is time-consuming, labor-intensive, expensive, and unable to localize DNA in histologic specimens, it is primarily a research tool. In situ hybridization utilizes similar techniques but the tissue sample is not consumed in processing. In situ hybridization can be applied to cytologic or histologic preparations. It can localize HPV in a current biopsy or archival specimen and the association of HPV genetic material with the neoplastic process can be studied with precision. It is significantly

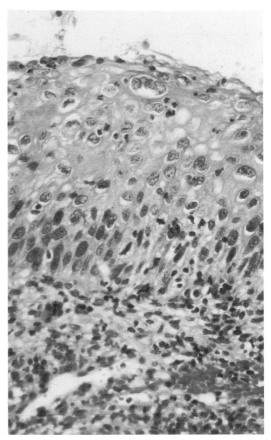

FIG. 43–2. Histologic section of cervix infected with human papillomavirus, showing typical koilocytes.

faster and cheaper than the Southern blot and only slightly less sensitive. It too is primarily a research tool.

Dot blot hybridization is fundamentally similar to the Southern blot. This technique decreases the expense and time of the test with only minimal loss of sensitivity. The technique requires specific complementary probes for each HPV type and does not rely on comparing a band pattern to a standard. Only one method (ViraPap) is FDA-approved and commercially available.

The polymerase chain reaction (PCR) is a relatively new technique that amplifies the amount of viral DNA more than 100,000 times prior to the component of HPV typing involved in the actual detection. It is extremely sensitive, permitting detection of portions of the HPV genome. Special laboratory procedures must be employed to prevent contamination by poorly cleaned glassware and fingers.

Although the clinical utility of HPV typing is still somewhat controversial, the technique is the only objective method of identifying DNA of HPV. It is clearly valuable in quality control in cytology and histology laboratories. Specifically, minor-grade lesions (CIN I and condylomatous atypia) that contain HPV 16 and HPV 18 DNA are more likely to progress to higher-grade lesions. This information may be useful in clinical management.

HPV types 6 and 11 are less likely and types 16, 18, and 31 are more likely to be associated with lesions that progress to cancer. Atypical mitotic figures in the biopsy are associated with higher rates of progression and more commonly with HPV type 16. Patients with condylomas and atypical mitotic figures and those with condylomas and CIN should be treated promptly with laser, cryotherapy, electrocautery, conization, or hysterectomy. About 80 to 90% of the male partners of women with condylomas demonstrate similar lesions on the penis when examined with the colposcope (androscopy).

Dysplasia connotes nuclear atypia of the cervical epithelium without involvement of its entire thickness. True carcinoma in situ (intraepithelial, or preinvasive, cancer) usually involves the entire thickness of the cervical epithelium (Fig. 43−3). The histologic changes include loss of polarity, hyper-chromatism, abnormal mitoses, and increase in nuclear size and number of nucleoli.

The essential feature of intraepithelial carcinoma is the limitation of the abnormal cells by the basement membrane of the cervical epithelium. Involvement of the endocervical glands does not constitute invasion, because the glands are part of the cervical epithelium.

Microinvasion represents the transition between intraepithelial carcinoma and the invasive lesion (Fig. 43−4). The definition and the treatment of this stage of the disease are still somewhat controversial, although the earliest forms are now often managed in the same manner as carcinoma in situ.

The Society of Gynecologic Oncologists (SGO) defines a microinvasive lesion as one in which neoplastic epithelium invades the stroma in one or more places to a depth of 3 mm or less below the base of the epithelium and no lymphatic or vascular involvement is demonstrated. Lesions defined thus strictly are associated with a very low risk of lymph node involvement and recurrence.

Whereas most cases of FIGO Stage IA1 (Table 43−1) are consistent with the SGO definition of microinvasion, many cases of FIGO Stage IA2 are not. Thus, radical surgery or radiation therapy is required in some patients with Stage IA disease, as defined by FIGO.

Cervical lesions of strictly inflammatory or viral origin do not necessarily require treatment. Because all forms of cervical therapy are associated with a risk of stenosis or incompetency, treatment should ordinarily be restricted to squamous intraepithelial lesions (SIL) only.

Low-grade squamous intraepithelial lesions (SIL) comprise CIN I and HPV changes without associated dysplasia (p. 268). Because the likelihood of progression to high-grade SIL is only about 15%, a reliable, compliant patient may be monitored by cytology, colposcopy, and biopsy (if indicated) every 6 to 12 months. If the patient is unreliable, noncompliant, or anxious about having an untreated lesion, or if the laboratory support is marginal, the transformation zone may be destroyed by cryotherapy, electrosurgical loop excision, or laser (p. 241). The patient should be advised, fur-

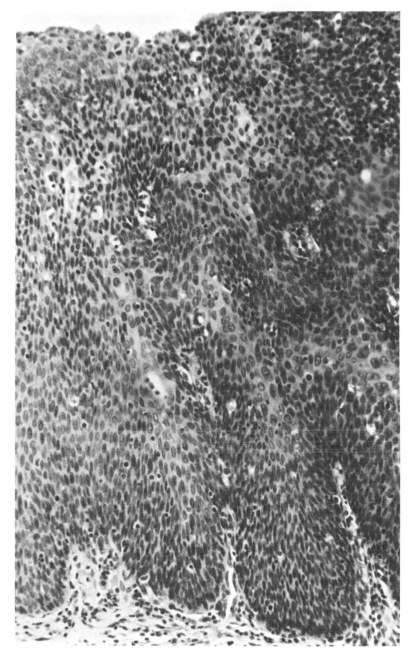

FIG. 43–3. Carcinoma in situ of the cervix (CIN III), showing replacement of entire epithelium by dysplastic cells.

thermore, that HPV lesions will persist after treatment and that no effective treatment for the viral infection is currently available.

High-grade squamous intraepithelial lesions include moderate dysplasia, severe dysplasia, and carcinoma in situ. Because rates of progression of these lesions vary from 30 to 60%, virtually all of them receive some form of therapy. Any method that reliably destroys the entire transformation zone is acceptable, including loop excision, cryotherapy, laser ablation, laser excision, or scalpel excision. Hysterectomy does not provide a higher rate of cure than the

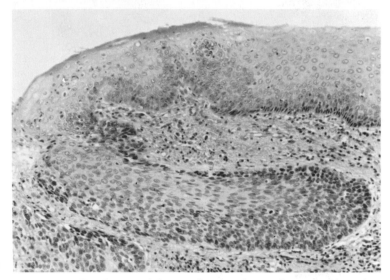

FIG. 43–4. Carcinoma of the cervix, showing early stromal invasion.

aforementioned conservative procedures. Because of its higher associated morbidity, hysterectomy is reserved for patients with additional indications for the procedure such as myomas or uterine prolapse. Cryotherapy is less effective than the other modalities for large CIN III lesions.

Treatment of microinvasive carcinoma depends on the patient's age, desire for further childbearing, and depth of penetration of the lesion. In young women with a tumor that penetrates to a depth of less than 1 mm and who desire retention of fertility, a therapeutic cone with clear margins is probably adequate therapy. Lesions that penetrate 1 to 3 mm are probably treated safely with simple hysterectomy. Lesions that invade more deeply than 3 mm, have multiple tongues of invading tissue, or invade lymphatics are treated more safely by radical hysterectomy. If such patients have medical complications that preclude radical hysterectomy, they may be treated effectively by cesium, external radiation, or both. The rationale for treatment of these early cancers is based on the finding that nodes are almost never involved when the total volume of microcarcinoma is less than 350 mm^3. Measuring the tumor in three dimensions is a very time-consuming procedure, but the current definition of Stage IA2, based on a two-dimensional examination (depth and horizontal spread), is roughly consistent with the volumetric criterion. Thus, Stage IA1 (Table 43–1) may be treated by conization in a patient of reproductive age or by simple hysterectomy in an older patient or one who no longer desires retention of fertility. Patients with Stage IA2 lesions usually are treated by simple hysterectomy or cesium implants.

Histologically, most carcinomas of the cervix (about 85%) are epidermoid (Fig. 43–5). About 15%, are adenocarcinomas (Fig. 43–6); carcinomas of mesonephric origin are rare. The epidermoid (squamous) tumor most commonly arises at the squamocolumnar junction. Chromosomal aneuploidy is found with increasing frequency as the lesion progresses from dysplasia through intraepithelial carcinoma to frankly invasive cancer. The tumor spreads locally into the vagina and parametria and then by regional lymphatics. A cervix that harbors an invasive lesion may be grossly normal, ulcerated, or replaced by a bulky exophytic tumor.

Adenocarcinoma of the cervix accounts for a larger proportion of cervical cancers than it did in the recent past. It is not entirely clear whether this increase is absolute or only relative, as the result of the more effective detection and treatment of precursors of the squamous variety. About 85% of adenocarcinomas arise within 1.5 cm of the squamocolumnar junction and are

TABLE 43–1 FIGO STAGING OF CARCINOMA OF THE CERVIX UTERI*

Stage 0	Carcinoma in situ, intraepithelial carcinoma	**Notes about the staging:**

Stage IA carcinoma should include minimal microscopically evident stromal invasion as well as small cancerous tumors of measurable size. Stage IA should be divided into those lesions with minute foci of invasion visible only microscopically as stage IA1 and macroscopically measurable microcarcinomas as stage IA2, in order to gain further knowledge of the clinical behavior of these lesions. The term "IB occult" should be omitted.

Stage I — The carcinoma is strictly confined to the cervix (extension to the corpus should be disregarded)

Stage IA — Preclinical carcinomas of the cervix, that is, those diagnosed only by microscopy

Stage IA1 — Minimal microscopically evident stromal invasion

Stage IA2 — Lesions detected microscopically that can be measured. The upper limit of the measurement should not show a depth of invasion of more than 5 mm taken from the base of the epithelium, either surface or glandular, from which it originates, and a second dimension, the horizontal spread, must not exceed 7 mm. Larger lesions should be classified as stage IB

The diagnosis of both stage IA1 and IA2 cases should be based on microscopic examination of removed tissue, preferably a cone, which must include the entire lesion. The lower limit of stage IA2 should be measurable macroscopically (even if dots need to be placed on the slide prior to measurement), and the upper limit of stage IA2 is given by measurement of the two largest dimensions in any given section. The depth of invasion should not be more than 5 mm taken from the base of the epithelium, either surface or glandular, from which it originates. The second dimension, the horizontal spread, must not exceed 7 mm. Vascular space involvement, either venous or lymphatic, should not alter the staging but should be specifically recorded, as it may affect treatment decisions in the future.

Stage IB — Lesions of greater dimensions than stage IA2, whether seen clinically or not. Preformed space involvement should not alter the staging but should be specifically recorded so as to determine whether it should affect treatment decisions in the future

Lesions of greater size should be classified as stage IB.

Stage II — The carcinoma extends beyond the cervix but has not extended to the pelvic wall. The carcinoma involves the vagina but not as far as the lower third

Stage IIA — No obvious parametrial involvement

Stage IIB — Obvious parametrial involvement

As a rule, it is impossible to estimate clinically whether a cancer of the cervix has extended to the corpus or not. Extension to the corpus should therefore be disregarded.

A patient with a growth fixed to the pelvic wall by a short and indurated but not nodular parametrium should be allotted to stage IIB. It is impossible, at clinical examination, to decide whether a smooth and indurated parametrium is truly cancerous or only inflammatory. Therefore, the case should be placed in stage III only if the parametrium is nodular on the pelvic wall or if the growth itself extends to the pelvic wall.

Stage III — The carcinoma has extended to the pelvic wall. On rectal examination, there is no cancer-free space between the tumor and the pelvic wall.
The tumor involves the lower third of the vagina.
All cases with a hydronephrosis or nonfunctioning kidney are included unless they are known to be due to other causes.

Stage IIIA — No extension to the pelvic wall

Stage IIIB — Extension to the pelvic wall and/or hydronephrosis or nonfunctioning kidney

The presence of hydronephrosis or nonfunctioning kidney due to stenosis of the ureter by cancer permits a case to be allotted to stage III even if, according to the other findings, the case should be allotted to stage I or stage II.

The presence of bullous edema, as such, should not permit a case to be allotted to stage IV. Ridges and furrows in the bladder wall should be interpreted as signs of submucous involvement of the bladder if they remain fixed to the growth during palpation (ie, examination from the vagina or the rectum during cystoscopy). A finding of malignant cells in cytologic washings from the urinary bladder requires further examination and a biopsy from the wall of the bladder.

Stage IV — The carcinoma has extended beyond the true pelvis or has clinically involved the mucosa of the bladder or rectum. A bullous edema as such does not permit a case to be allotted to stage IV

Stage IVA — Spread of the growth to adjacent organs

Stage IVB — Spread to distant organs

*International Federation of Gynecology and Obstetrics. Annual report on the results of treatment in gynecological cancer. Vol 20. Stockholm: FIGO, 1988.

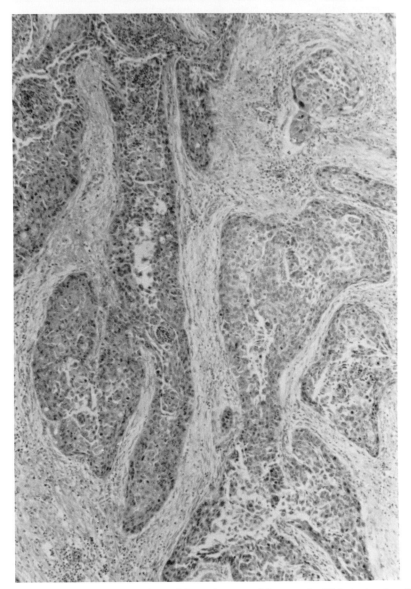

FIG. 43–5. Invasive epidermoid carcinoma of the cervix. This lesion is often designated squamous cell carcinoma.

therefore detectable cytologically. Use of a cervical brush or "broom" facilitates endocervical sampling. HPV, especially type 18, is implicated in adenocarcinoma also.

The peak incidence of carcinoma in situ occurs at about 37 years, whereas that of invasive cancer occurs about 10 years later (45 to 48 years). Because clinical signs of cervical cancer occur relatively late, success in the early detection and cure of this tumor depends on its identification in the preclinical stages. The most important means of

achieving this goal is the routine use of the Papanicolaou smear in conjunction with colposcopy and directed biopsy of suspicious lesions (see Chapter 38).

The earliest clinical signs of carcinoma of the cervix are blood-tinged leukorrhea and postcoital or contact bleeding. Pelvic pain, edema of the lower extremity (lymphatic involvement), irritability of the bladder, and rectal discomfort are late signs. Cachexia and genital tract fistulas indicate advanced disease. The tumor ultimately obstructs the

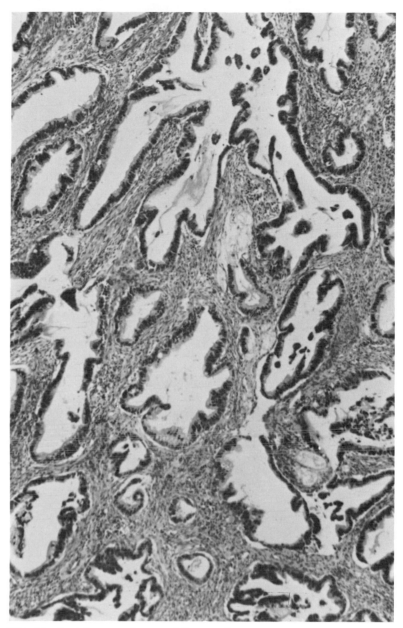

FIG. 43–6. Adenocarcinoma of the cervix.

ureters, producing uremia, the most common cause of death from carcinoma of the cervix. In advanced cases infection is often superimposed.

Successful management of carcinoma of the cervix depends on the detection of the preinvasive lesion, for intraepithelial carcinoma is curable in virtually 100% of cases. Once frank invasion occurs, the 5-year cure rate drops to about 85%. The mainstay of detection of the earliest stages of cervical cancer is the Papanicolaou smear followed by colposcopy, as indicated. A single Papanicolaou smear is only about 70% effective in detecting desquamated malignant cells from the cervix and vagina. The specimens should be obtained from the endocervical canal and portio vaginalis of the cervix. The squamocolumnar junction should be adequately sampled. Any clinically suspicious lesion should be subjected to biopsy regardless of the cytologic findings. Even during pregnancy, a colposcopically high-grade lesion requires histologic confirmation (Chapter 38).

The possibility of rendering carcinoma of the cervix a preventable disease is still far from realized because many women in the United States are not routinely screened cytologically. These women, furthermore, often belong to groups with a high prevalence of cervical carcinoma. For details of cytologic, colposcopic, and histologic terminology, refer to the respective sections of Chapter 38.

Because cytology is only a screening method, no therapy is to be based on the cytologic findings alone. Instead, a suspicious or positive smear must be investigated further. Treatment is based only on a histologic diagnosis. The management of the abnormal Papanicolaou smear is diagrammed in (Figure 43–7). Any gross lesion must be subjected at once to biopsy. A clinically normal cervix should be investigated by colposcopically directed biopsy with endocervical curettage, or cone biopsy if necessary. The number of diagnostic conizations performed has been greatly reduced by the wide use of colposcopy.

The colposcope provides a magnification of 6 to 40 times and helps determine the site for biopsy. Because colposcopy cannot detect a lesion in the endocervical canal, endocervical curettage or conization is required to rule out a lesion in that location. If the entire squamocolumnar junction cannot be visualized, conization is necessary to exclude invasive carcinoma. Colposcopy depends largely on the interpretation of vascular and epithelial patterns. A satisfactory colposcopic examination requires complete visualization of the entire squamocolumnar junction and all suspicious lesions (p. 237).

If the punch biopsies reveal invasive cancer, it is not necessary to perform a diagnostic cone. If they reveal a lesion less extensive than invasive cancer, a satisfactory colposcopy or a cone is required to rule out the coexistence of a more advanced lesion. Microinvasion on punch biopsy requires conization to rule out frank invasion.

The complications of conization include bleeding, parametritis, and injury to the internal os. Where no other method of excluding invasion is available, however, the cone is still required for diagnosis and treatment.

Staging of carcinoma of the cervix is crucial for decisions about treatment and for comparison of the results of treatment in various centers. Table 43–1 shows the current classification.

Any patient with a cervical carcinoma that may require radical surgical procedures or radiotherapy should have a diagnostic

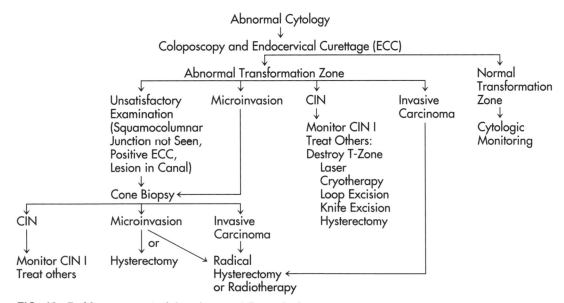

FIG. 43–7. Management of the abnormal Papanicolaou smear.

investigation that includes as a minimum the following: complete blood count, chest roentgenogram, intravenous pyelogram, cystoscopy, proctoscopy, and hepatic and renal function tests.

Although the involvement of lymph nodes does not affect the staging of carcinoma of the cervix, it does affect the prognosis. The frequencies of involvement of the lymph nodes in the various stages of cervical carcinoma are as follows: Stage I, 15%; Stage II, 30%; Stage III, 45%; and Stage IV, 60%.

The treatment of preinvasive and microinvasive carcinomas of the cervix is discussed on pp. 270 to 272. Invasive cervical cancer is treated by radical surgical procedures or radiation, depending on the stage. Surgical treatment is required for radioresistant lesions and for recurrences after full radiation. Radiation is employed in patients who present poor operative risks and for some recurrences after surgical treatment. In most cases, almost identical cure rates are obtained by surgical or radiotherapeutic means.

Stage I lesions may be treated by radical hysterectomy and pelvic lymphadenectomy or by radiation. Because the likelihood of lymph node involvement is Stage Ia lesions is less than 2%, it may be safe to treat these minimally invasive lesions as though they were intraepithelial carcinomas. Some Stage IIa lesions may be treated by radical hysterectomy, but most Stage IIb lesions are better treated by radiation. Stage III lesions are treated best by radiation. Stage IV lesions occasionally are cured by ultraradical surgical procedures such as exenteration. This drastic treatment should be employed in advanced lesions or recurrences only for cure and not for palliation.

Radiation therapy of cervical carcinoma usually involves an internal and an external source. The internal treatment typically consists of intrauterine and intravaginal radium, cesium, or other radioactive sources. ^{60}Cobalt or gamma radiation is used for the external source to increase the dose to the pelvic side walls. In certain circumstances the external therapy is delivered before the intravaginal radiation.

Radiation therapy is frequently administered by afterloading techniques. Hollow applicators designed to carry a radioactive source are implanted or inserted into the area to be treated. Their position is checked before any of the radioactive material is inserted. The advantage of this technique is the minimization of exposure of the personnel to the radiation.

Understanding the principles of radiotherapy of gynecologic cancer, particularly carcinoma of the cervix, requires definition of certain terms. A curie is a special unit of radioactivity equal to 3.70×10^{10} disintegrations per second. The curie (Ci) is based on the rate of disintegration of one gram of radium. A gamma ray is a photon emitted from the nucleus of a radioactive atom, differing from an x-ray photon only with respect to origin. A roentgen (R) is a special unit of the radiation quantity "exposure," equal to an electrical charge (produced by ionization) of 2.58×10^{-4} coulomb/kg of air. A rad is a unit of the radiation quantity "absorbed dose." One rad is equal to an energy absorption of 0.01 joule/kg. The rem (Roentgen-Equivalent-Man) is a special unit of the radiation protection quantity "dose equivalent." Dose equivalent is obtained by multiplying absorbed dose by a "quality factor." When dose is expressed in rads, dose equivalent is in rems.

Point A is an imaginary point lying 2 cm lateral to the cervical canal and 2 cm above the external cervical os. Point B lies 3 cm lateral to point A and is used as a means of evaluating the dosage to the pelvic wall.

Complications of radical surgical procedures include fistulas, hemorrhage, and immediate operative death. Blood volume should be measured before any radical procedures and the central venous pressure monitored during and after operation. Complications of radiation include urinary frequency (cystitis), diarrhea (frequently bloody), and bowel fistulas. Stenosis of the vagina and dyspareunia may also result.

Carcinoma of the cervix complicated by pregnancy requires special consideration. Carcinoma in situ may be managed conservatively, provided every effort has been made to rule out invasion. The pregnancy may be carried to term and the patient delivered vaginally. Definitive treatment may be performed post partum. Invasive cancer must be treated during pregnancy as in the nonpregnant state. In the first trimester, the patient may be subjected to radical hysterectomy or radiation treatment (which produces abortion). In the third trimester, maximal delay of a few weeks to ensure reasonable likelihood of fetal survival may be justified before cesarean section and definitive treatment are performed. In the second trimester, it is usually necessary to treat the carcinoma despite the nonviability or immaturity of the fetus. The patient must be involved in the decision to treat at this stage of gestation.

The survival in carcinoma of the cervix depends on the staging, which in turn is influenced by the success of the screening program. A successful program will result in a higher proportion of intraepithelial and early invasive lesions. The 5-year prognosis by stage is as follows: Stage 0—almost 100%, Stage I—85–90% (approximately equal by radiation or radical surgery); Stage II—65–75%, and Stage III—35–40% (these stages are generally better treated by radiation); and Stage IV—approximately 5–15% (by ultraradical surgical procedures).

44
CHAPTER

UTERINE MYOMAS AND OTHER BENIGN DISEASES OF THE CORPUS

The uterine corpus has a thick muscularis, the myometrium. Its internal surface is lined by mucous membrane, the endometrium, composed of columnar epithelium and simple tubular glands that extend deep into the lamina propria. Under the influence of the hypothalamus, the hypophysis, and the ovary, the endometrium undergoes the changes of the menstrual cycle.

The lamina propria of the uterus consists of three layers: a superficial stratum compactum, a middle stratum spongiosum, and a deep stratum basale. The compactum and spongiosum are made of cellular connective tissue and are nourished by coiled arteries. The stratum basale is made of dense cellular connective tissue and is vascularized by straight arteries. The stratum compactum and stratum spongiosum together form the stratum functionale, most of which is sloughed during the menstrual period. During menses, pieces of the endometrium are discarded irregularly; the entire endometrium does not slough simultaneously. While parts of it are degenerating, other areas already have begun to regenerate.

MENSTRUATION

At the time of menstruation, the hypothalamus signals the hypophysis to secrete FSH, which initiates the development of immature follicles and stimulates the production of estrogen. Under the influence of estrogen, the regenerative phase begins with proliferation of the epithelium lining the glands embedded in the stratum basale. The epithelium spreads over the surface denuded by the sloughing of the stratum functionale. Initially it is flat, but later in the cycle it changes to low cuboidal and then simple columnar, with some of the cells ciliated and others secretory.

As levels of estrogen rise, the hypothalamus secretes gonadotropin-releasing hormone (GnRH), which stimulates the adenohypophysis to produce and release LH. The midcyclic surge of LH and FSH appears to trigger ovulation. LH stimulates the resulting corpus hemorrhagicum to develop into the corpus luteum.

If implantation does not occur, the high titers of progesterone cause the pituitary to stop producing LH; as a result, the corpus luteum degenerates. As the blood level of progesterone falls, the coiled arteries that supply the stratum compactum and stratum spongiosum contract, with resulting ischemia and endometrial sloughing (menstruation). The falling levels of estrogen stimulate the hypophysis to secrete FSH, and a new group of immature follicles begins to develop.

THE ENDOMETRIAL CYCLE

In the early proliferative phase, the mucosa is low and the glands are short, narrow, and straight (Fig. 44–1). As the proliferative

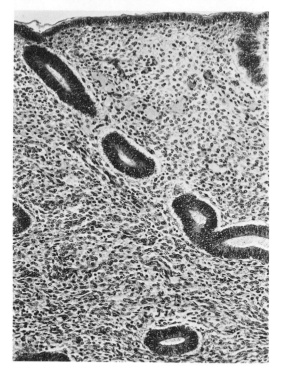

FIG. 44–1. Early proliferative endometrium, showing short, straight, narrow glands.

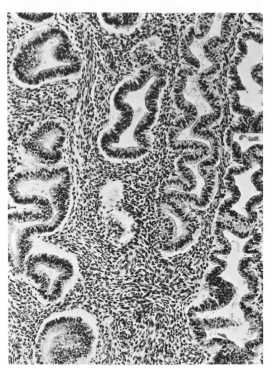

FIG. 44–2. Late proliferative endometrium, showing elongated, tortuous glands with pseudostratified nuclei.

phase advances, the glands become longer, thicker, and more tortuous (Fig. 44–2). Mitotic figures are seen in the endometrial epithelium throughout the proliferative but not in the secretory phase. The first sign of ovulation that can be detected with the light microscope is the subnuclear vacuole, on approximately the sixteenth day of a typical 28-day cycle (Fig. 44–3). During the first few days of the postovulatory (secretory) phase, the subnuclear vacuoles move past the nuclei to reach the lumina of the endometrial glands. By about day 21 (midsecretory phase), the glandular epithelium has become low and the endometrial secretions and stromal edema have provided an ideal bed in which the ovum may implant (Fig. 44–4). By day 25 (late secretory), the cytoplasmic borders of the glandular cells have become ragged and secretory exhaustion occurs (Fig. 44–5). The second half of the secretory phase, or the last week of the menstrual cycle, is concerned with changes in the stroma. In a cycle in which pregnancy does not occur, the secretory (premenstrual) endometrium regresses and menstruation

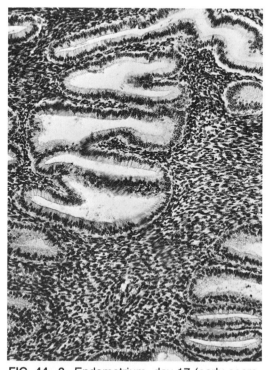

FIG. 44–3. Endometrium, day 17 (early secretory), showing subnuclear vacuoles.

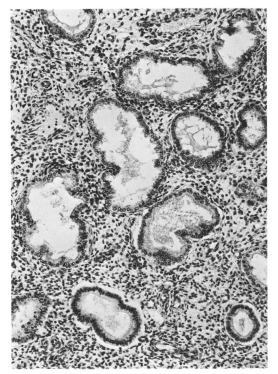

FIG. 44–4. Endometrium, day 21 (midsecretory), showing glands with intraluminal secretion and loose stroma.

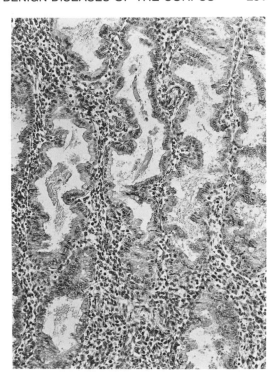

FIG. 44–5. Endometrium, day 25 (late secretory), showing serrated glands with inspissated secretion.

follows. If pregnancy occurs, the stromal changes progress to form a decidua, which begins first around the endometrial arteries (Fig. 44–6).

Morphologic signs of ovulation can be detected with the electron microscope almost 2 days earlier than with the light microscope. A subnuclear accumulation of glycogen is ultrastructurally evident on day 14. Additional electron microscopic features of the early postovulatory endometrium are the giant mitochondria (Fig. 44–7) and the characteristic nuclear channel system (Fig. 44–8).

MYOMAS

Myomas are the commonest benign tumors of the uterus. About 25% of women over 30 have palpable myomas. They are found most commonly in women in their thirties and forties and are larger and more common in black patients. The lesion consists of interlacing bundles of smooth muscle with

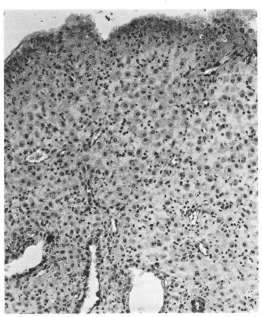

FIG. 44–6. Decidua parietalis, showing round and polygonal stromal cells.

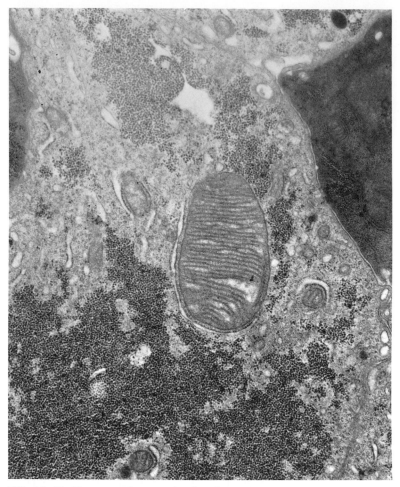

FIG. 44–7. Electron micrograph of endometrium on day 17, showing giant mitochondrion adjacent to deposit of glycogen.

only rare mitotic figures (Fig. 44–9). For this reason, the tumors should be termed myomas or leiomyomas rather than fibroids. Since myomas are surrounded by a pseudocapsule of condensed uterine tissue, unlike adenomyomas or sarcomas, they may be enucleated from the normal myometrium, usually with minimal loss of blood.

The tumors range in size from microscopic lesions to huge masses filling the abdomen. They may be located within the myometrium (intramural); they may protrude from the external surface of the uterus (subserous); or they may project into the uterine cavity (submucous). The subserous and submucous varieties may be sessile or pedunculated. Tumors may grow between the leaves of the broad ligament (intraligamentous), displacing the ureters and subjecting them to danger of injury during hysterectomy. Occasionally a myoma may detach from the uterus and obtain a new blood supply from another organ (parasitic myoma).

Large myomas frequently outgrow their blood supply and undergo degeneration, including hyalinization, liquefaction, calcification (detectable radiologically), formation of bone and fat, and necrosis (occasionally characterized by pain and leukocytosis). Carneous, or red, degeneration, usually occurring during pregnancy, is one of the few changes in a myoma (other than torsion) that is associated with pain. Sarcoma occurs in only a fraction of 1% of myomas.

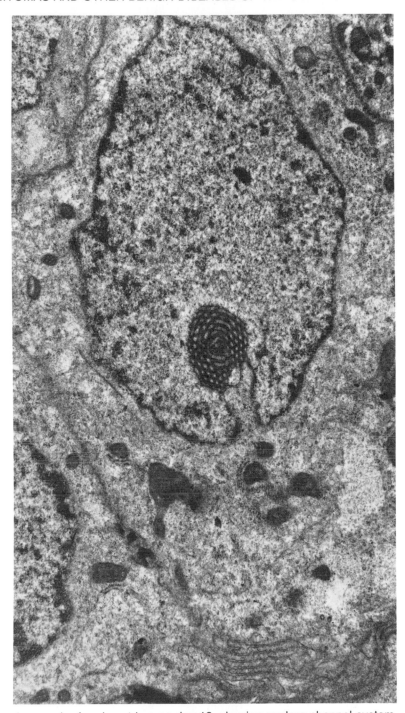

FIG. 44-8. Electron micrograph of endometrium on day 19, showing nuclear channel system.

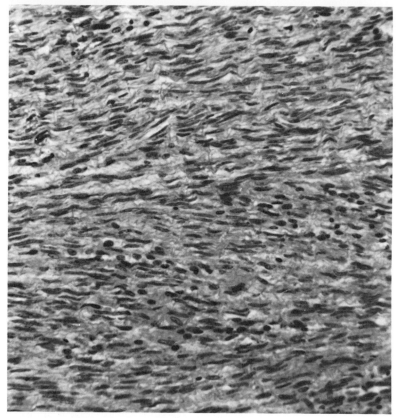

FIG. 44–9. Benign cellular myoma of the uterus.

Myomas appear to be under estrogenic control. They are tumors of the reproductive years and may be associated with other endocrine-dependent lesions such as endometrial hyperplasia and polyps, adenomyosis, and endometriosis. They may grow during pregnancy and with use of oral contraceptives that contain large amounts of estrogen.

Myomas do not grow after the menopause in the absence of exogenous estrogen. Tumors that appear after the menopause and all cases of postmenopausal bleeding must be attributed to other causes. The most prominent sign of myomas is abnormal uterine bleeding. The bleeding typically begins as prolonged menses (hypermenorrhea, or menorrhagia), which may be sufficiently severe to cause anemia. Intermenstrual bleeding may occur with extensive myomas but should suggest another lesion. The abnormal bleeding may be a result of increased surface area of the endometrium or interference by the myomas with normal uterine hemostasis.

Myomas may cause dysmenorrhea and a sensation of bearing down. Only rarely, even if large, do they obstruct the urinary tract or the bowel. A myoma protruding through the cervix may cause uterine cramps. Except when complicated by torsion, infarction, or carneous degeneration, myomas usually do not cause pain, which should therefore be attributed to another lesion, often pelvic inflammatory disease or endometriosis.

Myomas have often been implicated in infertility, although associated lesions such as pelvic inflammatory disease or endometriosis are more often the cause. Myomas may lead to infertility by blocking the ascent of spermatozoa, occluding the oviduct, or interfering with implantation. If a pregnancy occurs, there is a greater likelihood of premature labor and delivery, abnormal presentations, dystocia, dysfunctional labor, and postpartum hemorrhage.

Diagnosis of myomas is made by history; an irregular, firm, nodular uterus on pelvic examination; and if necessary hysterosalpingography or hysteroscopy to demonstrate a filling defect (submucous myomas). Differential diagnosis includes pregnancy, ovarian tumors, and uterine anomalies. The pregnant uterus is usually softer and more symmetrical and the chorionic gonadotropin test is positive. It is impossible on physical examination to distinguish myomas from ovarian tumors with certainty after the aggregate pelvic mass has reached 12 weeks' gestational size. By that time, the tumor has risen above the pelvic brim and the ovaries can no longer be palpated separately. Ultrasound may be helpful in differential diagnosis in such cases.

It is most important that the cause of bleeding in a patient with myomas be ascertained before hysterectomy. Bleeding in a patient with myomas does not necessarily stem from the myomas. It may be the result of a less serious lesion, such as an endometrial polyp, or a more serious disease such as carcinoma of the cervix or corpus. A Papanicolaou smear should therefore precede definitive therapy of myomas. If there is abnormal bleeding, a fractional curettage is also required.

Management of myomas may be conservative or may entail myomectomy or hysterectomy. No treatment is required in a woman of reproductive age if the tumors do not cause bleeding, pain, or infertility, and if they are less than 12 weeks' gestational size. In a patient near the menopause, conservative therapy may be employed after a curettage has ruled out a malignant lesion. Postmenopausal bleeding requires immediate diagnosis and treatment.

The usual treatment of symptomatic myomas has been hysterectomy, although hormonal manipulation with GnRH agonists is often effective. Myomectomy is logically performed only in a woman of reproductive age who desires children and in whom there is no other factor preventing pregnancy. Laparotomy is indicated for any mass greater than 12 weeks' size to rule out an ovarian tumor. A smaller myoma in a patient near the menopause may be managed conservatively if asymptomatic. Rapid growth in the absence of pregnancy or oral contraceptives requires investigation.

The gonadotropin-releasing hormone (GnRH) agonists (Synarel and Lupron) block pituitary stimulation of the ovary and stop production of estrogen. In some patients, the drug may cause complete disappearance of the tumor or at least significant diminution in its size so that myomectomy with preservation of the uterus may be accomplished more easily. If hysterectomy is still required, the smaller uterus is removed more readily through the vagina or through a transverse abdominal incision. Suppression of ovarian function by GnRH agonists may be so severe as to cause hot flashes, vaginal atrophy, and osteoporosis. Such treatment therefore should not exceed 6 months in duration.

A small uterus may be removed by the vaginal route, but very large myomas are best removed by total abdominal hysterectomy. The decision to remove the ovaries is based on their condition and the patient's age.

POLYPS

Endometrial polyps are finger-like projections of the endometrium into the uterine cavity. They consist of glands and stroma and vary from microscopic size to several centimeters in length (Fig. 44–10). In only a small percentage of cases does malignant change occur. Polyps are found in all age groups, but mostly in older women. They present with intermenstrual or postmenopausal bleeding. Diagnosis is made by fractional curettage, which may also be therapeutic. The differential diagnosis includes endocervical polyps, myomas, and carcinomas of the cervix and endometrium.

A placental polyp may occasionally simulate the more common endometrial polyp. It is a cause of delayed postpartum bleeding and it is recognized histologically by remnants of chorionic villi overgrown by regenerating endometrium.

HYPERPLASIAS

Endometrial hyperplasia entails glandular crowding and is generally associated with chronic unopposed estrogenic stimulation. The hyperplasias are classified according to the severity of their architectural disturbance and the degree of cytologic abnormality (atypia). A simple and clinically useful classification of hyperplasias of the endometrium is: simple, complex, simple atypical,

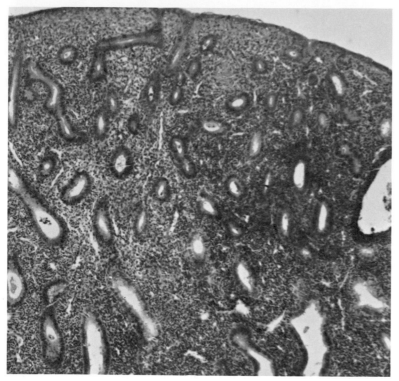

FIG. 44–10. Endometrial polyp, showing numerous glands and inflammatory cells.

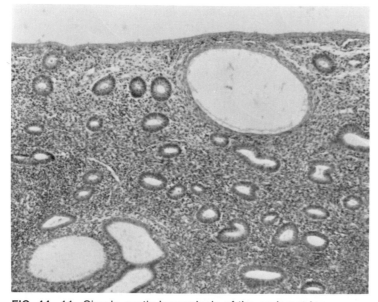

FIG. 44–11. Simple cystic hyperplasia of the endometrium.

and complex atypical. These four hyperplasias are said to progress to carcinoma in the following percentages of cases: Simple—1%; complex—3%; simple atypical—8%; and complex atypical—29%. An even simpler classification has been proposed by the International Society of Gynecological Pathologists: simple hyperplasia, complex hyperplasia, and atypical hyperplasia (regardless of architectural complexity).

Simple hyperplasia, with or without formation of cysts (Fig. 44–11), has very little if any malignant potential. It is essentially a benign proliferation of endometrial glands unassociated with cytologic or architectural abnormalities. Complex hyperplasia refers to lesions in which marked structural abnormality with back-to-back crowding of glands is seen but without cytologic atypia. In complex atypical hyperplasia, in addition to the architectural crowding, there is cytologic abnormality, such as nuclear atypia and loss of polarity.

Most patients with endometrial hyperplasia present with abnormal uterine bleeding. Diagnosis is made by formal curettage or endometrial sampling as an office procedure. Simple and complex hyperplasias without atypia generally respond to treatment with a progestational agent and revert to normal. Atypical hyperplasia may also respond to hormonal therapy and, if it does, it requires no further treatment. If atypical hyperplasia persists, hysterectomy is the treatment of choice.

45
CHAPTER

MALIGNANT NEOPLASMS OF THE CORPUS

CARCINOMAS

Carcinoma of the corpus accounts for almost half of all gynecologic cancers. In recent years, it has become the most common gynecologic cancer in the United States. Carcinoma of the corpus (endometrial cancer) affects predominantly menopausal and postmenopausal women. Its peak incidence is at age 55, or 10 years later than that of carcinoma of the cervix. In white patients of low parity and high socioeconomic status, carcinoma of the cervix is less common than carcinoma of the corpus, whereas in black patients of low socioeconomic status and high parity, the ratio of cancer of the cervix to cancer of the corpus may be as high as 10:1.

There is abundant evidence to support the relation of unopposed estrogen and anovulation to carcinoma of the corpus. The risk of carcinoma of the corpus in postmenopausal women receiving replacement therapy with estrogens is increased between threefold and eightfold (p. 342), although it can be minimized by the use of a progestin for 10 to 14 days each month. Carcinoma of the corpus is found more commonly in the obese nullipara and the patient with a late menopause and poor fertility. Hypertension, diabetes, and cardiovascular disease are often associated. Obesity appears to be the most significant risk factor in endometrial

carcinoma. Adrenal androstenedione is converted to estrone in adipose tissue; the estrone, in turn, is converted to estradiol, a potent stimulator of the endometrium.

Cancers of the endometrium are usually adenocarcinomas (Fig. 45–1). The in-situ form may be indistinguishable from severe complex atypical hyperplasia. The glands are crowded back to back, with individual cells exhibiting the criteria of malignancy.

A significant proportion of adenocarcinomas of the endometrium exhibit some form of squamous metaplasia. In cases in which the squamous component appears benign, the tumor is called adenocanthoma. When the squamous component appears to be malignant, the tumor is called adenosquamous carcinoma. A rare pure form of squamous carcinoma of the endometrium is also found. The prognosis of the carcinoma is related to the histologic grade of the glandular component. Endometrial carcinomas may also be of the clear cell type. A particularly aggressive form of adenocarcinoma is the papillary serous carcinoma, which spreads early to distant sites and has a poor prognosis.

Carcinoma of the endometrium may remain localized in the uterus for a long while and then may spread widely by the vascular route. Extension may occur also along the peritoneum or by penetration of the myometrium. Pyometra is an occasional compli-

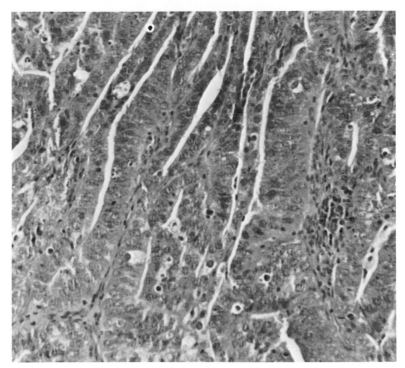

FIG. 45–1. Well differentiated adenocarcinoma of the endometrium.

cation. About 10% metastasize early to the ovary. When spread occurs to the cervix, the behavior and treatment of the tumor resemble those of carcinoma of the cervix. Prognosis of endometrial carcinoma is adversely affected by poor differentiation of the tumor and vascular involvement.

The main sign of carcinoma of the corpus is metrorrhagia (intermenstrual bleeding). Older women usually present with postmenopausal bleeding. In some series, about one third of all cases of postmenopausal bleeding are caused by carcinoma of the corpus.

The Papanicolaou smear is less reliable for diagnosis in this disease than in carcinoma of the cervix. Results may be improved by several techniques that sample the endometrium directly, such as the aspiration curettage, but the mainstay of diagnosis is conventional curettage. A fractional curettage may be performed to distinguish adenocarcinoma of the corpus from that of the cervix. A hysterosalpingogram should not be performed in the presence of suspected carcinoma of the corpus. Hysteroscopy to locate the lesion precisely and describe its intrauterine extent is not yet standard practice for this purpose, but it appears promising.

Carcinoma of the endometrium is now staged surgically, in much the same way as carcinoma of the ovary. Surgical staging minimizes the importance of preoperative fractional curettage and increases reliance on careful examination and histologic sampling of the corpus, cervix, ovaries, and lymph nodes after hysterectomy. Although imaging techniques are not included in the surgical staging, they may be helpful in evaluating certain selected patients. The techniques include computed tomography (CT), lymphangiography, and especially, magnetic resonance imaging (MRI). The new FIGO classification of endometrial carcinoma is shown in Table 45–1.

The standard treatment for nonserous carcinomas of the endometrium includes total abdominal hysterectomy, bilateral salpingo-oophorectomy, sampling of lymph nodes, and postoperative radiation that is based on the surgical stage of the disease. Papillary serous carcinoma requires, in addition, omentectomy followed by che-

TABLE 45–1. FIGO STAGING OF CARCINOMA OF THE CORPUS UTERI*

Stage IA G123	Tumor limited to endometrium	G2 = 6–50% of a nonsquamous or nonmorular solid growth pattern
Stage IB G123	Invasion to less than one-half the myometrium	G3 = more than 50% of a nonsquamous or nonmorular solid growth pattern
Stage IC G123	Invasion to more than one-half the myometrium	**Notes on pathologic grading:**
Stage IIA G123	Endocervical glandular involvement only	1) Notable nuclear atypia, inappropriate for the architectural grade, raises the grade of a grade 1 or grade 2 tumor by 1.
Stage IIB G123	Cervical stromal invasion	
Stage IIIA G123	Tumor invades serosa and/or adnexa, and/or positive peritoneal cytology	2) In serous adenocarcinomas, clear-cell adenocarcinomas, and squamous cell carcinomas, nuclear grading takes precedence.
Stage IIIB G123	Vaginal metastases	3) Adenocarcinomas with squamous differentiation are graded according to the nuclear grade of the glandular component.
Stage IIIC G123	Metastases to pelvic and/or paraaortic lymph nodes	**Rules related to staging:**
Stage IVA G123	Tumor invasion of bladder and/or bowel mucosa	1) Because corpus cancer is now staged surgically, procedures previously used for determination of stages are no longer applicable, such as the findings from fractional D&C to differentiate between stage I and stage II.
Stage IVB	Distant metastases including intraabdominal and/or inguinal lymph nodes	2) It is appreciated that there may be a small number of patients with corpus cancer who will be treated primarily with radiation therapy. If that is the case, the clinical staging adopted by FIGO in 1971 would still apply, but designation of that staging system would be noted.
Histopathology—degree of differentiation:		
Cases of carcinoma of the corpus should be classified (or graded) according to the degree of histologic differentiation, as follows:		3) Ideally, width of the myometrium should be measured along with the width of tumor invasion.
GI = 5% or less of a nonsquamous or nonmorular solid growth pattern		

*International Federation of Gynecology and Obstetrics. Annual report on the results of treatment in gynecological cancer. Int J Gynecol Obstet 1989; 28:189–190.

motherapy and radiation to the entire abdomen.

Stages IA and IB are generally managed by total abdominal hysterectomy, bilateral salpingo-oophorectomy, sampling of nodes, and cytologic washings. No further therapy is required for most well-differentiated lesions. Stage IC requires postoperative radiotherapy with or without vaginal cesium. Stage II is managed most commonly by pelvic radiotherapy with or without vaginal cesium. Stage III A is managed with pelvic radiotherapy with or without P^{32}, Stage III B with pelvic radiotherapy with or without vaginal cesium, and Stage III C with pelvic and paraaortic radiotherapy. Stage IV disease is managed by palliative radiotherapy with or without progestins or by chemotherapy.

The prognosis for disease-free survival of patients with well-differentiated Stage I lesions should be close to 100%. The prognosis for all Stage I lesions is close to 80%. In Stage II, the cure rate drops to about 60%. In Stage III, it is about 30%, and in Stage IV, it is less than 10%. The total 5-year survival in carcinoma of the corpus is between 60 and 70% The prognosis for papillary serous carcinoma is poorer in all stages.

SARCOMAS

Sarcoma of the corpus is much less common than carcinoma of the endometrium in the United States. Leiomyosarcoma is the commonest of the pure homologous sarcomas (Fig. 45–2). It may arise from the normal

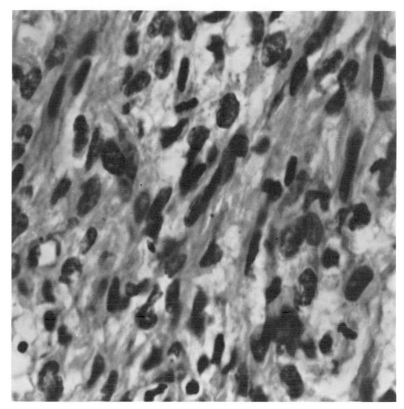

FIG. 45—2. Leiomyosarcoma of the uterus, showing numerous malignant cells with bizarre nuclei.

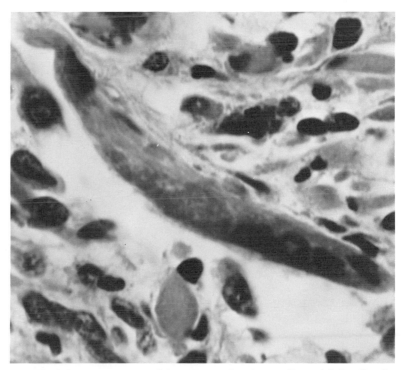

FIG. 45—3. Rhabdomyosarcoma of the uterus, showing malignant "strap" cell.

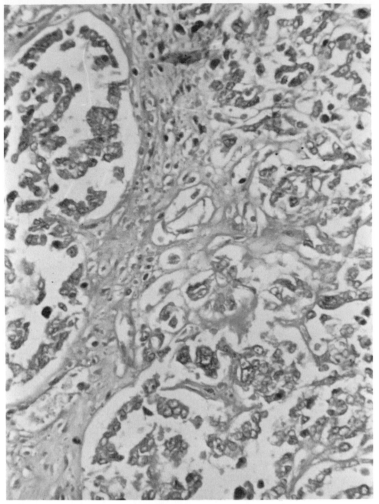

FIG. 45–4. Malignant mixed müllerian tumor of the uterus, showing malignant stromal and epithelial components.

myometrium or from a myoma. It presents with bleeding and vaginal discharge and may be suspected when an apparent myoma grows rapidly. The treatment is total abdominal hysterectomy and bilateral salpingo-oophorectomy. The additional benefit of radiation is questionable. Cellular myomas may be difficult to distinguish histopathologically from low-grade leiomyosarcomas. Generally, if the lesion contains 10 or more mitotic figures/10 high-power fields, it is considered a sarcoma. If there are only 5 to 9 mitotic figures/10 high-power fields but there is associated moderate to marked atypia, that lesion is also considered a sarcoma.

TABLE 45–2. SIMPLIFIED CLASSIFICATION OF UTERINE SARCOMAS

Pure sarcomas
  Pure homologous
    Leiomyosarcoma
    Endometrial stromal sarcoma
    Angiosarcoma
  Pure heterologous
    Rhabdomyosarcoma
    Chondrosarcoma
    Osteosarcoma
Mixed sarcomas (homologous or heterologous)
Mixed müllerian tumors
    Adenosarcoma (epithelial component benign)
    Malignant mixed müllerian (adenocarcinoma with homologous or heterologous sarcoma)
Malignant lymphoma

Sarcomas may also arise from the endometrial stroma or from heterologous elements (Fig. 45–3). These tumors, as well as malignant mixed müllerian lesions (Fig. 45–4), which are currently being reported in greater numbers, are treated by total abdominal hysterectomy and bilateral salpingo-oophorectomy. The effect of radiation is small and the prognosis is generally poor. Adjunctive chemotherapy with Adriamycin has proved helpful in patients with Stage I and Stage II sarcomas. In parts of Africa, malignant mixed müllerian tumors are much more common than they are in the United States. A simplified classification of uterine sarcomas is shown in Table 45–2.

46

CHAPTER

TUMORS OF THE OVIDUCT

Adenomatoid tumors (benign mesotheliomas) are the most common benign neoplasms of the oviduct. Benign neoplasms of the fallopian tube include myomas, hemangiomas, and fibromas, all very uncommon lesions. The more common parovarian cysts (Fig. 46–1), such as the hydatid of Morgagni, are of little clinical significance. Many of these structures, formerly considered to be of mesonephric origin, are now believed to be paramesonephric. Walthard rests, which may be found in the perisalpinx and elsewhere in the female genital tract, consist of the same epithelioid cells (Fig. 46–2) that are found in the Brenner tumor of the ovary (p. 304).

The fallopian tube is the least common site of carcinoma of the female genitalia. On physical examination, tubal neoplasms are commonly confused with ovarian masses.

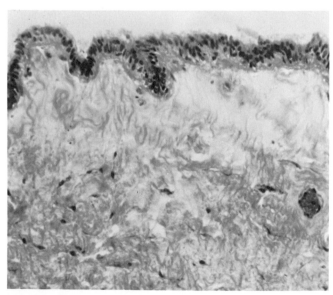

FIG. 46–1. Parovarian cyst with cuboidal epithelial lining.

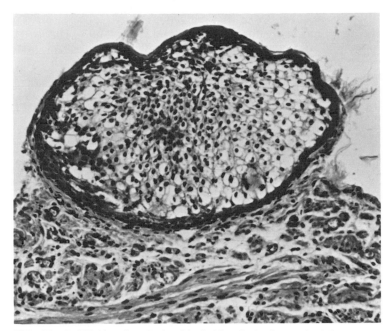

FIG. 46–2. Walthard rest of epithelioid cells in the perisalpinx.

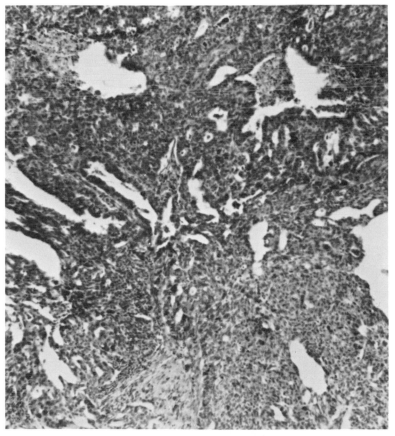

FIG. 46–3. Adenocarcinoma of the fallopian tube.

Histologically, cancer of the oviduct is usually an adenocarcinoma (Fig. 46–3), which spreads locally and by lymphatics. The lesion may present with vaginal bleeding, lower abdominal pain, and watery vaginal discharge (hydrorrhea). It should be suspected when curettings are negative in women with postmenopausal bleeding, particularly if there is an adnexal mass. The lesion is often found accidentally at laparotomy. Treatment is total abdominal hysterectomy and bilateral salpingo-oophorectomy, followed by chemotherapy with several agents (e.g., Cytoxan, Adriamycin, and cis-platinum) according to the pattern of spread. Carcinoma in the fallopian tube is more often metastatic, usually from the ovary or corpus.

47
CHAPTER

THE OVARY AND OVULATION

The gross anatomy of the ovary is discussed on page 19. The mesovarium is covered by squamous mesothelium. At the point where it attaches to the ovary, the epithelium, becomes cuboidal, the so-called germinal epithelium. On section, the ovary consists of an outer cortex and an inner medulla. The cortex comprises dense cellular connective tissue and many follicles and corpora lutea in various stages of maturity or degeneration. The medulla comprises loose connective tissue, large blood vessels, and degenerated corpora lutea (corpora albicantia).

The ovary at birth contains huge numbers of germ cells (Fig. 47–1). Immature ovarian follicles consist of an ovocyte I (primary ovocyte, or primary oocyte) surrounded by a layer of follicular cells. As it matures, the ovocyte I develops a thick membrane, the zona pellucida. As development continues, a cellular and highly vascular theca interna forms around the zona pellucida. The fibrous layer separating the theca interna from the surrounding stroma of the ovary is the theca externa.

After each menstrual period, 15 to 20 immature follicles begin to develop under the influence of FSH from the anterior lobe of the pituitary. Development is arrested in most of these follicles at various stages, and each collapses and degenerates into a corpus atreticum surrounded by a characteristic glassy membrane. Each month, however, one of the follicles continues to grow. The follicular cells multiply and small intercellular spaces appear. Coalescence of these spaces forms an antral cavity, which is lined with follicular cells (the stratum granulosum) and filled with liquor folliculi. The ovocyte I surrounded by the zona pellucida is coated by one or more layers of follicular cells, the corona radiata (Fig. 47–2). This complex is embedded in follicular cells on one side of the antral cavity, the cumulus oophorus. As liquor folliculi accumulates, the follicle enlarges to such an extent that it produces a bulge on the surface of the ovary. The theca interna surrounding the follicle produces estrogen.

At about midcycle, there is a surge in FSH and LH from the hypophysis. The first meiotic division occurs at this time, producing the ovocyte II (secondary ovocyte) and the reduced body I (polocyte I, or first polar body). Shortly thereafter, the follicle ruptures at the stigma, and the ovocyte II inside its zona pellucida and surrounded by the corona radiata is shed into the peritoneal cavity or extruded directly into the fimbriated end of the oviduct, where it begins its journey towards the uterus. At the time of ovulation, the ovocyte II begins its second meiotic division, but this process is arrested at metaphase. The reduced body II and the

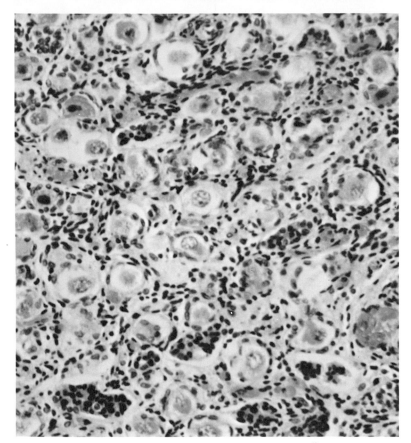

FIG. 47–1. Ovary at birth, showing numerous germ cells.

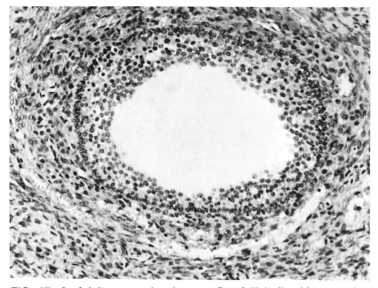

FIG. 47–2. Adult ovary, showing graafian follicle lined by granulosa cells.

ovum are not produced unless fertilization, which usually takes place in the ampulla of the oviduct, occurs.

Rupture of the ovarian follicle is accompanied by some bleeding. The resulting blood clot and remaining follicular cells are organized into a corpus hemorrhagicum, which in turn gives rise to the corpus luteum. The follicular cells of the stratum granulosum develop into an inner cell mass of large vacuolated cells, the granulosa lutein cells, which produce progesterone. The cells of the theca interna continue to produce estrogen. If fertilization occurs, the corpus luteum enlarges and helps maintain pregnancy during the first trimester. If fertilization does not occur, the corpus luteum degenerates into a fibrous corpus albicans.

48

CHAPTER

TUMORS OF THE OVARY

All adnexal masses must be considered potential ovarian neoplasms until proved otherwise. Of all ovarian tumors, about 30 to 40% are malignant. As the detection and treatment of early carcinomas of the cervix and corpus improve, carcinoma of the ovary becomes increasingly important. In some series, the ovary is the most common site of gynecologic cancer, but in general ovarian carcinoma accounts for about 25% of all female genital cancers although it may be the leading cause of death from gynecologic cancer. Ovarian cancer affects all age groups, with the greatest frequency in the 50- to 60-year-old group.

The ovary is unusual in that it is a common site of both primary and metastatic lesions. The poor prognosis is related to several factors: there is no detectable in-situ form of ovarian cancer; spread occurs rapidly by peritoneal implantation as well as vascular and lymphatic channels; and there are no early signs and symptoms. Routine vaginal cytology has not been effective in detecting preclinical ovarian carcinoma.

The clinical manifestations of ovarian cancer suggest an advanced lesion. They include abdominal pain, increase in abdominal girth, palpable abdominal and pelvic masses, gastrointestinal and urinary tract complaints, ascites, and thrombophlebitis. Nonspecific lower abdominal complaints and dysmenorrhea are more common than irregular vaginal bleeding. Anorexia and

cachexia occur still later. Any ovarian tumor may cause an acute surgical emergency through accidents such as rupture, torsion, hemorrhage, infection, infarction, and incarceration.

Differential diagnosis includes carcinoma of the rectum or sigmoid, diverticulosis, retroperitoneal tumors, ectopic pregnancy, pelvic kidney, endometriosis, pelvic inflammatory disease, and pregnancy. The lesion with which a solid tumor of the ovary is most commonly confused is a uterine myoma. An enlarging pelvic mass of gynecologic origin in the postmenopausal patient must be assumed to be an ovarian cancer, because myomas do not grow after the menopause (p. 284). An ovarian cyst may be differentiated from ascites by physical findings (p. 31).

MANAGEMENT

Detection of an ovarian tumor is followed by laparotomy without delay except in special circumstances: in a woman in the reproductive years, a cystic unilateral mass less than 5 cm in diameter may be managed conservatively because it may well be a functional cyst of the ovary. Proper management in such cases involves reexamination of the patient in about 6 weeks. Ovulation may be suppressed by oral contraceptives during the period of observation to avoid confusion resulting from the formation of a new functional cyst. If the mass has regressed, no further treatment is required. If it has remained stationary or enlarged, laparotomy is indicated. In all other cases, prompt laparotomy is required for ovarian tumors, including all solid or bilateral masses and all tumors greater than 5 to 6 cm in diameter. A palpable ovary of normal size or larger in a postmenopausal woman should be regarded as a possible malignant tumor.

Diagnostic measures before laparotomy often include computed tomography with contrast, sonography, proctoscopy, and upper or lower gastrointestinal roentgenograms, depending on the symptoms and signs. A scout film of the abdomen may identify the opacity characteristic of a benign cystic teratoma or may visualize a tooth or piece of bone.

STAGING

Staging of ovarian carcinoma is done at the time of laparotomy (surgical staging). Because of the enormous variety of histologic types and the individualization of management required, operations on patients with suspected carcinoma of the ovary should be performed only by the gynecologist who is thoroughly familiar with the surgical pathology. The laparotomy for ovarian cancer should include inspection and biopsy of the undersurface of the diaphragm and the retroperitoneal lymph nodes, with biopsy of other suspicious lesions, cytologic examination of peritoneal washings, omentectomy, and aggressive removal of all grossly visible tumor. A vertical incision should be used.

Staging of ovarian carcinoma is based on findings during surgical exploration. The histologic features of the tumor and the cytologic findings in the effusions require consideration in the staging. Biopsies of suspicious areas outside the pelvis are desirable. The current FIGO classification is shown in Table 48–1.

TREATMENT

Enucleation of the tumor or unilateral oophorectomy is acceptable treatment only for well-encapsulated benign tumors or possibly Stage Ia grade 1 carcinomas in young women. The basic surgical treatment for malignant tumors of the ovary is total abdominal hysterectomy with bilateral salpingo-oophorectomy. Aggressive removal of masses of tumor (debulking) and the omentum (to remove microscopic metastases) is indicated and even ultraradical procedures are sometimes justified. The amount of residual cancer after definitive surgical treatment is negatively correlated with ultimate survival. Occasionally, postoperative radiation may be used to treat a technically inoperable lesion. This radiation may shrink the tumor sufficiently to allow a second, more successful operation. Because most ovarian tumors are not highly radiosensitive, the role of radiotherapy as primary treatment for ovarian carcinoma is controversial. Its success is related to accuracy of staging, adequacy of fields of treatment, and time-dose relations.

Chemotherapy is the primary means of treating persistent or recurrent ovarian cancer. Rates of response as high as 85% and long-term survival approaching 30% even in Stage III disease have been reported. The effectiveness of chemotherapy depends on the volume of residual tumor after surgical resection, the histologic type and grade of the tumor, and the original stage of the disease. A second laparotomy with biopsy of suspicious areas should be performed before discontinuing chemotherapy. If microscopic disease is found at the time of the "second look," intraperitoneal P^{32} may be instilled to increase salvage.

Combined chemotherapy involves use of several classes of drugs, including alkylating agents such as Cytoxan, antimetabolites such as methotrexate, and antibiotics such as Adriamycin. Cisplatinum and hexamethylmelamine, especially when used in combination with Adriamycin and Cytoxan, are beneficial. Although these drugs may prolong life, serious side effects may occur, including leukopenia and gastrointestinal disturbances. During chemotherapy, the leukocyte and platelet counts must be monitored carefully. Intraperitoneal administration of chemotherapeutic agents is still investigational, but shows great promise. This technique provides high local concentrations of drug with minimal systemic toxicity. Management of incurable cancer of the

TABLE 48–1. FIGO STAGING OF CARCINOMA OF THE OVARY*

Staging of ovarian carcinoma is based on findings at clinical examination and by surgical exploration. The histologic findings are to be considered in the staging, as are the cytologic findings as far as effusions are concerned. it is desirable that a biopsy be taken from suspicious areas outside of the pelvis.

Stage I	Growth limited to the ovaries
Stage IA	Growth limited to one ovary; no ascites present containing malignant cells. No tumor on the external surface; capsule intact
Stage IB	Growth limited to both ovaries; no ascites present containing malignant cells. No tumor on the external surfaces; capsules intact
Stage IC[†]	Tumor classified as either stage IA or IB but with tumor on the surface of one or both ovaries; or with ruptured capsule(s); or with ascites containing malignant cells present or with positive peritoneal washings
Stage II	Growth involving one or both ovaries, with pelvic extension
Stage IIA	Extension and/or metastases to the uterus and/or tubes
Stage IIB	Extension to other pelvic tissues
Stage IIC[†]	Tumor either stage IIA or IIB but with tumor on the surface of one or both ovaries; or with capsule(s) ruptured; or with ascites containing malignant cells present or with positive peritoneal washings
Stage III	Tumor involving one or both ovaries with peritoneal implants outside the pelvis and/or positive retroperitoneal or inguinal nodes. Superficial liver metastasis equals stage III. Tumor is limited to the true pelvis but with histologically proven malignant extension to small bowel or omentum
Stage IIIA	Tumor grossly limited to the true pelvis with negative nodes but with histologically confirmed microscopic seeding of abdominal peritoneal surfaces
Stage IIIB	Tumor of one or both ovaries with histologically confirmed implants of abdominal peritoneal surfaces none exceeding 2 cm in diameter. Nodes are negative
Stage IIIC	Abdominal implants greater than 2 cm in diameter and/or positive retroperitoneal or inguinal nodes
Stage IV	Growth involving one or both ovaries, with distant metastases. If pleural effusion is present, there must be positive cytologic findings to allot a case to stage IV. Parenchymal liver metastasis equal stage IV.

†**Notes about the staging:** To evaluate the impact on prognosis of the different criteria for alloting cases to stage IC or IIC, it would be of value to know whether the rupture of the capsule was spontaneous or caused by the surgeon and if the source of malignant cells detected was peritoneal washings or ascites.

*International Federation of Gynecology and Obstetrics. Annual report on the results of treatment in gynecological cancer. Int. J. Gynecol. Obstet. 28:189–190, 1989.

ovary includes antibiotics for urinary tract infections, paracentesis for relief of ascites, and narcotics for pain in the terminal stages.

The rationale for combination chemotherapy, the cornerstone of postoperative treatment of ovarian cancer, is the ability of the drugs to kill a constant proportion of the remaining cells with each dose. Between doses, some regrowth of cells occurs, but with successful therapy the number of cells killed is greater than the number that regrow. The percentage of cells killed depends on the efficacy of the drug chosen and the sensitivity of the cells to that drug. Chemotherapy is based on the principle that neoplastic cells are killed at a rate greater than that of normal cells because they are dividing more actively and their cell cycle time is shorter than that of normal cells.

Combination chemotherapy involves use of drugs that act differently (cycle-specific or cycle-nonspecific) or inhibit cellular division at different points in the cell cycle. For example, certain alkylating agents (chlorambucil, cyclophosphamide, melphalan, and cisplatin) as well as certain antibiotics (actinomycin D and doxorubicin) are cell cycle-specific. Other alkylating agents are cell cycle-nonspecific. Of the cell cycle phase-specific chemotherapeutic agents in common use in gynecology, prednisone exerts its greatest activity on Gap 1 (G_1), whereas the antimetabolites fluorouracil and methotrexate affect the phase of DNA synthesis (S). Bleomycin and etoposide exert their main effects on Gap 2 (G_2), whereas vinblastine and vincristine affect mitosis (M) primarily.

Combination chemotherapy has undergone empiric evolution as different combinations and schedules have been tested in large clinical trials, which compare efficacy and toxicity. Drugs with different types of side effects are more desirable than those with additive toxicities. Platinum and Cytoxan delivered as a rapid infusion over about 45 minutes and repeated every 21 days is a standard regimen of chemotherapy for ovarian carcinoma. Carboplatinol, which is less toxic than the parent compound Platinol, and Taxol are two new promising drugs in the treatment of ovarian carcinoma.

The 5-year cure rate in ovarian cancer is still only about 20 to 30% because 50 to 80% of the tumors have spread beyond the ovary at the time of laparotomy. The survival drops from about 70% in Stage I to less than 60% in Stage II, and only about 20% in Stages III and IV. The histologic type is an important determinant of the prognosis. In general, the more poorly differentiated the lesion, the worse is the prognosis. Mucinous and endometrioid carcinomas, for example, have a generally better prognosis than do serous carcinomas.

CLASSIFICATION OF OVARIAN TUMORS

Although it is virtually impossible to construct a classification of ovarian tumors that satisfies all gynecologists and pathologists, the scheme shown in Table 48–2, which lists only the most common tumors, has the advantage of simplicity. A more detailed classification appears on page 305 (Table 48-3).

Of all primary ovarian neoplasms, about 80 to 85% are of coelomic epithelial origin, 10 to 15% are of germ-cell origin, 3 to 5% are of specialized gonadal stromal origin, and fewer than 1% are of nonspecific mesenchymal origin.

NONNEOPLASTIC CYSTS

Follicle cysts of the ovary signify failure of ovulation and may be a cause of dysfunctional uterine bleeding (Fig. 48–1). They

TABLE 48–2. SIMPLIFIED CLASSIFICATION OF COMMON OVARIAN TUMORS

I. Nonneoplastic (functional, physiologic) Ovarian Cysts
   A. Follicle cyst
   B. Corpus luteum and theca lutein cysts
   C. Endometrial cysts
II. True Neoplasms
   A. Benign
     1. Cystic
       a. Serous
       b. Mucinous
       c. Teratoma (dermoid cyst)
     2. Solid
       a. Fibroma
       b. Brenner tumor
     3. Hormonally active*
       a. Granulosa-theca tumors (estrogen-producing)
       b. Androblastoma (androgen-producing)
   B. Malignant
     1. Primary
       a. Adenocarcinoma
       b. Serous cystadenocarcinoma
       c. Mucinous cystadenocarcinoma
       d. Endometrial adenocarcinoma
       e. Solid teratoma
       f. Dysgerminoma[†]
     2. Metastatic

*These tumors are often considered to be of low-grade malignancy.

[†]This tumor is often of low-grade malignancy.

rarely exceed 6 cm in diameter and regress in 1 or 2 months. The polycystic ovary associated with the Stein-Leventhal syndrome is discussed on page 333.

A corpus luteum cyst is lined by luteinized granulosa cells, which secrete progesterone (Fig. 48–2). Since the associated clinical features include delay of menses and a unilateral adnexal mass, the lesion is often confused with ectopic pregnancy (p. 94).

Theca lutein cysts form in response to high levels of chorionic gonadotropin. They are commonly associated with trophoblastic growths (p. 250), but are occasionally found with normal pregnancy. They regress after the gonadotropic stimulus is removed and should not be excised surgically. Endometrial cysts, a manifestation of endometriosis (p. 216), also are classified as nonneoplastic cysts. Because they often contain old blood, they are a common variety of "chocolate cyst."

Parovarian cysts rarely reach large size. When palpable, they are often misdiagnosed as ovarian cysts.

The World Health Organization (WHO) classification of ovarian tumors is shown in Table 48—3.

BENIGN NEOPLASMS

Serous cystadenoma is the most common true neoplasm of the ovary, accounting for 20 to 25% of all ovarian tumors (Fig. 48—3). It is commonly multicystic and is bilateral in 20% or more of cases. It occurs in the reproductive and postmenopausal age groups. Histologically, the epithelial lining resembles that of the fallopian tube, and calcareous concretions called psammoma bodies may be found. As may all pedunculated tumors, the serous cystadenoma may undergo torsion. The papillary variety is more likely to undergo malignant change. About 25% of the papillary serous cystadenomas are potentially or actually malignant. Bilateral tumors and those in which the capsule has been penetrated are more likely to be malignant.

The mucinous cystadenoma accounts for about 10% of all ovarian tumors (Fig. 48—4). It is often multilocular, and about 5% are bilateral. The likelihood of malignant change is about 5 to 10%. The epithelial lining of the cyst resembles that of the endocervix or the small intestine. These tumors may attain very large size. Rupture of the cyst may produce the condition known as pseudomyxoma peritonei, which may be fatal.

Mesonephroid tumors of the ovary may be benign, borderline, or malignant (Fig. 48—5).

The benign cystic teratoma (dermoid cyst) is the second most common benign ovarian tumor, accounting for about 15% of all ovarian tumors. It contains derivatives of all three germ layers, although skin and its appendages usually predominate (Fig. 48—6). The tissues found in the benign teratoma are mature and well differentiated. They commonly occur in the third decade of life. About 25% of benign cystic teratomas are bilateral. Rupture of this tumor may produce a severe chemical peritonitis. Diagnosis of such a cyst may occasionally be made preoperatively by roentgenologic demonstration of teeth or bone.

A special variety of teratoma, in which thyroid tissue predominates, is the struma ovarii (Fig. 48—7). This tumor may produce hyperthyroidism, which regresses after removal of the neoplasm. The risk of malignant change in a benign cystic teratoma is only about 1%. The most commonly associated cancer is squamous cell carcinoma.

The most common benign solid tumor of the ovary is the fibroma (Fig. 48—8). This neoplasm accounts for about 5% of all ovarian tumors. About 90% are unilateral, and they occur more commonly after the menopause. There is less than a 1% likelihood of malignant transformation. In about 25% of cases, the tumor is complicated by ascites and hydrothorax (Meigs' syndrome). The effusions regress after removal of the tumor. The cause of the hydrothorax and ascites is not clear.

The Brenner tumor (Fig. 48—9), which is usually unilateral, accounts for about 1 to 2% of all ovarian tumors. It is a solid benign neoplasm with a very small likelihood of malignant change and is usually found in women above the age of 40. Histologically it consists of a fibrous stroma surrounding epithelioid cells with longitudinally grooved nuclei.

SEX CORD-STROMAL TUMORS

Endocrinologically active tumors of the ovary are difficult to classify. They are generally of a low degree of malignancy and are therefore often considered with both the benign and the malignant tumors. They may be classified according to histologic type or endocrine effects. The interconvertibility of the steroid hormones adds to the difficulty in classification. Sex cord-stromal tumors are often described as gonadal stromal tumors or mesenchymomas. In the granulosa-theca cell tumors, one or the other element may predominate or occur exclusively. In general, these are estrogen-producing lesions, which account for about 10% of all solid ovarian tumors.

The granulosa cell tumor accounts for between 1 and 3% of all ovarian tumors (Fig. 48—10). About 95% are unilateral, and all are generally small. Histologically, the granulosa cells form a columnar or folliculoid pattern. The poorly differentiated tumors may appear sarcomatoid. Granulosa cell tumors may cause precocious puberty in the child or postmenopausal bleeding in the

TABLE 48-3. WHO CLASSIFICATION OF OVARIAN TUMORS

I. Common Epithelial Tumors
  A. Serous tumors
    1. Benign
      a. cystadenoma and papillary cystade-
        noma
      b. surface papilloma
      c. adenofibroma and cystadenofibroma
    2. Borderline malignancy (carcinomas of
      low malignant potential)
      a. cystadenoma and papillary cystade-
        noma
      b. surface papilloma
      c. adenofibroma and cystadenofibroma
    3. Malignant
      a. adenocarcinoma, papillary adenocar-
        cinoma, and papillary cystadenocarci-
        noma
      b. surface papillary carcinoma
      c. malignant adenofibroma and cystade-
        nofibroma
  B. Mucinous tumors
    1. Benign
      a. cystadenoma
      b. adenofibroma and cystdenofibroma
    2. Borderline malignancy (carcinomas of
      low malignant potential)
      a. cystadenoma
      b. adenofibroma and cystadenofibroma
    3. Malignant
      a. adenocarcinoma and cystadenocarci-
        noma
      b. malignant adenofibroma and cystade-
        nofibroma
  C. Endometrioid tumors
    1. Benign
      a. adenoma and cystadenoma
      b. adenofibroma and cystadenofibroma
    2. Borderline malignancy (carcinomas of
      low malignant potential
      a. adenoma and cystadenoma
      b. adenofibroma and cystadenofibroma
    3. Malignant
      a. carcinoma
        i. adenocarcinoma
        ii. adenocanthoma
        iii. malignant adenofibroma and
          cystadenofibroma
      b. endometrioid stromal sarcomas
      c. mesodermal (müllerian) mixed tu-
        mors, homologous and heterologous
  D. Clear cell (mesonephroid) tumors
    1. Benign: adenofibroma
    2. Borderline malignancy (carcinomas of
      low malignant potential)
    3. Malignant: carcinoma and adenocarci-
      noma
  E. Brenner tumors
    1. Benign
    2. Borderline malignancy (proliferating)
    3. Malignant
  F. Mixed epithelial tumors
    1. Benign
    2. Borderline malignancy
    3. Malignant
  G. Unclassified carcinoma
  H. Unclassified epithelial tumors

II. Sex Cord Stromal Tumors
  A. Granulosa-stromal cell tumors
    1. Granulosa cell tumor
    2. Tumors in the thecoma-fibroma group
      a. thecoma
      b. fibroma
      c. unclassified
  B. Androblastomas; Sertoli-Leydig cell tumors
    1. Well differentiated
      a. tubular androblastoma; Sertoli cell tu-
        mor (tubular adenoma of Pick)
      b. tubular androblastoma with lipid stor-
        age; Sertoli cell tumor with lipid stor-
        age (folliculome lipidique)
      c. Sertoli-Leydig cell tumor (tubular ade-
        noma with Leydig cells)
      d. Leydig cell tumor; hilus cell tumor
    2. Intermediate differentiation
    3. Poorly differentiated (sarcomatoid)
    4. With heterologous elements
  C. Gynandroblastoma
  D. Unclassified
III. Lipid (Lipoid) Cell Tumors
IV. Germ Cell Tumors
  A. Dysgerminoma
  B. Endodermal sinus tumor
  C. Embryonal carcinoma
  D. Polyembryoma
  E. Choriocarcinoma
  F. Teratomas
    1. Immature
    2. Mature
      a. solid
      b. cystic
        i. dermoid cyst (mature cystic ter-
          atoma)
        ii. dermoid cyst with malignant
          transformation
    3. Monodermal and highly specialized
      a. struma ovarii
      b. carcinoid
      c. struma ovarii and carcinoid
      d. others
  G. Mixed forms
V. Gonadoblastoma
  A. Pure
  B. Mixed with dysgerminoma or other form of
    germ cell tumor
VI. Soft Tissue Tumors Not Specific to Ovary
VII. Unclassified Tumors
VIII. Secondary (Metastatic) Tumors
IX. Tumor-like Conditions
  A. Pregnancy luteoma
  B. Hyperplasia of ovarian stroma and hyperthe-
    cosis
  C. Massive edema
  D. Solitary follicle cyst and corpus luteum cyst
  E. Multiple follicle cysts (polycystic ovaries)
  F. Multiple luteinized follicle cysts, corpora
    lutea, or both
  G. Endometriosis
  H. Surface-epithelial inclusion cysts (germinal
    inclusion cysts)
  I. Simple cysts
  J. Inflammatory lesions
  K. Parovarian cysts

older patient; furthermore, they may stimulate the development of endometrial cancer. In a woman in the reproductive years, they are likely to cause abnormal uterine bleeding or endometrial hyperplasia. About 10 to 30% undergo malignant change. In the young patient, unilateral oophorectomy may be attempted, but in the older patient, the treatment of choice is total abdominal hysterectomy with bilateral salpingo-oophorectomy. Granulosa cell tumors have a tendency to recur years or even decades after initial treatment.

Thecomas are also estrogen-producing tumors of the ovary (Fig. 48–11). They too account for a small percentage of all ovarian tumors. In general, they are small and unilateral. Not more than 1% of these tumors have malignant potential. The tumors histologically resemble fibromas, from which they may be distinguished by appropriate lipid stains. Luteinization of an estrogen-producing tumor may be associated with a progestational endometrium. According to some investigators, there is an increased risk of endometrial carcinoma in patients with these tumors. Treatment of thecomas is based on the same principles as that of granulosa cell tumors.

A typical masculinizing tumor of the ovary is the androblastoma (arrhenoblastoma). About 95% of these uncommon tumors are unilateral, and the majority occur in women under the age of 35. The malignant potential is about 20 to 25%. A well-differentiated form of the tumor is the Pick, or testicular, adenoma (Fig. 48–12). The Leydig cells, which are the source of androgen, are not prominent in the highly differentiated testicular adenoma. Treatment is usually total abdominal hysterectomy and bilateral salpingo-oophorectomy. Defeminization is followed by masculinization, or virilization. The usual sequence is amenorrhea, involution of the breasts and uterus, and infertility, followed by hirsutism, acne, deepening of the voice, and hypertrophy of the clitoris.

Still less common masculinizing tumors of the ovary are the hilus cell and the adrenal rest tumors. The hilus cell tumor has about a 1% malignant potential. Microscopically, the hilus cells resemble Leydig cells and may contain crystalloids of Reinke.

MALIGNANT NEOPLASMS

Of all epithelial ovarian cancers, about 35 to 40% are serous, 15 to 20% are endometrioid, 6 to 10% are mucinous, 5% are clear cell, fewer than 1% are of the Brenner type, and 15 to 30% are undifferentiated. Primary adenocarcinoma of the ovary is basically a solid tumor, which may contain cystic or necrotic areas. It is relatively undifferentiated, commonly bilateral, and highly malignant. Since the tumor spreads rapidly by seeding of the peritoneum and omentum, the patient with this lesion often presents with ascites.

Serous cystadenocarcinoma is the most common cancer of the ovary, accounting for about half of all ovarian carcinomas (Fig. 48–13). In more than 50% of cases, it presents as bilateral cystic or loculated ovarian masses with ascites. The papillary projections may detach and implant widely in the peritoneal cavity. Several authors believe that carcinoma of this histologic variety is a manifestation of generalized abdominal carcinomatosis rather than primary ovarian disease.

Mucinous cystadenocarcinoma accounts for about 10 to 15% of all ovarian cancers. The tumors are often large and multilocular, with numerous areas of hemorrhage. About 25% are bilateral.

The cure rate of endometrioid (endometrial) adenocarcinoma of the ovary is better than that of the other cystic ovarian cancers.

Solid teratomas of the ovary usually contain poorly differentiated derivatives of all three germ layers. They are found more commonly in the young patient. The degree of malignancy is high and the prognosis is poor.

GERM CELL TUMORS

The dysgerminoma arises from the undifferentiated germ cell and is histologically identical with the seminoma of the testis (Fig. 48–14). The tumor is found in young adults, about 75% occurring before the age of 26. The dysgerminoma is bilateral in 10 to 20% of cases. Microscopically, it consists of large ovoid cells separated by delicate septa of connective tissue with a sprinkling of lymphocytes. The degree of malignancy is variable. Bilateral tumors and those in which the capsule has been broken have a poorer prognosis. The tumor occasionally produces chorionic gonadotropin (with or without associated teratoid trophoblast) and is sometimes found in intersexes. The usual treatment in the patient who has completed her family is total abdominal hysterectomy and bilateral salpingo-oophorectomy. Occasionally in the young patient, a well-encapsulated unilateral tumor may be treated by unilateral oophorectomy. This tumor, unlike most ovarian neoplasms, is highly radiosensitive.

The endodermal sinus (yolk sac) tumor is a highly aggressive extraembryonal teratoma (Fig. 48–15). Alpha-fetoprotein is a useful marker for this neoplasm. New regimens of chemotherapy (e.g., Vincristine, Bleomycin, and cisplatinum) have produced high rates of cure, with frequent preservation of fertility.

METASTATIC TUMORS

About 20 to 25% of all ovarian tumors are metastatic. Common primary sites are the endometrium, the gastrointestinal tract, and the breast. A Krukenberg tumor is usually metastatic from the gastrointestinal tract (Fig. 48–16). Microscopically, it consists of signet-ring (fat-containing) cells in a dense fibrous stroma.

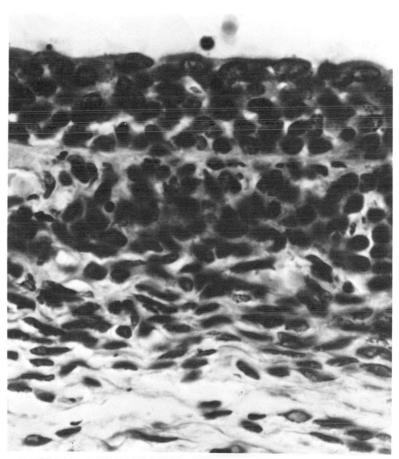

FIG. 48–1. Follicle cyst lined by granulosa cells.

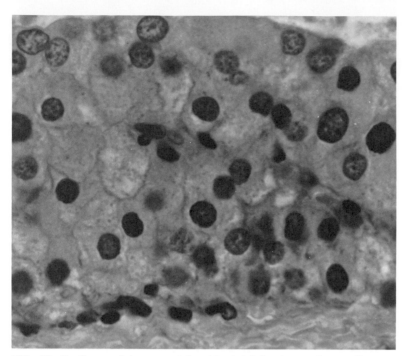

FIG. 48—2. Corpus luteum cyst lined by luteinized granulosa cells.

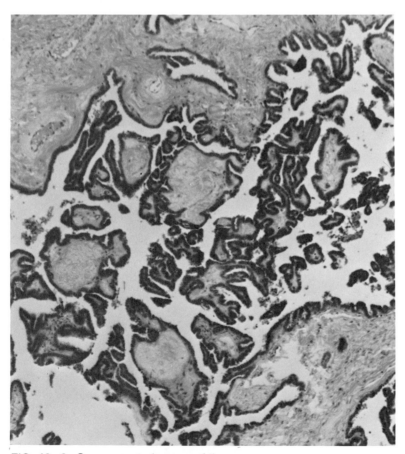

FIG. 48—3. Serous cystadenoma of the ovary.

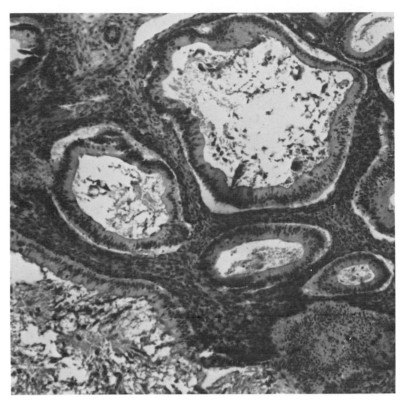

FIG. 48-4. Mucinous cystadenoma of the ovary.

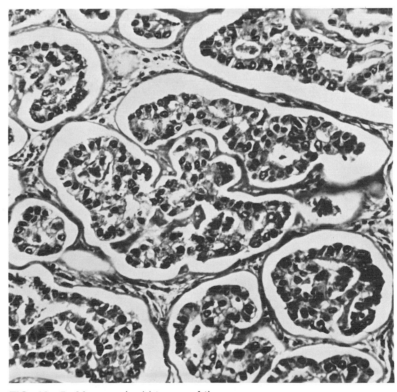

FIG. 48-5. Mesonephroid tumor of the ovary.

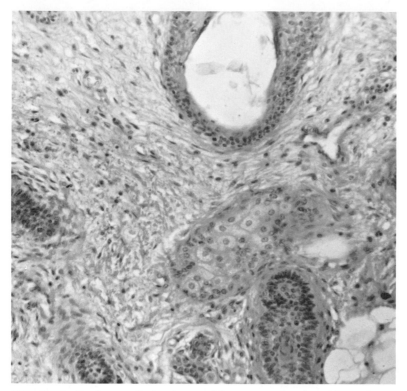

FIG. 48–6. Benign cystic teratoma of the ovary, showing skin and epidermal appendages.

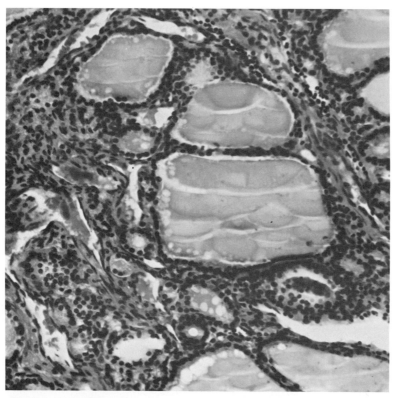

FIG. 48–7. Benign cystic teratoma with preponderance of colloid-containing thyroid tissue (struma ovarii).

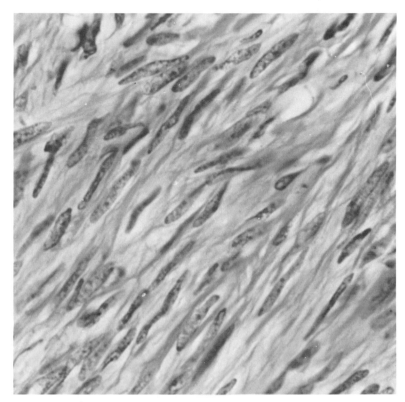

FIG. 48–8. Fibroma of the ovary.

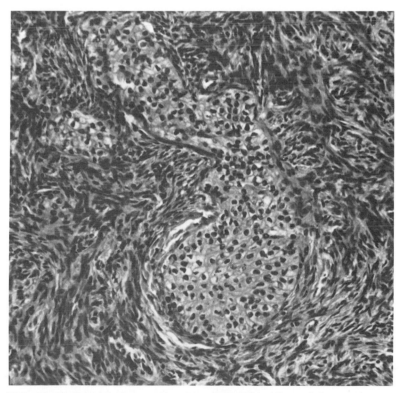

FIG. 48–9. Brenner tumor, showing epithelioid cells and dense stroma.

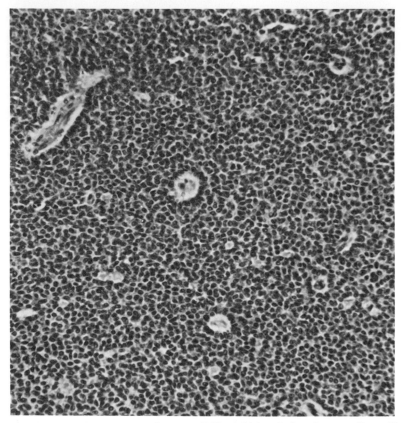

FIG. 48–10. Granulosa cell tumor (folliculoid type), forming rosettes with Call-Exner bodies.

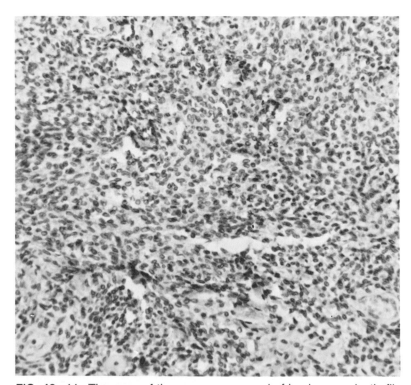

FIG. 48–11. Thecoma of the ovary, composed of benign neoplastic fibrocytes.

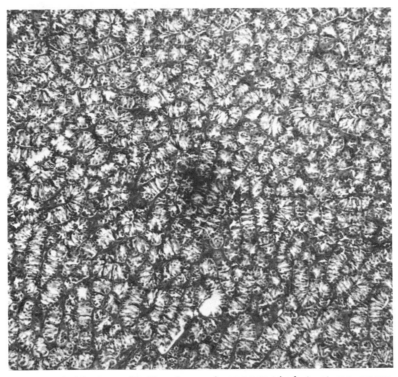

FIG. 48–12. Well differentiated androblastoma (Pick's adenoma), composed of structures resembling testicular tubules.

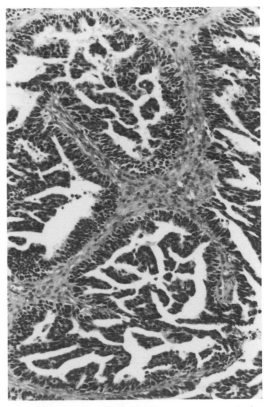

FIG. 48–13. Invasive papillary serous cystade-nocarcinoma of the ovary.

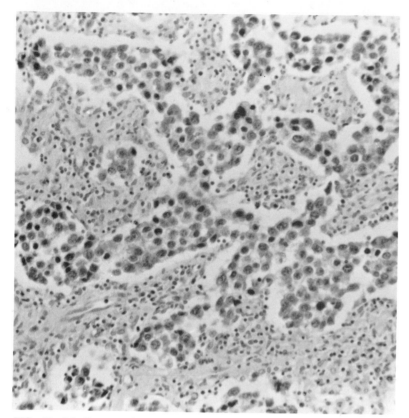

FIG. 48–14. Dysgerminoma (germinoma, or seminoma), showing clusters of germ cells separated by septa containing lymphocytes.

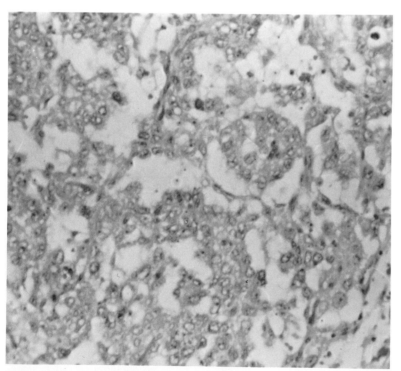

FIG. 48–15. Endodermal sinus (yolk sac) tumor of the ovary, an extraembryonal teratoma, showing small cystic spaces (sinuses) lined by irregular layers of flattened endothelium into which project glomeruloid tufts with central vascular cores.

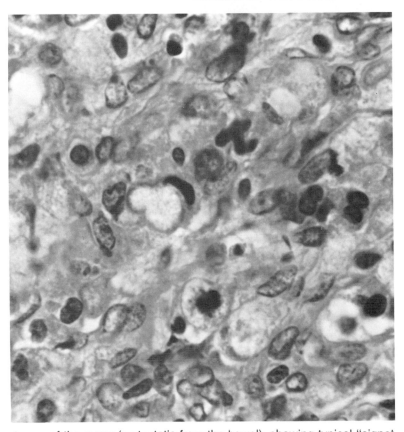

FIG. 48–16. Krukenberg tumor of the ovary (metastatic from the bowel), showing typical "signet ring" cells.

V

REPRODUCTIVE ENDOCRINOLOGY, INFERTILITY, AND RELATED TOPICS

49
CHAPTER
ACTION OF HORMONES

Basic understanding of gynecologic endocrinology requires knowledge of general endocrinology, for lesions of the central nervous system, hypothalamus, pituitary and other endocrine glands directly affect the function of the ovary and uterus. Furthermore, reproductive endocrine function is affected by metabolic disorders, systemic diseases, and psychogenic factors. The information in this unit is helpful in understanding further the physiologic changes in pregnancy (p. 61) and the mode of action and side effects of steroidal contraceptives (p. 171).

The most common endocrine problems are menopause; a delay in menarche or puberty; amenorrhea; virilization and hirsutism; and ambiguous genitalia, or intersexuality. In addition, management of infertility often includes endocrinologic diagnosis and therapy.

Abnormal uterine bleeding frequently results from endocrine dysfunction, but it is mandatory to rule out all other causes, especially neoplasms, before instituting hormonal therapy.

Dysmenorrhea and premenstrual tension are common problems that may have an endocrine component.

Patients with complicated problems should be referred to a specialist in gynecologic endocrinology for diagnosis and therapy.

Finally, a knowledge of normal endocrine function is requisite to a rational discussion of human sexuality (Unit VI).

The hypothalamus is controlled by neurohumoral secretions (neurotransmitters) from higher areas in the central nervous system. Several that play a role in reproduction are dopamine, norepinephrine, and serotonin, which originate in the nerves of the limbic system. These substances cause the hypothalamus to produce releasing hormones, which inhibit or stimulate the release of tropic hormones from the adenohypophysis (anterior lobe of the pituitary gland).

The neurotransmitters stimulate the cells of the anterior hypothalamic area; the preoptic, arcuate, and ventromedial nuclei; and the prechiasmatic area and median eminence. The gonadotropin-releasing hormone (GnRH), a decapeptide, originates in the preoptic, prechiasmatic, and anterior hypothalamic areas. It stimulates synthesis and release of LH and FSH from the gonadotropic cells of the pituitary.

A major advance in reproductive endocrinology was the discovery of the pulsatile release of GnRH and the subsequent pulses of LH and FSH. In fact, most hormones are thought to be secreted episodically. Menstrual function, for example, is dependent not only on the mean plasma values of FSH and LH but also on the pulse frequency of these gonadotropins and of GnRH.

In the rhesus monkey, destruction of the arcuate nucleus results in complete cessation of secretion of GnRH (and therefore of LH and FSH) and of menstrual function. Replacement of GnRH by constant infusion of physiologic amounts of the decapeptide fails to restore the expected pituitary secretion of gonadotropin, and no menstruation results. Only when GnRH is replaced in pulsatile fashion (hourly) are normal secretion of FSH and LH and menses restored.

Many previously unexplained phenomena of reproductive physiology, including the initiation of puberty, several causes of infertility, and the onset of menopause, are understood more clearly in this context.

FSH and LH attach themselves to specific portions of the membranes (receptor sites) of the target cells. After the hormone is bound to the receptor, the resulting complex is brought into the cell membrane. The internalized hormone-receptor complex then activates the adenylate cyclase system and generates cyclic AMP, which acts as a second messenger to initiate the biochemical processes that culminate in synthesis of protein. Ovarian follicles and seminiferous tubules produce a polypeptide hormone, inhibin, which exerts negative feedback on secretion of gonadotropins, primarily FSH. Polyacrylamide gel electrophoresis of highly purified preparations of inhibin has shown that it is a dimer, composed of two subunits. Comparison of the structures of subunits of inhibin from various species has revealed a high degree of homology. In women, inhibin is thought to be produced primarily by the granulosa cells and possibly by the corpus luteum as well. Inhibin and inhibin-related peptides are believed to exert long-loop feedback effects on the secretion of FSH as well as local paracrine or autocrine actions within the ovary.

The lipid-soluble, free steroid hormones of the end organs diffuse across the plasma membrane of the target cell into the cytoplasm. Free estradiol (E_2), for example, binds to its receptor in the endometrial cell. Receptor proteins are believed to be of nuclear origin. The hormone-receptor complex (E_2-R) is then translocated into the nucleus, where it binds to DNA. The resulting complex activates the genome, causing transcription, or production of messenger RNA, which enters the cytoplasm and binds to the ribosome, where synthesis of protein is translated. The effects include mitosis and synthesis of enzymes and proteins, among which are receptors for estrogen and progesterone, which provide additional capacity for binding. The complex dissociates in the nucleus after activating DNA. Free hormones are metabolized or excreted from the cell and the receptor is recycled back into the cytoplasm. Progesterone reduces the replenishment of new cytoplasmic estrogen or progesterone receptors, thus exerting an antiestrogenic action.

The secretion of pituitary gonadotropins is modulated by hormonal signals originating in the target organs, the pituitary, and the hypothalamus itself through feedback mechanisms. In the case of positive feedback, increased secretion of a hormone stimulates secretion by the pituitary; with negative feedback, the secretion of a hormone inhibits the output of the pituitary.

Through the long feedback loop, estrogens may exert negative feedback on secretion of both FSH and LH, as well as positive feedback on secretion of LH (as with the preovulatory surge, which precedes the LH peak at midcycle). LH itself may exert negative feedback on the hypothalamus, resulting in decrease in GnRH and subsequent lowering of LH through a short feedback loop. It is also possible that LH may exert positive feedback with respect to its own secretion. In the ultrashort feedback loop, the synthesis, storage, and release of the hypothalamic releasing hormones are influenced by changes in their own titers. A negative ultrashort feedback has been demonstrated to affect GnRH.

Masculinization of the hypothalamus and perhaps other parts of the central nervous system during fetal life causes the male, or tonic, pattern of secretion of FSH or LH. In the male, only negative feedback of sex steroids occurs, which results in rather constant secretion of FSH and LH. If the fetus is not exposed to androgens, it develops a female, or clonic, pattern of secretion of gonadotropins, in which both negative and positive feedback occur.

The sex steroids produced by the gonads are classifiable physiologically into three groups: progestins, estrogens, and androgens. Progestins have 21 carbon atoms (C21), androgens have 19 (C19), and estrogens have 18 (C18). In estrogens, furthermore, the A ring of the steroid nucleus is aromatized. The biosynthetic pathways leading to formation of the principal gonadal hormones are diagrammed in Figure 49–1.

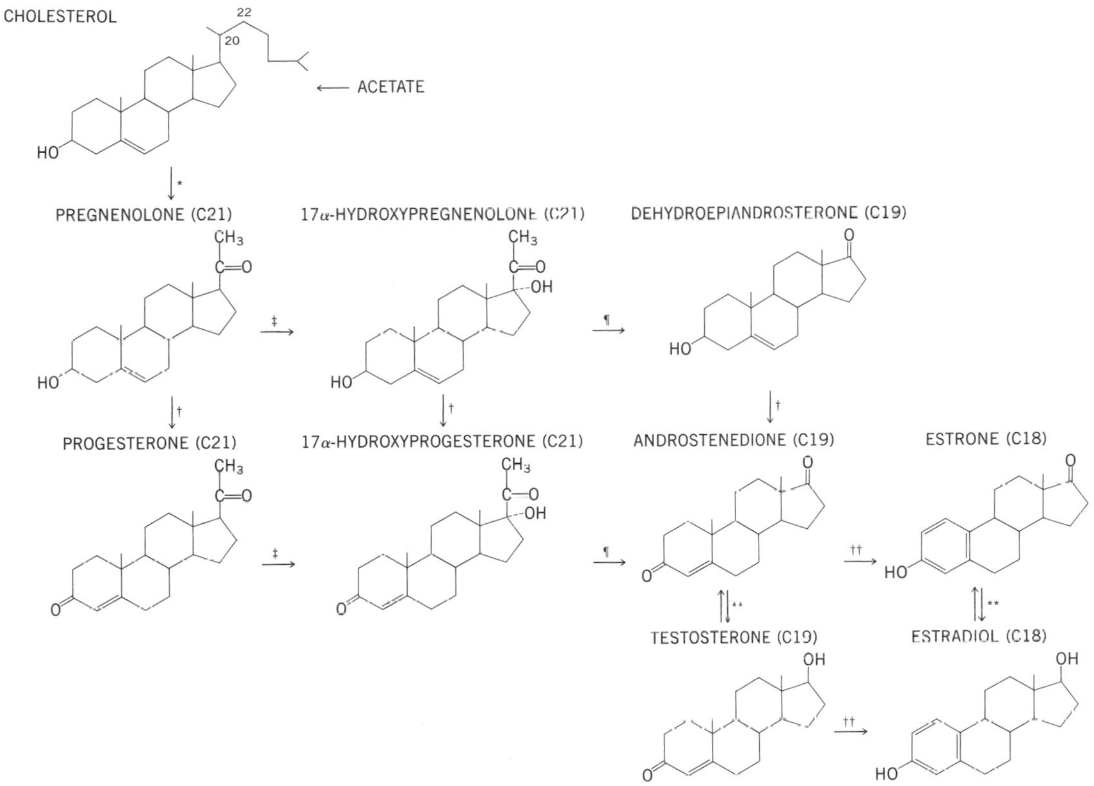

FIG. 49–1. Biosynthetic pathways of gonadal steroids. Enzymes involved are as follows:
* = 20-hydroxylase, 22-hydroxylase, and 20,22-desmolase
† = 3β-ol-dehydrogenase and Δ^4-Δ^5 isomerase
‡ = 17α-hydroxylase
¶ = 17,20-desmolase
** = 17β-ol-dehydrogenase
†† = aromatizing enzyme system

50

CHAPTER

PUBERTY

Puberty is the period when a person becomes sexually mature, the reproductive organs become functional, and the secondary sexual characteristics become developed. Its onset varies somewhat with racial, hereditary, social, and nutritional factors. Menarche, or the onset of menses, occurs about 2 years after the onset of puberty, which normally lasts between 4 and 8 years. Puberty begins about 2 years earlier in girls than in boys. Menarche in industrialized countries normally occurs between 9 and 18 years of age, with an average of 12.8 years in North America. The average age of menarche in the United States appears to have stabilized, halting its trend in this century to occur in progressively earlier adolescence. Since the first few cycles are usually anovulatory, fertility is ordinarily not established until about 2 years after menarche. The changes accompanying puberty normally occur in a well-defined sequence: development of the breasts (thelarche), growth of pubic hair (adrenarche or pubarche), growth of axillary hair, and finally menses.

The first sign of puberty is usually the appearance of downy pubic hair. A small growth spurt in height and weight is then followed by elevation of the nipples and the growth of coarse and curly pubic hair. Budding of the breasts and enlargement of the areolae precede the marked growth spurt. Enlargement of the labia, further growth of pubic hair, and filling out of the breasts accompany the development of axillary hair. Menarche then occurs, followed by further growth of the labia and a decrease in the rate of general growth. The distribution of pubic hair is now of the adult type. Axillary hair is more abundant and the breasts approach the adult configuration. Labia are now of the adult type, annual growth decreases, and menstruation is well established.

Generally, the growth spurt in puberal girls is maximal between 11 and 12 years of age. The growth rate then declines and ceases about 2.5 years after menarche. The epiphyses close at 16 to 17 years of age.

PRECOCIOUS PUBERTY

Precocious puberty is defined as puberty before the age of 8 in girls (or 10 in boys). It is more common in girls. Another definition is menarche before the age of 10 and adrenarche before the age of 9 in girls.

True precocious puberty, the premature initiation of the appropriately sequenced events of puberty, is thought to result from dysfunction at the level of the hypothalamus. Gonadotropin levels, if measured, reflect mature feedback dynamics. It is always isosexual; in girls it culminates in ovulation. Its cause is usually unknown (idiopathic, or constitutional), but it may result from a variety of rare disease of the central nervous system or from polyostotic fibrous dysplasia (Albright's syndrome).

Precocious pseudopuberty (pseudopubertal precocity) implies the premature appearance of one or more secondary sexual characteristics without the development of normal reproductive capabilities. It may result from abnormal hormonal (steroidal) stimulation or abnormal sensitivity of the end organs to normal levels of steroidal hormones. In the isosexual variety, estrogenic effects are evident in the female, and androgenic effects in the male; in the heterosexual variety, estrogenic effects are evident in the male, and androgenic effects in the female. Pseudoprecocious puberty implies premature manifestation of sex-steroid-dependent sexual characteristics without a consistent elevation in pituitary gonadotropins.

In all forms of sexual precocity, the patients are initially tall for their age, but because their epiphyses close prematurely, they are ultimately shorter than average for their age. Diagnosis requires expert evaluation. Gonadotropins and gonadal steroidal hormones should be measured to distinguish true precocity from pseudoprecocity. In true precocity, all hormonal levels are within normal adult limits. In pseudoprecocity, the levels of serum estrogens or androgens are elevated or, if the end organs are abnormally sensitive, within the normal range for children. The requirement for additional tests depends upon the preliminary diagnosis.

Investigation of true precocity requires evaluation of the central nervous system with neurologic examination and radiologic techniques such as computed tomography (CT scan) and cerebral angiography. Investigation of pseudoprecocity requires techniques to localize the site of origin of the steroids. An estrogen-producing neoplasm in the young girl should be easily palpable on physical examination.

Treatment of precocious puberty depends on the cause. True precocity without an organic lesion requires no direct treatment, but pregnancy must be prevented if the patient is ovulating. Counseling is helpful to aid the girl in her psychosexual adjustment.

In the pseudosyndrome, treatment may be directed toward removing the tumor or suppressing the hyperplastic adrenal cortex. (p. 331).

ONSET OF PUBERTY

The onset of puberty occurs when the hypothalamus begins to secrete gonadotropin-releasing hormone in periodic bursts, which stimulate the pituitary gland to produce gonadotropins. These hormones, in turn, stimulate the gonads to produce the sex steroids, which induce the changes that characterize puberty. Unless the releasing hormone is secreted intermittently, the pituitary will not release enough gonadotropin to stimulate production of sex steroids. If it is secreted continuously, the pituitary becomes desensitized and ceases to release gonadotropin. With the use of a synthetic analog of gonadotropin-releasing hormone that is more potent and longer acting than the natural hormone, the pituitary may be desensitized. This promising technique may be the most effective method of arresting precocious puberty.

RETARDED PUBERTY

Retarded puberty may be associated with low or elevated gonadotropins and arise from dysfunction of the ovary, pituitary, or central nervous system or from genetic causes. It should be evaluated by the age of 15. Gonadal dysgenesis, testicular feminization, and diencephalic lesions must be excluded. Any associated emaciation or obesity should be corrected.

Causes associated with low gonadotropins include: constitutional delay, tumors and malformations of the central nervous system, gonadotropin deficiencies, and miscellaneous syndromes such as Prader-Willi and Laurence-Moon-Biedl.

Causes associated with elevated gonadotropins include: gonadal dysgenesis, cytotoxic drugs and radiation, galactose intolerance, gonadotropin resistance, and deficiencies of steroidal enzymes such as cholesterol desmolase, 17α-hydroxylase, and 17-20 lyase.

51
CHAPTER
AMENORRHEA

Of all the stigmata of endocrine disorders, amenorrhea has the greatest diversity of causes. It figures prominently in the differential diagnosis of defeminization, intersexuality, and infertility. An entirely satisfactory simple classification of the amenorrheas is therefore almost impossible to construct because the various etiologic subgroups are often interrelated. Investigation and treatment of amenorrhea require basic knowledge of developmental and chromosomal abnormalities and general endocrinology.

Primary amenorrhea is lack of menarche by the age of 18. Amenorrhea should be investigated by the age of 16, and preferably earlier. Secondary amenorrhea is the cessation of menstruation for at least 6 months in a woman who has had her menarche.

The causes of amenorrhea may be considered physiologic or pathologic. Amenorrhea is normal (physiologic) in childhood, pregnancy, lactation, and the menopause. By far the commonest cause of amenorrhea in a woman in the reproductive years is pregnancy. Amenorrhea may persist normally from 6 weeks to 6 months after pregnancy and may be prolonged somewhat by breastfeeding or stimulation of the nipples. Amenorrhea lasting longer than 6 months post partum may reflect a significant underlying disorder.

Pathologic amenorrhea may stem from anatomic, congenital, or chromosomal defects or may reflect dysfunction of the central nervous system, hypothalamus, pituitary, ovary, or uterus. It may also follow in the wake of systemic diseases, dysfunction of the other endocrine glands, or psychogenic factors (Table 51–1). Before a diagnosis of amenorrhea is undertaken, pregnancy must be excluded. When the cause of amenorrhea cannot be ascertained, the disorder is often termed idiopathic (Fig. 51–1).

Developmental anomalies occasionally cause primary amenorrhea. In such cases, the diagnosis is usually obvious, as with an imperforate hymen. This lesion and vaginal atresia may result in uterine bleeding that cannot escape from the body (cryptomenorrhea).

EMBRYOLOGY OF THE GENITAL SYSTEM

Knowledge of normal development of the genitourinary system is prerequisite to understanding the numerous anatomic malformations that may cause amenorrhea or otherwise interfere with reproductive function. The urinary and reproductive systems develop from the intermediate mesoderm (p. 49). During folding, the intermediate mesoderm migrates ventrally and forms two longitudinal masses named the nephro-

TABLE 51–1. ETIOLOGY OF AMENORRHEA

I. Physiologic
   A. Prepuberal state
   B. Pregnancy
   C. Postpartum lactation
   D. Menopause

II. Congenital Anatomic
   A. Imperforate hymen
   B. Developmental anomalies of vagina, cervix, or corpus

III. Chromosomal and Genetic
   A. Gonadal dysgenesis
   B. Testicular feminization
   C. True hermaphroditism
   D. Other forms of pseudohermaphroditism and intersexuality

IV. Central Nervous System-Hypothalamic-Pituitary
   A. Hypothalamic dysfunction
   B. Pituitary insufficiency
   C. Tumors and other organic lesions

V. Psychogenic
   A. Psychosis and anxiety
   B. Emotional shock
   C. Pseudocyesis
   D. Anorexia nervosa

VI. Systemic
   A. Chronic disease
   B. Nutritional disorders
   C. Drugs

VII. Other Endocrine Causes
   A. Adrenal hyperplasia, tumors, or insufficiency
   B. Hyperthyroidism or hypothyroidism
   C. Steroidal contraceptives

VIII. Ovary
   A. Insensitive ovocytes
   B. Destructive lesions
   C. Estrogen-producing and androgen-producing tumors
   D. Premature ovarian failure

IX. Uterus
   A. Endometrial destruction (Asherman's syndrome)
   B. Cervical stenosis

genic cords, which produce the urogenital ridges.

Three sets of excretory organs develop in human embryos. The first is the pronephros, which appears in human embryos as a few small cords or tubules on day 22. Its regression is complete by the beginning of the fifth week and it probably is never functional. It consists of several pairs of tubules and a pronephric duct. Caudad to the pronephros, the blind end of the pronephric duct continues to grow toward the cloaca, which it perforates on about day 30. The mesonephros appears during the fourth week, caudad to the pronephros. Clusters of cells within the nephrogenic cord differentiate into S-shaped mesonephric tubules, which be-

come continuous with the pronephric duct, which at this stage is designated the mesonephric duct. The medial end of each tubule expands, is invaginated by capillaries, and forms a glomerulus. Although they are functional in some mammals, the tubules are not believed to function in man. Their importance is in formation of part of the male reproductive system. By the tenth week, most of these tubules have degenerated. A few caudal tubules persist as genital ducts in men or as vestigial structures in women. The metanephros, or adult kidney, develops from the ureteric bud and the metanephrogenic mass. The ureteric bud, which arises during the fifth week from the mesonephric duct, gives rise to the ureter, renal pelvis, calyces, and all the collecting ducts of the adult kidney. Mesenchymal cells from the metanephrogenic mass form a cap over the blind end of each newly formed collecting duct. Clusters of cells in each cap differentiate into Bowman's capsule and its associated tubules to form a nephron. Communication is then established between nephron and collecting duct. By early in the third month, the fetal kidney has become functional. The mature fetus may void as much as 450 mL/day into the amnionic sac (Fig. 51–2).

The cloaca, a common endodermal chamber, is divided into a dorsal rectum and a ventral region comprising bladder and urogenital sinus. The apex of the bladder tapers to form an elongate tube, the urachus, which is the proximal remnant of the allantois. After birth, the urachus persists as the median umbilical ligament.

Sex cannot be ascertained in the human embryo except by chromosomal analysis until approximately the sixth to seventh week. In early development, the genital systems in both sexes are similar and potentially bisexual. This indifferent stage persists until the seventh week of development.

The gonads are derived from three sources: the coelomic epithelium of the urogenital ridge, the underlying mesenchyme, and the primordial germ cells. A bulge on the medial side of the mesonephros forms the gonadal ridge. The coelomic epithelium gives rise to primary sex cords, which grow into the underlying mesenchyme. The primordial germ cells are first seen early in the fourth week in the wall of

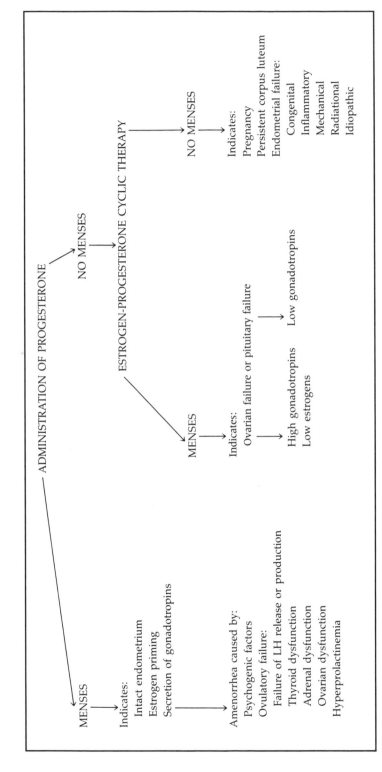

FIG. 51–1. Diagnosis of Amenorrhea

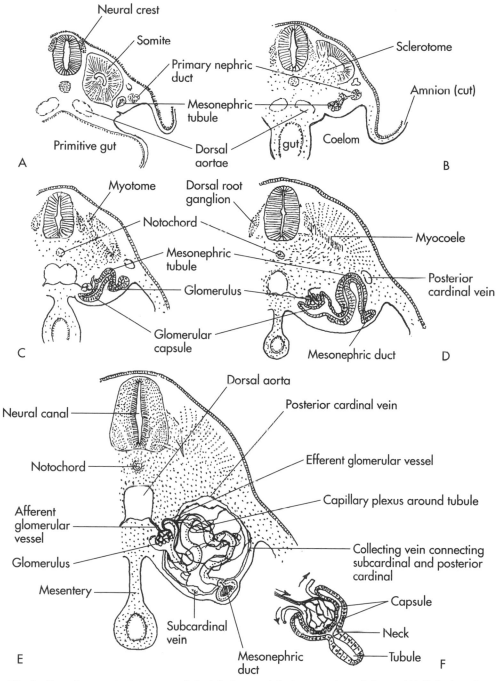

FIG. 51–2. Development of mesonephric tubules and their vascular relations. (A) Tubule primordium still independent of duct. (B) Union of tubule with primary nephric duct. (C) Early stage in development of glomerulus and capsule. (D) Further development of capsule and lengthening of tubule. (E) Relations of blood vessels to well-developed mesoepehric tubule. (F) Glomerulus and capsule, enlarged. (With permission from Patten B.M.: Human Embryology, 3rd ed. New York, McGraw-Hill Co (Blakiston Div.)

the yolk sac near the origin of the allantois. They migrate along the dorsal mesentery of the hindgut into the gonadal ridge. During the sixth week, they are incorporated into the primary sex cords.

In embryos with a Y chromosome, the seminiferous cords form branches, the ends of which anastomose to form the rete testis. Mesonephric tubules that communicate with the mesonephric (wolffian) duct give rise to the efferent ductules, whereas the mesonephric duct forms the epididymis and ductus (vas) deferens. Mesenchymal elements give rise to the interstitial cells of Leydig.

In embryos that lack a Y chromosome, gonadal development occurs slowly. The primary sex cords do not become prominent but form a rudimentary rete ovarii. During the fourth month, the definitive cortex of the ovary first appears. The germinal epithelium produces the secondary sex cords, or cortical cords, which incorporate primordial germ cells.

The paramesonephric (müllerian) duct first appears during the sixth week as a dimple or groove in the thickened epithelium on the lateral aspect of the urogenital ridge. The groove never closes at its cephalic end but remains open to the coelomic cavity. Distally, the edges of the groove fuse to form the paramesonephric duct, which runs parallel to the mesonephric duct. Caudally, the paramesonephric ducts cross ventrad to the mesonephric ducts, fusing in the midline into a Y-shaped uterovaginal primordium. This primordium reaches the urogenital sinus during the eighth week, producing an elevation named the müllerian tubercle.

In the absence of testes, and the müllerian duct inhibitor, the paramesonephric ducts develop into the female genital tract. The cranial longitudinal segments form the oviducts, their ostia becoming the fimbriated extremities. The uterus develops from the middle transverse portion of the paramesonephric duct as a result of proliferation of cells in this region and elevation of the cranial aspect of the uterovaginal primordium. The cervix and part of the vagina develop from the caudal longitudinal segment of the paramesonephric duct. The caudal tip of the uterovaginal primordium

proliferates to produce a solid vaginal cord. Paired sinovaginal bulbs grow from the urogenital sinus and fuse with the vaginal cord. This solid cord of endodermal and mesodermal cells forms the vaginal plate. The central cells of this plate subsequently break down and form the lumen of the vagina, part or all of which is lined by endodermal cells derived from the sinovaginal bulbs.

In the female, buds grow out from the urethra into the surrounding mesenchyme to form the urethral and paraurethral (Skene's) glands. Similar outgrowths from the urogenital sinus form the greater vestibular (Bartholin's) glands.

The entire mesonephric system undergoes atrophy in the female in the absence of male hormone. The cranial group of tubules persists as a functionless vestige, the epoophoron, which is located within the mesosalpinx. The caudal group of mesonephric tubules forms the small paroophoron, which usually disappears before adult life. Vestiges of the caudal portion of the mesonephric duct (Gartner's duct) may be found anywhere between the epoophoron and the hymen.

During the indifferent stage of genital development, the mesoderm surrounding the cloacal membrane undergoes proliferation (at about the fourth week), producing, cranially, the genital tubercle, and, laterally, the labioscrotal swellings and urogenital folds. The phallus develops as the genital tubercle elongates. The rectouterine septum fuses with the cloacal membrane at the end of the sixth week. Rupture of this membrane forms the anus and the urogenital opening.

The external female genitalia develop during the ninth to twelfth weeks. The phallus develops into the clitoris, with glans and prepuce. The urogenital folds, which form the labia minora, do not fuse except in front of the anus. Laterally, the labioscrotal folds, which form the labia majora, remain unfused except posteriorly, to form the posterior labial commissure, and anteriorly, to form the mons pubis.

Of the numerous malformations of the genital tract from the external genitalia to the uterus, only a few prevent or conceal menstruation. In children, agglutination of the labia may be confused with an imperforate hymen. The simplest effective treatment is gentle digital separation of the adhesions and the local use of petrolatum or estrogen creams.

A true imperforate hymen at the onset of menses results in retention of blood within the vagina (hematocolpos), uterus (hematometra), fallopian tube (hematosalpinx), and even the peritoneal cavity. Treatment is incision of the hymen and sometimes excision of a wedge of tissue. Ultimate fertility is preserved if the tubes are not damaged by the collections of blood.

Aplasia of the vagina may be associated with absence of the uterus and anomalies of the urinary tract. If the corpus and cervix are normal, fertility may be restored after reconstruction of a vaginal canal.

A transverse septum of the vagina may be mistaken for congenital absence of the vagina. A longitudinal septum has no effect on menses or fertility in general. Aplasia of the vagina results from agenesis of the vaginal cord. Atresia results from failure of canalization.

Most anomalies of the uterus result from aplasia, abnormalities of differentiation, regression, or fusion of the müllerian ducts. In the case of aplasia, a cord of connective tissue replaces the uterus. This malformation is usually accompanied by vaginal anomalies. Only a few of the uterine malformations are clinically significant.

A unicornuate uterus, which results from aplasia of one müllerian duct, is not clinically important. A noncommunicating rudimentary horn may collect blood to form an enlarging mass. In a septate uterus, fusion is complete but the septum persists. In a bicornuate uterus, fusion occurs only in the lower portion of the müllerian ducts, resulting in a single cervix and a single vagina. With complete duplication of the müllerian ducts (uterus didelphys), the uterus and cervix are double and the vagina is septate. The ovaries are normal, however, and there is no disturbance of menstruation.

GONADAL DYSGENESIS

Chromosomal and genetic causes of amenorrhea include several fairly common disorders such as gonadal dysgenesis and testicular feminization and a great variety of rare hermaphroditic and intersexual syndromes, some of which reflect specific biochemical defects.

Patients with gonadal dysgenesis typically have "streak gonads." The müllerian ducts form, but the uterus and oviducts remain prepuberal. The external genitalia are female and the children are usually reared as girls, although they fail to manifest secondary sexual characteristics.

Diagnosis is suspected on clinical grounds and confirmed by karyotype and laparoscopy. The levels of FSH and LH are elevated but those of other hormones are usually normal. Differential diagnosis includes ovarian hypoplasia, delayed puberty, and pituitary dwarfism.

The common forms of gonadal dysgenesis are Turner's syndrome and pure gonadal dysgenesis. Patients with Turner's syndrome classically are short, with low-set ears, webbed neck, shield chest, coarctation of the aorta, nevi, and edema at birth. The karyotype is classically 45,X, but mosaics have been described as well as chromosomal patterns containing an iso-X or a ring chromosome. Of all fetuses with a single X chromosome, fewer than 3% are born alive.

Patients with pure gonadal dysgenesis are of normal stature or may even be taller than average and they have no somatic abnormalities other than the absence of secondary sexual characteristics. The karyotype is usually 46,XX, but mosaics have been described in this syndrome also.

In the rare condition of gonadal agenesis, the entire gonadal anlage is missing. These patients may have an XX or an XY chromosomal pattern, but they are amenorrheic and their gender role is female.

Treatment of all patients with gonadal dysgenesis or agenesis comprises cyclic estrogen and progestin. Estrogen alone may be given for the first several months. Treatment should be delayed until around age 14 to prevent premature closure of the epiphyses. Patients with Turner's syndrome do not achieve normal height, and development of the breasts may be suboptimal even after treatment.

Klinefelter's syndrome is the commonest sex chromosomal anomaly. These phenotypic males have a chromosomal pattern of

47,XXY, atrophic testes, and oligospermia or azoospermia. They frequently have gynecomastia and some degree of mental retardation.

The 47,XXX "superfemale" may be a phenotypically normal woman. There is an increased incidence of mental retardation, but the patients are sometimes fertile.

HERMAPHRODITISM

TESTICULAR FEMINIZATION

Testicular feminization is a fairly common cause of amenorrhea in phenotypic females with an XY chromosomal constitution. This disorder may be considered a form of intersexuality or pseudohermaphroditism and it tends to be familial. The patients have scanty sexual hair (pubic and axillary) but may have moderately well developed breasts. Because müllerian development is lacking, the uterus is absent or rudimentary, and oviducts are missing. Testes may be abdominal, inguinal, or vulvar. The vagina commonly ends in a short blind pouch. Levels of serum estrogen and androgen are in the normal male range.

The main cause is probably a defect in androgen receptors or androgen receptor-effector mechanisms in the end organs. The testes should be removed because of the increased incidence of neoplasia in these ectopic gonads. Estrogen therapy should be initiated preoperatively and continued permanently. It may be necessary to construct a functional vagina when the patient indicates a desire to initiate coitus. These patients should not be told that they are genetic males, for their psychologic orientation and sex of rearing are female. Great care must be taken to give them sufficient psychologic support so that they can perceive themselves as sexually adequate women. In incomplete forms of the syndrome, the external genitalia are ambiguous.

TRUE HERMAPHRODITISM

True hermaphrodites have both ovarian and testicular tissue, either in the form of one ovary and one testis or as bilateral mixed gonads containing both tissues. The hermaphrodite may have associated anomalies of the urinary tract. The most common chromosomal pattern is 46,XX and the sex chromatin is usually positive, but the phenotype depends on the predominant tissue. The external genitalia are usually ambiguous. Although these patients may menstruate, they are usually infertile.

PSEUDOHERMAPHRODITISM

The female pseudohermaphrodite has ovaries, but the genital ducts and external genitalia differentiate to some extent along male lines. The male pseudohermaphrodite has testes, but the genital ducts, external genitalia, or both differentiate to some extent in the female direction.

Sexual differentiation depends on genetic and environmental factors. A discrepancy among the various criteria of sexual identification results in intersexuality.

CRITERIA OF SEXUALITY

Criteria of sexuality include chromosomal pattern, sex chromatin, gonadal structure, differentiation of the genital ducts (internal genitalia), external genitalia, hormonal status, sex of rearing, and gender role (psychologic orientation). Since the sex of rearing is crucial to the psychologic development of the child and is well established after the second year of life, it is important to assign sex definitively as early as possible.

SEXUAL DEVELOPMENT

All fetuses are potentially bisexual. In the fourth week of gestation, an indifferent gonad appears in both sexes. Gonadal differentiation occurs at about the sixth week. Normally a Y chromosome leads to the development of a testis, which in turn produces a male phenotype, with certain exceptions such as testicular feminization. The primordia differentiate into the internal genitalia, or genital ducts, at about the seventh week. Testes produce an androgenic steroid, which stimulates the wolffian ducts and induces the development of male external genitalia. The Sertoli cells of the testes normally produce a polypeptide, müllerian-inhibiting factor (MIF), or antimüllerian hormone (AMH), which inhibits the development of the müllerian ducts. Animal models suggest that this phenomenon is the result of an induced local response to hyaluronidase, which removes the hyaluronate in the periductal regions. As a consequence, mesenchymal condensation occurs, inhibiting the development of the müllerian ducts. In normal female differentiation, the wolffian ducts regress and the müllerian ducts develop into uterus, oviducts, and possibly a portion of the upper vagina. Normal sexual development requires appropriate stimulation of one ductal system and repression of the other. Development of the external genitalia is hormonally determined. In brief, androgen (usually testosterone) causes development of the male external genitalia. In the absence of androgen, female genitalia develop.

The mammalian Y chromosome plays a dominant role in the initiation of fetal testicular differentiation. Testicular differentiating genes on the Y chromosome can be detected serologically as H-Y antigen. The correlation of numeric and structural abnormalities of the sex chromosomes combined with reactivity of the H-Y antigen, gonadal histology, and phenotype has led to mapping the loci of these genes on the Y chromosome. Genes on the X chromosome may regulate the activity of testicular differentiating genes on the Y chromosome.

AMBIGUOUS GENITALIA

Clinical investigation of the child with ambiguous genitalia should occur in a systematic sequence. A history of the pregnancy with special references to drugs or hormones ingested by the mother should be obtained. Physical examination of the infant should detect associated anomalies, as in Turner's syndrome, or small testes, as in Klinefelter's syndrome. Small testes in a virilized male infant may suggest the adrenogenital syndrome. A karyotype should be performed to ascertain genetic sex and to detect aneuploidy and mosaicism. Urethroscopy or injection of contrast medium into the "vagina" or urogenital sinus may be necessary to reveal the internal genitalia.

Hormonal studies may provide diagnostic information. Urinary 17-ketosteroid as well as serum DHEA-S and 17α-OH progesterone concentrations are elevated in the congenital adrenogenital syndrome, whereas they are normal if the masculinization results from exogenous androgens transferred from the maternal circulation. In certain cases, laparotomy with biopsy of the gonads may be required for definitive diagnosis. Intravenous pyelography should be performed to detect associated anomalies of the urinary tract.

In the adult, two primarily psychiatric problems should be distinguished from hermaphroditism. The transsexual patient has no discrepancies among the anatomic criteria of sex but feels "trapped in the body of the wrong sex." Such patients may request surgical change of gender. These extensive operations should be performed only after psychiatric evaluation.

A transvestite is a person who derives pleasure from wearing the clothes of the opposite sex. These patients do not request operations to change their sex. When their behavior conflicts with the law, they require psychiatric care. Neither transvestites nor transsexuals are necessarily homosexual.

Female pseudohermaphrodites have a 46,XX karyotype but external genitalia that do not develop in the normal female direction. Female pseudohermaphroditism usually results from either congenital adrenal hyperplasia in the fetus or excessive maternal androgen arising from exogenous hormones or a masculinizing tumor of the ovary. The external genitalia are ambiguous or masculinized but the internal genitalia are normal.

Congenital adrenal hyperplasia is the most common cause of female pseudohermaphroditism. It results from an absolute or relative deficiency in one of several enzymatic steps in hydroxylation in the zona fasciculata of the adrenal cortex. As a result, there is a deficiency in production of cortisol. Negative feedback promotes an increase in ACTH. In turn, there results a relative increase in several precursors of cortisol, including androgenic steroids produced in the zona reticularis. The most common form of this syndrome results from a relative block in 21-hydroxylase activity. Genetic linkage studies involving human lymphocyte antigen (HLA) pedigrees have clarified the relationship between homozygous and heterozygous 21-hydroxylase-deficient syndromes. Additionally, synthetic-ACTH stimulation tests have suggested that the two less common adrenogenital syndromes, 11-hydroxylase deficiency and 3-β-hydroxysteroid dehydrogenase deficiency, may be more prevalent than formerly believed.

Patients usually first come to the attention of the physician either as newborns with ambigúous external genitalia, which present a problem in gender identity, or as adolescents with amenorrhea and a somewhat masculine habitus. Because it is difficult to change a gender role from female to male in later life, in cases of doubt the children should be raised as girls.

Adolescents with congenital adrenal hyperplasia frequently demonstrate precocious growth until age 10 or 11, when they cease to grow. They manifest signs of puberty but fail to menstruate. Manifestations of excessive androgen, such as masculine habitus, hirsutism, and clitoromegaly, also may appear.

Diagnosis often can be made from tests performed on serum or urine, involving single or serial measurements of precursor: product ratios of hormones requisite to the synthesis of cortisol. Serum dehydroepiandrosterone, 17α-hydroxyprogesterone, deoxycorticosterone, or other intermediates may be abnormally low or high. Occasionally, transient pharmacologic stimulation of the adrenal gland with synthetic ACTH is necessary to confirm the diagnosis. Plastic surgical procedures may be required if the external genitalia are significantly masculinized.

HYPOTHALAMIC-PITUITARY DYSFUNCTION

Amenorrhea may be caused by a variety of abnormalities in the central nervous system, hypothalamus, or pituitary. The most common cause is hypothalamic dysfunction. If the dysfunction first appears when puberty is expected, the manifestations will be delay of puberal changes and primary amenorrhea. If it first appears after menarche, a secondary amenorrhea results. The essential common dysfunction in these patients is lack of cyclic hypothalamic stimulation of the pituitary. The levels of FSH and LH are normal or only slightly depressed but they do not undergo the periodic elevations that are characteristic of the normal female reproductive cycle. Inasmuch as stimulation of the pituitary by releasing hormones causes a normal response, the primary dysfunction cannot be attributed to the pituitary. Because of the lack of stimulation by gonadotropin, the ovaries are hypoplastic and the levels of estrogen are low or at least slightly depressed. Most patients with amenorrhea of this cause do not bleed after withdrawal of progestin.

A variety of neoplastic, inflammatory, and destructive lesions in the hypothalamus or pituitary may be associated with amenorrhea. The most common lesion is a prolactin-secreting tumor of the pituitary. Galactorrhea may or may not accompany the amenorrhea. The elevation of the level of prolactin in the serum is positively correlated with the size of the tumor. If the lesion is smaller than 1 cm in diameter, it is a microadenoma; if larger, it is a macroadenoma. Most patients with these lesions have no abnormalities other than amenorrhea, elevated levels of prolactin, and possibly galactorrhea.

Diagnosis of the lesion is made by history, elevated levels of prolactin, and radiologic identification of a sellar or suprasellar mass. The most accurate radiographic technique is magnetic resonance imaging (MRI), which can identify a lesion smaller than 3 mm in diameter. Arteriography may occasionally be useful. Neurologic findings such as changes in the visual fields are uncommon because most of the tumors are small, but they can occur with larger lesions.

Possible methods of management of pituitary prolactinomas include observation alone, medical management with dopamine agonists, and surgical removal. Longitudinal follow-up of surgically treated patients with microadenomas and macroadenomas confirms the recurrence of hyperprolactinemia in a significant number of cases.

Pituitary insufficiency may manifest itself as an inability to produce one or more tropic hormones. Isolated or partial deficiencies are more common than complete hypopituitarism (panhypopituitarism). Although the causes are usually unknown, etiologic factors include pituitary tumors, cysts, and necrosis. Hypopituitarism may follow hemorrhage and shock. When it occurs in association with pregnancy, it is called Sheehan's syndrome. Hypopituitarism unassociated with pregnancy is known as Simmond's disease. A selective deficiency of gonadotropins produces hypogonadotropic hypogonadism.

A deficiency of gonadotropins that results in anovulation and infertility is the classic indication for gonadotropin therapy. Complications of the therapeutic use of these hormones for any cause include ovarian cysts and plural gestations.

POLYCYSTIC OVARY SYNDROME

The polycystic ovarian (Stein-Leventhal) syndrome is characterized by obesity, hirsutism, ovulatory dysfunction, and bilaterally enlarged ovaries that contain multiple small follicular cysts. Physical manifestations of this syndrome are highly variable, however. Diagnosis may be confirmed by the finding, at laparoscopy or laparotomy, of large white ovaries with numerous small cysts under a thickened capsule. Assessment of random gonadotropin values often reveals that FSH falls within the lower range of normal for women, and that LH levels are usually elevated, with a resulting LH:FSH ratio greater than 2 but rarely greater than 4. The differential diagnosis includes polycystic ovarian syndrome, idiopathic hyperandrogenism, late-onset congenital adrenal hyperplasia (LOCAH), and Cushing's syndrome. Medical treatment by stimulation of ovulation with clomiphene is the method of choice. Wedge resection of the ovary is rarely used today because it may result in ovarian adhesions and subsequent infertility.

INDUCTION OF OVULATION

Clomiphene citrate (Clomid or Serophene) is a nonsteroidal estrogen agonist: antagonist. It provides a primary option for treatment of the anovulatory patient who has ovarian follicular function with production of basal endogenous estrogen, as demonstrated by either serum estradiol measurements or appropriate endometrial withdrawal bleeding after the administration of progestins. Although clomiphene citrate binds to all estrogen receptor sites, its primary effect is at the level of the hypothalamus. Successful ovulation is preceded by significant changes in the pattern of gonadotropin-releasing hormone pulses, concurrent with the oral ingestion of the medication. A majority of patients respond to

low-dosage regimens of clomiphene citrate; increasing dosages must be monitored carefully to minimize the likelihood of cystic ovarian enlargement and other side effects. The incidence of twin pregnancies is trebled among patients conceiving on clomiphene citrate.

In patients with deficiencies in pituitary gonadotropins (serious hypothalamic-pituitary disease), human menopausal gonadotropin (hMG) is effective in inducing ovulation. This substance, which is purified from the urine of postmenopausal women, consists of both FSH and LH, but its effect is mainly that of FSH. Overstimulation of the ovaries with hMG (Pergonal) is a serious drawback to the use of this hormone.

Clomiphene is administered in an initial oral dose of 50 mg a day for 5 days. The dose may be increased to 100 mg or 150 mg a day for 5 days if necessary. Ovulatory function improves with this drug alone in about 75% of women, but pregnancies usually occur in only half of the women who ovulate consistently. Some patients require an intramuscular injection of 5000 or 10,000 units of hCG to induce ovulation.

Polycystic ovarian disease is now considered to result from primary dysfunction of the hypothalamus and pituitary rather than the ovary. Overstimulation by gonadotropins is found in association with an excess of ovarian steroids, indicating that the sex hormones do not suppress the gonadotropins, as in normal feedback mechanisms. As a result, there is an exaggerated response to gonadotropins. As does Cushing's disease, the Stein-Leventhal syndrome represents increased pituitary activity in conjunction with a paradoxical excess of the target hormone. The rationale for use of clomiphene citrate is the blockage of the action of estrogen at the level of the hypothalamus.

The elevated level of LH may result from an increased pituitary response to estradiol (increased positive feedback). There may be in addition an increased pituitary response to gonadotropin releasing hormone. The histologic changes in the ovaries are related to increased levels of androgens.

Amenorrhea attributable to discontinuation of oral contraceptives may occur in 1% of women. This complication may not be different statistically from the prevalence of secondary amenorrhea in the population of all women of reproductive age. If spontaneous menstruation does not resume within 6 to 12 months after discontinuation of the oral contraceptives, the patients should be evaluated in the manner appropriate for any patient with secondary amenorrhea.

PSYCHOGENIC AMENORRHEA

Psychogenic causes of amenorrhea include psychosis, severe emotional shock, anxiety, pseudocyesis (false, or spurious, pregnancy), and anorexia nervosa. Although general anterior pituitary function is preserved, patients with anorexia may exhibit a wide variety of metabolic and endocrine disturbances, which suggest significant derangement of hypothalamic function. Clinical evaluation reveals hypotension, faulty regulation of temperature, bradycardia, abnormal gonadotropin responses to short-term GnRH stimulation, mild hypercortisolemia, and altered thyroid metabolism. Their amenorrhea is caused by profound hypogonadotropic hypogonadism. In anorexia nervosa, unlike Sheehan's syndrome, no organic lesion of the pituitary is found, but in some patients with anorexia, dysfunction of thyroid and adrenal metabolism may be detected.

CHRONIC DISEASES

A variety of chronic diseases such as tuberculosis and nutritional deficiencies may cause oligomenorrhea or amenorrhea. Diabetes mellitus, particularly if untreated, also adversely affects menstrual function. Hepatic or renal dysfunction may interfere sufficiently with the metabolism of hormones to prevent normal menstruation. Many drugs in addition to hormones may depress menstrual function. The commonest etiologic agents are phenothiazines and narcotics.

ADRENAL AND THYROID DYSFUNCTION

Dysfunction of the other endocrine organs may also interfere with menstrual function. Adrenal hyperplasia, neoplasms, or insufficiency (Addison's disease) may lead to amenorrhea.

Unlike congenital adrenal hyperplasia, Cushing's syndrome represents hyperfunction of the zona fasciculata as well as the zona reticularis. Cushing's syndrome classically includes obesity, amenorrhea, hirsutism, and hypertension. In this syndrome, overreaction to ACTH occurs, corticosteroids are elevated, and the adrenal cortex cannot be suppressed with cortisone. Loss of diurnal fluctuation in the level of cortisol is found.

Hyperthyroidism as well as hypothyroidism may affect menstrual function unpredictably. Aside from pregnancy, perhaps the commonest endocrine cause of decreased menses is ingestion of oral contraceptives. The patient should always be asked whether she has used these agents before other endocrine causes of amenorrhea are considered.

OVARIAN DYSFUNCTION

The ovary itself may be the cause of amenorrhea as a result of biochemical defects, insensitivity to tropic hormones, or destructive lesions. Functioning tumors of the ovary also may produce menstrual abnormalities including amenorrhea. Androgen-producing tumors of the ovary or adrenal and estrogen-producing varieties (granulosa cell and theca cell tumors) may all cause amenorrhea or other menstrual abnormalities.

Premature menopause is the cessation of ovarian function before age 40. Ovarian failure results from premature aging of the ovaries.

UTERINE DYSFUNCTION

Finally, the uterus itself may be the cause of amenorrhea. Uterine trauma sufficient to destroy the endometrium may occur after infection or overly vigorous curettage, particularly after pregnancy (Asherman's syndrome). The intrauterine synechiae are best treated during hysterosopic visualization followed by mechanical division of adhesions.

Cervical stenosis, which may also result from trauma, prevents the escape of menstrual blood. It may be treated by cervical dilatation.

DIAGNOSIS

Diagnosis of the cause of amenorrhea can often be made by careful history and physical examination alone. After pregnancy, chronic disease, and drug-induced amenorrhea are ruled out, consultation with a gynecologic endocrinologist is desirable.

The next steps in the diagnosis of secondary amenorrhea are a progestin challenge and measurements of FSH, LH, and prolactin. Other tests that are sometimes useful include measurement of serum TSH, thyroxine, dehydroepiandrosterone sulfate, testosterone, and cortisol. Occasionally a karyotype of the patient is indicated as is radiologic evaluation of the pituitary. Laparoscopy, hysterosalpingography, endometrial curettage, and hysteroscopy may detect local lesions. Stimulation of the adrenal or pituitary glands less frequently provides diagnostic information in the initial evaluation of secondary amenorrhea.

The treatment of secondary amenorrhea is determined by the etiologic factor and the reproductive desires of the patient. Diagnosis and correction of the disorder rather than the induction of menstruation are the primary goals. It is not necessary to induce ovulation except in patients who want to become pregnant.

52
CHAPTER

HIRSUTISM AND VIRILIZATION

Defeminization, the relative loss of female sexual characteristics, usually precedes virilization, or masculinization. Defeminization involves diminution in mammary tissue and female distribution of fat, amenorrhea, and ovarian failure. Virilization is the development of male secondary sexual characteristics in a woman as a result of stimulation of the responsive tissues by excessive androgen. A common sequence of masculinization is deepening of the voice, hirsutism, a male pattern of baldness, increased secretion of sebaceous glands with occasional acne, hypertrophy of the clitoris, and increased muscle mass.

Hirsutism is the excessive growth of hair on the body or face of a woman, usually involving the upper lip, chin, chest, abdomen, or legs. The major causes are listed in Table 52–1. Genetic, familial, and racial predispositions are the most common etiologic factors in hirsutism. Hairiness, or hypertrichosis, is more common in Mediterranean races, for example. It is therefore necessary in such people to compare the patient with other members of her family. In this idiopathic form of hirsutism the levels of serum testosterone and dehydroisoandrosterone are within normal limits.

Hirsutism of some degree is noted in many syndromes involving amenorrhea of central, constitutional, or peripheral origin,

such as the polycystic ovary, Cushing, and adrenogenital syndromes. Most of the causes of hirsutism are discussed elsewhere in this unit under the appropriate syndromes. Masculinizing tumors of the ovary or adrenal almost always cause rapidly progressive signs. They should be suspected when the level of serum testosterone ex-

TABLE 52–1. ETIOLOGY OF HIRSUTISM

I. Genetic, Familial, or Racial
II. Pituitary-Hypothalamic
  A. Acromegaly
  B. Cushing's syndrome
  C. Polycystic ovary syndrome
III. Other Endocrine Defects
  A. Adrenogenital syndrome (congenital or acquired)
  B. Cushing's syndrome
  C. Adenoma and carcinoma of the adrenal
  D. Hypothyroidism in children
IV. Ovarian
  A. Masculinizing tumors
  B. Menopause
V. Systemic Physical and Emotional Illnesses
  A. Porphyria
  B. Anorexia nervosa
VI. Local Effects
  A. Plaster casts
  B. Roentgen therapy
VII. Drug-Induced
  A. Dilantin
  B. Androgens
  C. Corticosteroids
  D. Diazoxide

ceeds 250 ng/dL or that of dehydroisoandrosterone exceeds 700 ng/dL. Hirsutism caused by adrenal hyperplasia can be distinguished from that resulting from adrenal neoplasms in that the androgens from adrenal tumors are not suppressed by the administration of dexamethasone. Supraphysiologic production of adrenal androgens may be suppressed by low-dose corticosteroid therapy. Additionally, the effect of androgens on target tissues may be minimized by the administration of spironolactone, an antagonist of aldosterone, which binds competitively to androgen receptors.

Elevation of dehydroisoandrosterone or its sulfated metabolite suggests an adrenal source of excess androgens; elevation of testosterone suggests an ovarian source. Furthermore, a large number of patients with hirsutism may have a mixed pattern of androgenic excess. Catheterization of the ovarian and adrenal veins to measure concentrations of androgens confirms this pattern. Testosterone-producing tumors or areas of stromal hyperplasia of the ovary may be too small to visualize at laparoscopy or laparotomy and often are not distinguishable on ultrasonographic examination.

53
CHAPTER

ABNORMAL UTERINE BLEEDING

Abnormal or excessive uterine bleeding may result from endocrine dysfunction, but neoplasms and other anatomic causes and complications of pregnancy must be ruled out before hormonal therapy is initiated. Dysfunctional uterine bleeding (bleeding without an obvious anatomic abnormality) is usually anovulatory and is associated with a nonsecretory endometrium. It is most common shortly after the menarche or just before the menopause, but it may occur at other times as well.

Prolonged dysfunctional bleeding may result from a persistent graafian follicle. In such cases, withdrawal of estrogen leads to delayed endometrial shedding and irregular bleeding. The bleeding is caused by estrogenic overstimulation followed by withdrawal or diminution of estrogen, unopposed by progesterone. Estrogenic stimulation results in bleeding from a proliferative or hyperplastic endometrium, or occasionally from endometrial polyps or carcinoma. A related cause is "breakthrough bleeding" during the use of oral contraceptives.

Dysfunctional bleeding may result from disorders of the central nervous system, pituitary, or ovary, or from the effects of exogenous or endogenous steroids. Etiologic factors related to systemic metabolic disorders include hyperthyroidism, hypothyroidism, hepatic dysfunction, and a variety of chronic diseases. Anovulatory bleeding requires consideration of nutritional, metabolic, and emotional factors. Polycystic ovaries may be ruled out by measurement of FSH and LH or laparoscopy.

Bleeding from a secretory endometrium, which indicates ovulation, usually implies an anatomic lesion rather than an endocrine disorder. The investigation of ovulatory bleeding may include a hysterogram, hematologic studies, and diagnostic hysteroscopy.

Most important, any abnormal bleeding in an adult requires a Papanicolaou smear and endometrial sampling before treatment. For greatest accuracy of diagnosis, curettage is best performed just before menses. In an adolescent patient, presumptive dysfunctional bleeding may be treated without curettage.

Ovulatory bleeding may occasionally produce minimal midcyclic bleeding in the absence of an organic lesion. Abnormal uterine bleeding may result from organic lesions of the ovary, oviduct, corpus, cervix, or vagina. Complications of pregnancy include ectopic gestation, abortion, bleeding corpus luteum, hydatidiform mole, and choriocarcinoma.

Genital causes unassociated with pregnancy include myomas; carcinoma, polyps, or hyperplasia of the endometrium; chronic cervicitis; polyps and carcinomas of the cervix; carcinoma of the vagina; functional ovarian cysts; and functioning ovarian neoplasms.

Extragenital causes include blood dyscrasias, thrombocytopenia, deficient clotting factors, endocrinopathies, and, uncommonly, hypertension. In addition, bleeding from the urinary tract and rectum must be excluded.

Treatment of uterine bleeding depends on the cause. In adolescents, cyclic progestin or estrogen-progestin therapy may be instituted after a Papanicolaou smear without a preliminary curettage. If irregular bleeding persists after cyclic estrogen-progesterone therapy (medical curettage), a complete diagnostic investigation including formal curettage is required. In cases of recurrent apparently dysfunctional bleeding in younger patients, progesterone may be used while the investigation continues.

Attempts to induce ovulation are justified only when fertility is part of the goal of therapy. In premenopausal patients medroxyprogesterone acetate administered cyclically may induce regular withdrawal bleeding and preclude the need for further therapy. In patients who have completed their families, recurrent irregular uterine bleeding that is unresponsive to progestin therapy may be treated by hysterectomy.

54
CHAPTER

DYSMENORRHEA

Dysmenorrhea, or painful menstruation, is a symptom and not a disease. Dysmenorrhea may be the commonest gynecologic symptom. It is the direct cause of the loss of countless woman-hours of work.

Primary dysmenorrhea occurs in the absence of a significant pelvic lesion. It is essential, or functional, dysmenorrhea and is caused by factors intrinsic to the uterus. Primary dysmenorrhea is the more common form of the symptom. Its onset is usually in adolescence, within two years of the menarche. It is generally associated with ovulatory cycles and appears to be caused by an excessive production of endometrial prostaglandins, which stimulate painful uterine contractions.

In secondary dysmenorrhea, pelvic disease can be demonstrated, for example, endometriosis, adenomyosis, and chronic pelvic inflammatory disease. Even if palpable findings are absent on pelvic examination, endometriosis may still be the cause of the dysmenorrhea. It should therefore be ruled out by laparoscopy. The secondary form begins in adult life, affecting a previously symptom-free woman.

The principal treatment of primary dysmenorrhea is administration of inhibitors or antagonists of prostaglandin. In more severe cases, ovulation may be inhibited by oral contraceptive drugs.

Psychotherapy and surgical procedures play small roles today in the management of primary dysmenorrhea . The principal drugs currently employed are nonsteroidal, anti-inflammatory agents that inhibit synthesis or activity of prostaglandins. Many are indoles, indole-like compounds, or arylpropionic acids. Effective compounds include indomethacin, various fenamates such as flufenamic acid and mefenamic acid, ibuprofen, and naproxen sodium. The fenamates inhibit synthesis and activity of prostaglandin and have an antagonistic effect on prostaglandin receptors. Ethanol and β-sympathomimetic agents, although tocolytic, are not highly effective in treating dysmenorrhea.

55
CHAPTER
MENOPAUSE

Menopause is the cessation of menstruation for a year or more. It is caused by ovarian failure and is frequently preceded by anovulatory bleeding. It occurs normally between the ages of 40 and 55 and is often accompanied by the symptoms of the climacteric, including hot flashes, excessive perspiration, and depression or agitation. Menopause is frequently followed by endocrine and metabolic changes. Secretion of estrogens by the ovary is decreased markedly, although peripheral conversion of adrenal steroids to estrone continues after the menopause. In obese women, there is greater production of estrone. Production of gonadotropin, mostly FSH, is high, particularly in the early postmenopausal years. Later, atrophy of the introitus and the vagina, with occasional dyspareunia and pruritus, occur. Involution of the breasts is common. Atrophy of the epithelia of the genitourinary tract may predispose to cystitis, and in some women osteoporosis and cardiovascular degeneration may occur. (See also Chapter 36 on the Aging Woman.)

The routine use of estrogen for all postmenopausal women remains controversial. The treatment of women with climacteric symptoms, however, is indicated. Estrogen should be used in the smallest dose that is sufficient to alleviate symptoms and should be combined with cyclic progestational therapy of at least 10 and preferably 13 days'

duration. One commonly employed regimen is estrogen on days 1 through 25 of the month and progestin on days 13 through 25.

The rationale for the replacement of estrogen in asymptomatic postmenopausal women is undergoing reassessment. The principal benefit of estrogen replacement may prove to be a reduction in the risks of myocardial infarction and cerebrovascular accidents. Currently popular regimens of exogenous estrogen replacement appear to have salutary effects on a woman's lipid profile. Longitudinal studies are required to correlate decreased cardiovascular risks in women with improved lipid profiles. Estrogen prevents the accelerated loss of bone in women who are estrogen-deficient; the hormone is most efficacious when it is started before loss of bone has occurred and when it is combined with increased intake of calcium and exercise. If the patient has her uterus, the estrogen should be given with a progestin. In evaluating and treating climacteric patients, environmental stresses associated with the postmenopausal era of life must be recognized, for not all the symptoms attributed to the menopause result from the decline in ovarian function. Mild discomfort may be managed with tranquilizers and mild sedation, or these drugs may be used to reduce the dose of estrogen. Symptoms of vasomotor instability and urogenital atrophy with pruritus are indications for estrogen replacement. Less vaginal atrophy has been reported in women who are sexually active than in those who are inactive. Women with less vaginal atrophy, furthermore, are reported to have higher levels of androgen and gonadotropins, particularly LH.

Low-dose estrogen given to postmenopausal women may decrease the risk of myocardial infarction and possibly cerebrovascular accidents. It is not certain whether estrogen given to postmenopausal women causes an increased incidence of mammary tumors, but it is clear that such treatment does not prevent these tumors. Baseline mammographic studies are appropriate prior to hormonal replacement. Treatment with unopposed estrogen does, however, increase the risk of endometrial carcinoma in postmenopausal women (p. 288), but the relation appears to be strongly dose-dependent.

Estrogen may be used in doses sufficient to treat climacteric symptoms without stimulating the endometrium or causing postmenopausal bleeding. The desired duration of therapy remains controversial. Although the duration of treatment of climacteric symptoms may be short, prevention of osteoporosis requires long-term therapy. A progestational agent administered cyclically for 10 to 14 days each month protects against the carcinogenic effect of estrogens on the endometrium but may produce adverse effects on serum lipids, with cardiovascular disease and reversal of the beneficial effect of estrogen on stroke.

Medroxyprogesterone acetate can be used to treat the vasomotor flushes in women to whom the administration of estrogen is undesirable. Certain complaints can be alleviated by psychotherapy and tranquilizers; several other substances, such as naloxone, bioflavonoids, and clonidine, may be effective in relieving climacteric vasomotor instability. Regular manual examination of the breast and mammography are required. Postmenopausal bleeding demands the prompt exclusion of neoplastic diseases, particularly carcinoma of the endometrium.

56

CHAPTER

INFERTILITY

Infertility is the involuntary inability to achieve a pregnancy in a reasonable interval of coital exposure. If a woman fails to conceive in 12 to 18 months, a diagnosis of infertility should be considered. If 100 couples voluntarily discontinue contraception, the cumulative pregnancy rate should approach 60% at 6 months, 85% at 12 months, and 90% at 18 months. A woman with primary infertility has never achieved a pregnancy; secondary infertility implies one or more earlier pregnancies with either normal or abnormal outcomes. Female sterility is the absolute inability to conceive, in contrast to a reduced capacity to conceive. There are many causes for a couple's infertility. Problems or factors related specifically to the female may be uncovered in one third of cases. The remaining two thirds of cases of infertility may be divided equally between male factors solely and problems shared by the couple.

Male causes include impotence; failure to ejaculate; and disturbances in number, motility, or maturation of spermatozoa. Common female causes of infertility include ovulatory dysfunction, tubal disorders, abnormalities of production or function of mucus, and distortion of pelvic structures by endometriosis or pelvic inflammatory disease.

Anovulation is evaluated by means of a daily morning temperature graph (basal body temperature, or BBT), progesterone assay or endometrial biopsy to demonstrate lack of a secretory endometrium, and inadequate cyclic changes in the cervical mucus or vaginal cytologic smear. The ovaries may be visualized directly by endoscopy.

Occlusion of the oviduct may be evaluated by several means. The most common technique is hysterosalpingography, in which sterile contrast medium is injected transcervically under fluoroscopic control, resulting in the visualization of the endometrial cavity and lumina of the fallopian tubes. A second technique, applied during laparoscopy, involves the retrograde injection of a colored dye through a cervical cannula. After injection, dye should be apparent in the pelvic cavity. Hysterosalpingography combined with laparoscopy may provide maximal information.

Abnormalities of cervical mucus are detected by careful examination of the amount and quality of mucus throughout the menstrual cycle. During the second week of a normal menstrual cycle, cervical mucus should show increasing Spinnbarkeit (the ability of the mucus to be drawn into a long thread) and, when allowed to dry on a microscopic slide, form increasingly complex patterns of deposition of salt (ferning). These properties can be demonstrated several days before midcycle but should be maximal at the approximate time of ovulation. If the cervical mucus is obtained 4 to 10 hours after intercourse, a Sims-Hühner (postcoital) test may be performed. Multiple microscopic (400X) fields are scanned to detect motile sperm. The consistent finding of 5 to 10 motile sperm/high power field is a reassuring postcoital result.

The couple should be interviewed together early in the work-up and an initial plan for evaluation prepared. Documentation of adequacy of production of sperm, patency of the fallopian tubes, and normalcy of ovulation should be confirmed before proceeding with more invasive or complicated testing or therapy.

MALE INFERTILITY

Semen for analysis should be collected after a period of abstinence of 2 to 4 days to help minimize the known variability of indices after either frequent ejaculation or prolonged storage within the male reproductive tract. Normal seminal values include a volume of 2.5 to 6 mL, with complete liquefaction of the sample within one hour of collection. More than 60% of the sperm should be motile at 1 hour, with some reduction in the motile fraction at 2 to 4 hours. A normal sperm count varies between 20 million and 200 million per mL. At least 60% of the cells should be normal morphologically. The concentrations of fructose and citric acid in the semen are indices of function of the seminal vesicles and prostate, respectively.

Common male factors are defects in number of spermatozoa (oligospermia), proportion of morphologically normal spermatozoa (teratospermia), or motility (asthenospermia). Although isolated deficits in a single criterion are well documented, more commonly the subfertile male shows deficits in all three categories—number, motility, and shape of spermatozoa.

In evaluation of the semen, the total ejaculate should be obtained, preferably by masturbation. In certain cases of oligospermia, a homologous insemination may be performed with the husband's semen. The use of a split ejaculate, in which only the first portion is used for insemination, is occasionally valuable in homologous insemination for oligospermia. The first por-

tion, containing fluid from the prostate and Cowper's glands, contains most of the viable spermatozoa and can be effectively separated from the third portion, which contains fluid from the seminal vesicles. With azoospermia, a heterologous (donor) insemination may provide an alternative to adoption.

Causes of male infertility include: congenital defects of the genitalia, such as cryptorchidism, testicular hypoplasia, absence of the vasa deferentia, hypospadias, and epispadias; acquired defects, such as varicocele, local infections and trauma, and neoplasms; physical and toxic factors, such as heat, radiation, and drugs; chromosomal aberrations, such as Klinefelter's syndrome with dysgenesis of the seminiferous tubules; retrograde ejaculation, of idiopathic or diabetic origin; neuropsychiatric problems; and nutritional and endocrine factors. Improved production of sperm often follows ligation of the spermatic veins in a man with a varicocele and oligospermia or asthenospermia.

FEMALE INFERTILITY

Normal ovulation is suggested by a history of predictable, regular menses at intervals of 26 to 33 days, associated with premenstrual molimina such as backache, fullness of the breasts, swelling of the hands and feet, bloating, acne, and irritability. After ovulation, the corpus luteum produces increasing amounts of progesterone, secreted in a pulsatile manner, which establishes a peak peripheral serum level approximately 1 week after ovulation. This hormone influences hypothalamic function to the extent that resting basal temperature is increased by approximately 0.5°C. Oral temperatures obtained early in the morning before activity may be graphed and suggest ovulation if the temperature rises and remains elevated during the luteal phase of the menstrual cycle. Abnormalities in production of luteal phase hormones or their effects are known collectively as luteal phase defect or luteal phase insufficiency. This heterogeneous disorder may result from inadequate folliculogenesis, inadequate preovulatory estrogen, or abnormalities in effect of progesterone on a principal target organ, the endometrium. The suspicion of luteal phase defect may be confirmed by means of a well-timed late-cycle endometrial biopsy or pooled progesterone values. Secretion of progesterone is pulsatile and its metabolism is influenced by physical activity, so that a random progesterone value may vary greatly during a single day. Advanced secretory changes in tissue obtained by endometrial biopsy (p. 244) or serial ultrasonic assessments of folliculogenesis (Fig. 56–1) and development of a corpus luteum are the best indirect indices of ovulation.

Several clinical and laboratory tests may be used to predict ovulation. Midcycle pelvic discomfort (Mittelschmerz) has been correlated ultrasonographically with the final maturational stages of the dominant follicle and tends to be maximal subjectively the day before ovulation. Serial changes in the cervical mucus are correlated well with increasing estrogen, resulting in an increased amount and decreased viscosity of mucus through midcycle. After ovulation, progesterone results in increased viscosity and decreased production of cervical mucus. The urinary clearance of LH after a nocturnal surge in the hormone can be detected with recently developed home-use assay kits to facilitate prediction of ovulation.

Anovulation may result from disturbances anywhere from the central nervous system to the ovary. Major causes are discussed in the section on amenorrhea (pp. 324 to 335). The treatment is induction of ovulation.

Less commonly, infertility may stem from lesions of the vagina (anomalies or stenosis) or cervix (trauma, inflammation, stenosis, and incompetent os). Abnormalities of the corpus that occasionally lead to infertility include congenital anomalies, submucous myomas, and traumatic scarring of the endometrium (Asherman's syndrome), which may be treated by gentle curettage.

Inflammatory occlusions of the oviduct or adhesions may be treated surgically with moderate success, especially if the fimbriae and tubal peristalsis remain unimpaired. Tuberculosis must be ruled out during the investigation of the woman. Immunologic causes, such as antibodies to components of the semen, are difficult to treat and require referral to specialized centers.

Psychogenic factors are said to cause spasm of the reproductive tract on occasion. In rare instances, psychiatric treatment may be helpful.

ASSISTED REPRODUCTIVE TECHNOLOGY

Couples with refractory infertility may benefit from a variety of types of assisted reproductive technology (ART). The techniques generally involve a sequence of con-

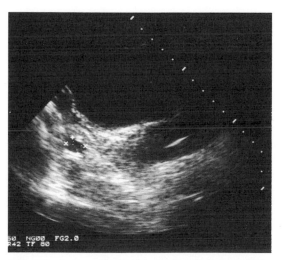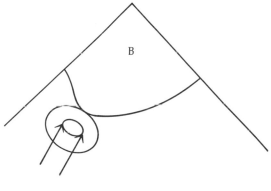

FIG. 56–1. Longitudinal sonogram demonstrating an ovarian follicle that measures approximately 12 × 13 mm, demarcated by arrows. Preovulatory follicles are usually about 20 mm in diameter. After ovulation, the follicle can be shown to collapse.

trolled hyperstimulation with mechanical retrieval of more than one mature preovulatory ovum, which is then combined with a sample of semen prepared in the laboratory for fertilization. In vitro fertilization with embryo transfer (IVF-ET) has achieved successful pregnancy for more than a decade. An alternative method, which does not involve extracorporeal fertilization, is gamete intrafallopian transfer (GIFT), in which ova and specially prepared sperm are mixed and placed directly into the ampulla of one or both oviducts. In zygote intrafallopian transfer (ZIFT), technologic features of IVF-ET and GIFT are combined, in that an extracorporeally fertilized ovum (zygote) is transferred to the oviduct for further development. Other promising options include freezing of embryos for repetitive transfer and micromanipulation of single spermatozoa and ova.

57
CHAPTER

PREMENSTRUAL SYNDROME

The premenstrual syndrome is a symptom complex occurring in the days or week before menstruation. It comprises tension, irritability, or depression, sometimes associated with tenderness or fullness of the breasts, abdominal bloating, headache, and edema. The onset of the syndrome is usually in the fourth decade of life.

Premenstrual tension is almost always associated with ovulatory cycles. In its severe form, it may cause psychic and physical incapacitation of the woman for one third of the month. It is temporally related to an increase in crimes committed by women, accidents, and suicides.

The syndrome may be associated with a variety of abnormal hormonal conditions, including secondary hyperaldosteronism, which results in retention of sodium and fluid and consequent edema and headaches. Abnormalities in production of progesterone, altered metabolism of progesterone, and elevation or decrease in prolactin have not been correlated consistently with symptoms in women who clearly exhibit cycle-dependent features of premenstrual syndrome. Regimens of treatment, which have been far from uniformly successful, include strong reassurance, antidepressant medication, diuretics including spironolactone, and programs of recreational exercise. Short-term suppression of ovulation with GnRH agonists has shown promise. Severe emotional disturbances may require referral to a psychiatrist.

VI

HUMAN
SEXUALITY

58
CHAPTER

SEXUALITY

Detailed discussions of human sexuality are beyond the scope of even large textbooks of gynecology, but awareness of the wide range of normal sexual behavior and recognition of common psychosexual problems are requisite to effective gynecologic diagnosis and therapy. The necessity for obtaining a complete factual history of sexual habits is discussed in Unit I. The same objectivity should be applied to this area of gynecology as to discussion of cardiovascular or gastrointestinal function. The criteria of sexuality are enumerated on p. 330.

The gynecologist is often the first physician to deal with female sexual inadequacies and is also required to exclude organic causes of sexual dysfunction in his patients. He or she must be competent to counsel young patients and avert psychiatric sexual problems. Control of conception is one important facet of sexual counseling, for fear of pregnancy may lead to sexual inadequacy.

The physician requires knowledge of sex-specific differences in the cycle of sexual response and the wide variations in psychologic attitudes and physical behavior in both sexes. The physician must differentiate sexual problems based on ignorance from true sexual psychiatric disorders and organic diseases. He or she must recognize the enormous variety of cultural mores and taboos and strive to prevent his or her own sexual inhibitions from interfering with effective rapport with the patient. He or she must expand the concept of normal sexual behavior, which is defined by some experts in the area as including any activity that mutually pleases two consenting adults without causing physical or psychologic harm.

Statistically, an act may be classified as normal if it is practiced without deleterious effects by large numbers of people. In this sense, orogenital activity, masturbation, and egosyntonic homosexual relations between consenting adults are not classified by psychiatrists as aberrations. The physician must help destroy psychologically harmful sexual myths. In particular, he or she must assure the patient that some form of masturbation is practiced almost universally at certain times of life and that it serves a useful function in relieving tension. The physician must also dispel the myths about the value, or indeed the existence, of specific aphrodisiacs. It is important that he or she distinguish love from sex and explain the differences to his or her patients.

The physician should be familiar with the basic Freudian concepts and recognize the need for psychiatric referral. He or she should be aware of changing patterns of sexuality and the sexual readjustments by men and women that are created by female liberation, the abolition of the double sexual standard, and the active role assumed by women in sexual encounters. The physician must be able to explain to the patient the changes in sexual response after major gynecologic operations and during the prenatal course and post partum. He or she should discourage unnecessary restriction of sexual activity in pregnancy that is based on unfounded fears of injuring the fetus or inducing prematurity. The physician should explain that the woman's libido may be increased or decreased during her pregnancy, whereas the man's is often unchanged. The physician should understand that sexual activity and sexual problems may involve patients of advanced age.

Sexual counseling requires time and patience. The first visit is often devoted simply to establishing confidence of the patients in the physician. Successful treatment requires a careful sexual history obtained independently from each partner. Difficult problems should be referred to expert sex counselors, often a team comprising a gynecologist and a psychologist. Deep-seated disorders should be referred to a psychiatrist.

At the first visit, the physician should elicit a sexual history in a routine, nonthreatening way. The physician must understand his or her own attitude toward sexuality before he or she can be sufficiently comfortable with the patient to advise her appropriately. Illnesses may interfere with the patient's normal sexual function through both physical and psychologic means. Informing a patient about the possible side effects of a particular illness may avert a sexual dysfunction or reveal a preexisting dysfunction, which may be managed promptly. Some neurologic, neuromuscular, and endocrine diseases have obvious direct impacts on sexual function. These diseases may affect the hypothalamus, hypophysis, gonads, or end organs. Brief illnesses that cause sexual dysfunction are usually of such short duration that they require no therapy. Sexual dysfunction caused by chronic illness can be managed most effectively by curing the illness or eliminating the cause of exacerbation of sexual symptoms. The evaluation and treatment of the dysfunction may be facilitated by classifying the problem as difficulty in desire, arousal, or orgasm.

The frequency of sexual activity varies enormously within any age group, although in general, frequency decreases with age. Libido in women increases between the early twenties and the middle thirties. In men, libido is greatest in the late teens, decreasing notably in the late twenties. In both sexes, libido may continue into advanced years. It is affected throughout life by general mental health, depression, and anxiety. It is influenced also by chronic alcoholism and by drugs such as morphine, heroin, and LSD. Medications have obvious effects on sexual function. Although most of the drug studies were performed primarily in men, it is assumed, but not proved, that the effects are similar in women, because both sexes exhibit the same four stages of sexual response, as described in Chapter 59. The physician must be sufficiently well informed about the current AIDS epidemic to advise his or her patients appropriately about safer sexual practices.

59
CHAPTER

HUMAN SEXUAL RESPONSE

Human sexual response is basically similar in both sexes. Sexual stimulation leads to vascular engorgement, muscular tension, and their physiologic consequences. The four phases of sexual response described by Masters and Johnson are excitement, plateau, orgasm, and resolution. The excitement phase is the longest. It may be induced by somatic or psychogenic stimuli and delayed or interrupted voluntarily.

Whereas the female may have multiple orgasms in rapid succession, the male undergoes a refractory period of 5 to 30 minutes, during which orgasm cannot be achieved by any means. Ordinarily, orgasm in the male is reached faster and more directly than in the female, in whom physical contact appears to be a less significant erotogenic factor. The feeling that the female is desired may in itself lead to heightened sexual response. The intensity of the female reaction may depend upon amount and type of foreplay. The physician should advise against attempts to attain simultaneous orgasms in both partners, for such a result is neither common nor necessarily desirable. He should also refute the concept of the superiority of vaginal over clitoral orgasm, since, despite Freud's teaching, the two means of stimulation produce identical orgasms. Direct contact with the clitoris is not usually achieved during intercourse in the "missionary position" (man over

woman), since the clitoris normally retracts under the symphysis. Effective stimulation of the clitoris is achieved more directly by digital manipulation.

Another myth concerns the advantage of the large over the small penis as an effective organ of copulation; nor does circumcision increase or decrease sensation or delay ejaculation. Most important, the physician should recognize that sexual incompatibilities are usually psychogenic rather than physical. He or she should identify serious psychosexual disorders and obtain psychiatric consultation at the first opportunity.

The details of human sexual response have been described in the writings of Masters and Johnson. In general, there is notable similarity in the genital and extragenital responses in both men and women during excitement, plateau, orgasm, and resolution.

During the excitement phase in women, there is tumescence of the glans of the clitoris, vasocongestion, and increase in diameter and length of the shaft. The vagina provides lubrication within 10 to 30 seconds of stimulation and the vaginal tube expands and assumes a darker purplish hue. The uterus is partially elevated and the corpus becomes irritable. The labia majora in the nullipara undergo flattening, separation, and anterolateral elevation away from the vaginal outlet; in the multipara, vasocongestion, increase in diameter, and slight movement away from the midline occur. The labia minora undergo slight thickening and expansion.

In the plateau phase, the clitoris retracts under the symphysis. The vagina forms an orgasmic platform at its outer third and undergoes further increase in width and depth. Corpus and cervix are fully elevated, and there is further increase in irritability of the corpus. The labia majora in the nullipara are severely engorged; in the multipara, further vasocongestion occurs. The labia minora undergo a striking change in color from bright red to deep wine, indicating impending orgasm. At this stage Bartholin's glands secrete a drop or two of mucoid material.

At orgasm, contractions of the orgasmic platform in the vagina are noted at intervals of 0.8 seconds, recurring 6 to 12 times. The uterus undergoes contractions, the extent of which parallels the intensity of the orgasm. In the multipara, there may be up to a 50% increase in uterine size.

During the phase of resolution, the clitoris returns to its normal position. Five to 10 seconds after orgasm, the platform ceases to contract and undergoes rapid detumescence. The vaginal walls relax and their normal color returns within 10 to 15 minutes. The uterus returns to its normal position, but the external os continues to gape for about 20 to 30 minutes. In the nullipara, the labia majora return to their normal thickness and midline position; in the multipara, the labial vasocongestion disappears. The labia minora change color from bright red to light pink within 15 seconds and their size decreases.

In addition, there are numerous extragenital reactions during the various phases of female sexual response. During excitement, several changes occur in the breasts. The nipples become erect and increase in size; concomitant tumescence of the areolae occurs. A maculopapular rash (sex flush) develops late in the phase of excitement, beginning over the epigastrium and spreading over the breasts. Myotonia, both voluntary and involuntary, increases. Tachycardia parallels the degree of sexual tension.

During the plateau phase, the nipples become turgid. The breasts increase further in size and the areolae undergo further erection. The sex flush is better developed and myotonia increases, accompanied by spastic contractions. Tachycardia increases to as high as 175/minute, accompanied by increases in systolic and diastolic blood pressures of 20 to 60 and 10 to 20 mm Hg, respectively.

At the time of orgasm, the sex flush parallels the intensity of the reaction. Myotonia is maximal, with loss of voluntary control, accompanied by involuntary contractions of the rectal sphincter. The respiratory rate increases to as high as 40/minute and tachycardia increases to between 110 and 180/minute. Blood pressure rises about 30 to 50 mm Hg systolic and 20 to 40 mm Hg diastolic.

During resolution, rapid detumescence of the nipples and areolae occurs. The decrease in volume of the breasts is slower. The sex flush disappears rapidly in the reverse order in which it appeared. Myotonia rarely continues for more than 5 minutes after orgasm. Hyperventilation and tachycardia return rapidly to normal. A widespread film of perspiration appears, unrelated to the extent of physical activity.

In the male, the genital and extragenital reactions are similar to those just described in the female. During excitement, the most obvious event is the rapid erection of the penis. Erection may be lost and regained or inhibited by numerous stimuli during this phase. There is tensing and thickening of the scrotal skin and elevation of the sac. The testes are elevated as a result of shortening of the spermatic cords.

During the plateau phase, the penis undergoes an increase in circumference at the coronal ridge and possibly a change in color of the corona. The testes are said to undergo an enlargement of 50% over their nonstimulated state. Full elevation of the testes indicates impending ejaculation. Cowper's glands provide a preejaculatory emission of a few drops of fluid containing numerous active spermatozoa.

At orgasm, the penis undergoes contraction along the entire length of the penile urethra. The contractions start at intervals of 0.8 second. After the first three or four contractions, the expulsive force is reduced.

During resolution, the penis undergoes detumescence in two stages, a rapid and a slow. The scrotum rapidly loses its congestion and its normal folds reappear. The testes return to normal size and position.

The male also undergoes certain extra-genital reactions. In excitement, there is occasional erection of the nipples, myotonia (including voluntary and involuntary components), and tachycardia and hypertension in proportion to the degree of sexual tension.

During the plateau phase, an inconsistent further increase in erection of the nipples occurs. A maculopapular rash develops late in this phase. The rash originates over the epigastrium and spreads to the chest wall, neck, forehead, and other locations. Myotonia is characterized by a further increase in voluntary and involuntary components. Hyperventilation occurs late in this phase, and tachycardia may range between 100 and 175/minute, with an increase in blood pressure from 20 to 80 mm Hg systolic and 10 to 40 diastolic.

At orgasm, a well-developed sex flush is seen in about 25% of men. Myotonia is characterized by loss of voluntary control and by involuntary contractions and spasm. The rectal sphincter undergoes contractions occurring at intervals of 0.8 second and the respiratory rate may rise to as high as 40/minute. Tachycardia ranges from 110 to 180, and a rise in blood pressure of 40 to 100 systolic and 20 to 50 diastolic occurs.

During resolution, there is involution of erection of the nipples and rapid disappearance of the sex flush in reverse order of its appearance. Myotonia disappears within 5 minutes after the end of orgasm. The increased blood pressure, heart rate, and respiratory rate return to normal. Perspiration in the male is inconsistent and involuntary and is usually confined to the palms and soles.

60
CHAPTER

DISORDERS OF SEXUAL FUNCTION AND SEXUAL ASSAULT

DISORDERS OF SEXUAL FUNCTION

Sexual dysfunction may result from disorders of sexual desire or arousal. Education and counseling are of great benefit in simple cases of ignorance of sexual function.

Disorder of sexual desire is the persistent disinterest in sexual activity. A primary lack of desire, in which no interest ever existed, is best treated by psychotherapy or sex therapy. A secondary lack of desire implies that the sexual interest present in the past has diminished greatly or disappeared. In this situation, an underlying organic or situational cause must be uncovered and treated.

Disorders of sexual excitement occur when lack of vasocongestion fails to provide adequate lubrication and engorgement during sexual activity. A thorough evaluation of organic and psychologic causes must be attempted in these cases. After an organic component is treated or ruled out, disorders of sexual excitement are best treated with behavioral and psychodynamic therapy.

Vaginismus is one of the disorders of sexual excitement and an obvious cause of dyspareunia. Patients with this disorder may be treated successfully with graduated dilators or lubricated fingers. When the vaginal opening is large enough to permit penile penetration, the patient is ready for intercourse.

Disorders of female arousal are sometimes treated effectively by so-called sensate focus exercises. With this technique, the male is asked to defer orgasm as he proceeds through three stages of sexual activity. The first stage avoids contact with either the female genitalia or breasts. In the second stage, the breasts are stimulated. In the third stage, coitus is permitted. The woman assumes a superior position, which increases her control of the coital act. She initiates intercourse and thrusts slowly while contracting her pubococcygeal muscles.

Some drugs, such as androgens, may increase libido or tendency to orgasm. In general, alcohol, marijuana, and other illicit drugs depress the central nervous system and tend to inhibit both sexual desire and sexual performance. Ethanol, since antiquity, and marijuana have been reported to increase desire in some cases, but the result is not improvement in sexual functioning.

Three groups of drugs frequently interfere with sexual function: antihypertensives, antihistaminies, and psychotropic drugs, especially antidepressants. Other medications such as antibiotics and anticholinergic drugs may cause sexual dysfunction indirectly by decreasing vaginal lubrication or predisposing to vaginitis so that penile penetration becomes painful.

Changing the schedule of medication so that the timing of coitus coincides with the nadir of the concentration of the drug in the blood and decreasing the dosage of the medication until sexual function returns (with subsequent increase in the dose slowly back to therapeutic values) are frequently helpful in alleviating the sexual problem. If these simple methods are unsuccessful, a change in medication to one with different side effects may be logical. Physicians should inform their patients of possible sexual side effects of their particular medications in order to decrease the likelihood of anxiety and frustration.

Orgasmic dysfunction may be treated by teaching the woman how to masturbate. If manual stimulation of the clitoris and breasts is ineffective, she may use a vibrator. Sexual reeducation in this disorder involves the woman's deferring coitus until she is close to orgasm, use of fantasy, contraction of the perineal and abdominal muscles, use of the stop-start technique, adjunctive stimulation of the clitoris during coitus, and rapid thrusting by the woman when she feels an impending orgasm.

Inhibition of orgasm may be either primary or secondary. Primary lack of orgasm is uncommon; it is a serious dysfunction involving patients who have never achieved orgasm. Treatment includes use of Kegel exercises and masturbation. The exercises involve contraction of the pubococcygeal muscles. Secondary inhibition of orgasm is a more common complaint and is often amenable to sex therapy. If the cause is a rather superficial immediate response, sex therapy alone may be adequate. If, however, deep intrapsychic conflict underlies the inhibition of orgasm in primary or secondary categories, psychotherapy is usually indicated.

Pelvic congestion is a vague syndrome that is thought to be of neurovascular origin. It may be a manifestation of psychosexual conflict, fear of pregnancy, inadequate sexual response, or failure of orgasm. The venous channels of the pelvis are congested and the uterosacral ligaments are indurated. Deep pelvic pain increases just before menses, and dyspareunia is common. Diagnosis is suggested by multiple complaints in an unusually tense patient. The uterus is often retroverted and enlarged to the size of a 10 weeks' gestation. Differential diagnosis includes endometriosis (p. 216) and chronic pelvic inflammatory disease (p. 201). In the pelvic congestion syndrome, unlike endometriosis, the tense ligaments seem to disappear under anesthesia. Treatment may include tranquilizers, psychotherapy, and adrenergic blocking agents.

Dyspareunia (painful or otherwise unsatisfactory intercourse) may result from organic causes such as atrophy of the introitus, scars, or severe vaginitis. Additional common causes include endometriosis of the uterosacral ligaments, the pelvic congestion syndrome, and purely psychogenic factors. Pain at the onset of intercourse may result from congenital malformations, injuries, or infections of the vulva, vagina, urethra, or bladder. Pain on deep thrusting usually indicates disease in the pelvis, such as endometriosis of the uterosacral ligaments or other structures, pelvic congestion, pelvic inflammatory disease, or, less likely, ovarian neoplasms or other tumors.

Vaginismus is painful involuntary spasm of the paravaginal and levator ani muscles. It occurs at the time of attempted penile penetration. In its milder form it causes dyspareunia, whereas in its severe form it prevents intromission entirely. This problem stems from a conditioned reflex, which may be triggered during an attempt to insert a vaginal speculum. Vaginismus often has a psychologic component and is the most common cause of unconsummated marriage. It is, however, easily treated with vaginal dilators and counseling.

Premature ejaculation is defined as failure to delay ejaculation for 30 seconds after penetration. It is a very common complaint, which only in its severe or chronic form may be termed a psychosexual disorder. A technique in which the penis is squeezed by the partner is frequently recommended to delay ejaculation.

Impotence is failure to achieve and maintain an erection during coitus. It is primarily a psychologic problem, in which fear of failure to perform well sexually may create a vicious cycle.

It was thought in the first half of this century that most sexual dysfunction had a single profound cause. More recently, the Kaplan triphasic model of sexuality, as developed in the 1960s, has gained wider acceptance. According to this concept, there are three phases, each with its associated dysfunction: sexual desire, excitement, and orgasm.

Treatment of these dysfunctions is based on the severity of the psychologic component. Sex therapy comprises education, behavioral modification, and psychodynamic therapy and is best accomplished with the participation of both partners whenever possible. It can be combined with medical treatment in cases of sexual dysfunction of organic origin.

In order for the physician to choose the mode of therapy most likely to be successful, the psychologic component should be categorized as either an immediate emotional response or a deeper intrapsychic conflict. An immediate emotional response by the patient at the initiation of physical intimacy affects the outcome of the entire sexual experience. Fear, anger, anxiety, distaste, ignorance, or apathy can result in a negative sexual event. These problems, however, usually respond to behavioral or supportive therapy.

Deeper psychic conflicts, which are more likely to have originated in childhood, are much more difficult to treat, for the specific cause is often subconscious. These patients require psychotherapy and possibly sex therapy.

If particular sexual practices cause distress, they must be examined more closely. Sexual variations such as homosexual activity and certain paraphilias do not require professional attention when such activity occurs in private between consenting adults and is not in conflict with the law.

Paraphilias include but are not limited to the following. Fetishism is sexual excitement or gratification derived from substitution of an inanimate object or part of the body for the other person. Transvestism is sexual excitement or gratification achieved through wearing the clothing and enacting the role of the opposite sex (cross-dressing). Zoophilia, or bestiality, is sexual gratification achieved through intercourse with animals. Pedophilia is pathologic sexual interest in children. Exhibitionism is exposure of the body, especially the genitalia, as a means of attracting sexual attention or achieving sexual excitement or gratification. Voyeurism is sexual pleasure derived from watching others, especially when they are nude. Masochism is sexual pleasure derived from physical or psychologic pain, self-inflicted or caused by others. Sadism is sexual excitement or gratification derived from inflicting pain on others. Pyromania is sexual excitement or gratification achieved through starting and watching fires.

SEXUAL ASSAULT

Rape is a sexual assault on a victim. One woman in four to six will be assaulted thus in her lifetime, but this proportion is probably an underestimate because many women fail to report the crime. Rape is not a crime of sexual passion but of violence. The primary goal of the rapist is to demonstrate dominance or to inflict abuse and degradation. A rapist may repeat the crime frequently, and the crimes often become increasingly violent.

Physicians should obtain a meticulous history from a rape victim and perform a thorough physical examination for medicolegal purposes. They should educate the patient and provide support. They should focus on the violent, nonsexual aspects of the rape and reassure the patient that she is indeed a victim.

The management of the victim of a rape in the immediate aftermath of the crime will influence her long-term adjustments. The immediate and long-term effects on the patient have been termed the "rape trauma syndrome." The initial emotional response of the victim may be expressive or controlled. The patient may express shock, disbelief, anger, fear, guilt, or shame, or may appear calm and subdued. Informing a patient that perverse sexual practices are common with rapists may avoid embarrassment and shame when the history is obtained.

When a physical examination is performed on a victim of rape, it is important to allow the patient to retain as much control as possible, because the objective of the rapist is to deprive the victim of all control. The examiner should therefore ask permission of the patient at each step in the examination and encourage the victim to talk and ask questions.

Victims of rape need treatment for injuries, sexually transmitted diseases, and prevention of pregnancy. The patient must be informed that risk of pregnancy from a single act of intercourse is 1 to 1.5%. She should be apprised of the methods of prevention and the risks of intervention. The victim also should be offered treatment for gonorrhea, chlamydial infection, and syphilis. There is, however, no method of prevention of the viral infections, such as those caused by herpes, human papillomavirus, and human immunodeficiency virus.

The immediate duty of a physician in cases of actual or alleged rape is to record the history as accurately as possible, preferably in the patient's own words, and to record objectively the physical findings. The first examiner should describe the condition of the clothing and record whether there are bruises or lacerations on the patient's body. The gynecologic consultant should perform an examination of the lower abdomen, buttocks, and external genitalia to record injuries. The throat and rectum should be examined as well. The condition of the hymen is then recorded. A speculum should be inserted, if possible, to expose the cervix, and a specimen of fluid from the vagina should be examined to detect spermatozoa. The possibility of sexually transmitted diseases and pregnancy should be discussed with the patient and appropriate treatment instituted. If the patient is not pregnant already, diethylstilbestrol, 50 mg per day, for 5 days, or a combination oral contraceptive such as Ovral, twice a day for 4 doses, may be given as a postcoital contraceptive (p. 177). Ideally, a counselor should be available at the time to minimize the likelihood of adverse psychologic sequelae.

The initial examination of the victim of rape should include cultures for *Neisseria gonorrhoeae* from any potentially infected sites; cultures, if possible, for *Chlamydia trachomatis* from those sites; examination of vaginal specimens for *Trichomonas vaginalis* by wet mount; a serologic test for syphilis; and a single sample of serum that is frozen and saved for future testing.

The risk of infection is not known precisely, but prophylaxis may be administered with tetracycline, 500 mg, by mouth, twice a day for at least 7 days, or doxycycline, 100 mg, by mouth, twice a day for at least 7 days, in addition to ceftriaxone, 250 mg, once intramuscularly. Spectinomycin, 2 g intramuscularly, or erythromycin may be substituted as necessary (p. 198). Medical follow-up is indicated in 7 days and the aforementioned studies, except for the serologic test for syphilis (STS), should be repeated. The STS should be repeated 6 weeks after the incident.

Any sexually transmitted infection in a child should be considered evidence of sexual child abuse until proved otherwise. Such cases should be reported promptly to the appropriate authorities. These children should be evaluated for sexually transmitted diseases as described for victims of rape, but with particular care to avoid physical and psychologic trauma. Treatment is indicated when disease is found, but prophylaxis is usually not administered unless there is evidence that the assailant is infected.

The "rape trauma syndrome" is divided into two phases: disorganization and reorganization. The phase of disorganization may last days to weeks and may include a variety of emotional and somatic symptoms. The emotions may range from shame, guilt, anger, revenge, and embarrassment to fear of injury, recurrence of rape, and death. The somatic complaints may include generalized or localized pain or soreness, nausea, disturbances of sleep, and loss of appetite.

During the phase of reorganization, the victim will attempt to restructure her personality and her life. She may attempt a change of address, appearance, or job. Sexual dysfunction is more likely to emerge at this stage, along with symptoms of paranoia, depression, insomnia, nightmares, and flashbacks. This phase may last for months to years. If a chronic state of maladaptive responses supervenes, a posttraumatic stress disorder must be considered. In this unfortunate case, referral to a qualified psychiatrist or clinical psychologist is indicated.

INDEX

In this index, page numbers in *italics* designate figures; page numbers followed by "t" designate tables. *See* cross-references designate the synonymous term where entries may be found; *See also* cross-references designate related topics or more detailed topic breakdowns.